ENCYCLOPEDIA OF VITAMINS, MINERALS AND SUPPLEMENTS

Tova Navarra, B.A., R.N.
and
Myron A. Lipkowitz, R.Ph., M.D.

Foreword by
John G. Navarra, Jr., J.D.

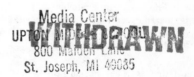

Facts On File, Inc.

Facts On File, Inc.
11 Penn Plaza
New York, NY 10001

Library of Congress Cataloging-in-Publication Data

Encyclopedia of vitamins, minerals, and supplements / Tova Navarra and
  Myron A. Lipkowitz.
     p.   cm.
   Includes bibliographical references and index.
   ISBN 0-8160-3183-5 (hardcover :alk. paper). — ISBN 0-8160-3241-6
(pbk. : alk. paper)
    1. Vitamins in human nutrition—Encyclopedias. 2. Minerals in
human nutrition—Encyclopedias. 3. Dietary supplements—
Encyclopedias. I. Navarra, Tova. II. Lipkowitz, Myron.
  QP771.E53   1996
  612.3′99′03—dc20   96-12645

To my dear friend
Margaret M. Ferrer, M.S.W.,
who nourishes my spirit.
—T.N.

To my new grandson, Zachary Patrick Burkey;
in loving memory of my parents, Irving J. and Rena Wineberg Lipkowitz;
Solomon and Irving Wineberg and Max H. Siegel;
and to journalist and dear friend Michael Dragovich.
—M.A.L.

Sickness is felt, but health not at all.
—French proverb

Prevention is better than cure.
—Latin proverb

Better is a dinner of herbs where love is,
than a stalled ox and hatred therewith.
—Proverbs 15:17

An apple a day keeps the doctor away.
—17th-century proverb

Der Mensch ist was er isst.
(Man is what he eats.)
—German philosopher Ludwig Feuerbach

"A loaf of bread," the Walrus said,
"Is what we chiefly need:
Pepper and vinegar besides
Are very good indeed."
—Lewis Carroll, from *Through the
Looking-Glass, And What Alice Found There*

CONTENTS

PREFACE

This plain-language reference book on vitamins, minerals and food supplements provides non-judgmental information on nutritional options, as opposed to books dedicated to one nutritional philosophy. As health professionals, we present positive, negative and neutral views, if appropriate, of the many substances known to have some effect upon human well-being.

We acknowledge freely that a good number of these substances have their detractors. Therefore, we do not advocate taking any particular substance or combination of substances unless you are well informed and have confidence in the substance's known effects. Many people report that eating raw garlic cloves cures them of a sore throat. But please keep in mind that not every sore throat is just a sore throat, and not everyone's metabolism and mindset are the same. If a sore throat is caused by cancerous lesions, or if a person is severely allergic to garlic, this choice of treatment may lead to tragic results.

The alternatives to the better-known vitamins and minerals, including substances used in traditional Chinese medicine, Ayurvedic (traditional Hindu) medicine, Native American and other herbal medicine and homeopathic medicine, were interesting to research and write about, and the more familiar substances, such as vitamin C and iron, took on a headier scientific glow as this book neared completion. We noted that the books, periodicals and other materials we used in our research each had valuable information, though none was truly complete in itself. Scientific opinions, such as the controversy over vitamin C's effectiveness, surprising media reports of liver damage caused by the herb chaparral and a death caused by an herbal tea, and political actions, such as the passing of the new law on supplements (see Appendix 7), often change the "supplement scene" unexpectedly in the public eye.

In addition to presenting entries on essential (that is, necessary to human life) and nonessential nutrients, we offer entries on herbal and other supplements that have long been considered nutritive and medicinal agents. We discovered, at times to our horror, that there are thousands upon thousands of herbs in use, so we decided to feature the ones we thought were the most widely used, the most broad-spectrum and the most fascinating. Many herbal preparations prescribed by homeopaths, naturopaths and others are believed to be effective against the most common ailments of many cultures. Therefore, some entries may seem repetitive as remedies for the same problems. But varying dosages and combinations with other herbs that are not addressed in this book create the possibility of treating several different illnesses, from a simple cold to catastrophic diseases such as cancer.

Our research uncovered a wealth of information. For example, without the mineral zinc, we would have a much-diminished sense of taste or smell; without salt, no neurotransmitters; without sugar, no energy; and so on. The study of vitamins, minerals and supplements seems to be in its infancy, even though Hippocrates, the Ancient Greek "father of medicine," used diet and herbs as the staples of his treatments. Many of the substances described are cross-referenced, and we included several appendices offering related information to the text.

We sincerely hope everyone who opens this volume will find something of personal interest, valuable information and perhaps a new attitude on nutrition, say, that your body is a sacred temple and deserves not to be inundated with garbage, but lovingly fed nature's "gold."

ACKNOWLEDGMENTS

I am most grateful to Susan Schwartz and the editorial staff of Facts On File, Inc., for conceiving and supporting this book; Eric Rosenthal and Denise da Marra, of the public relations department of Fox Chase Cancer Center in Philadelphia, for facilitating interviews and providing information with unflagging good nature; Dorothy Fox, R.N., M.S.N., Ed.S.; Madeline Herzlinger and Marilyn Gifford, reference librarians at the Monmonth County Library Headquarters, and Eastern Branch, respectively; Miss Sharp, my fifth-grade home economics teacher (wherever you may be); Faith Hamlin, my agent; and my husband, John, for his foreword and his very strange ability to live with me and my endless projects.

—Tova Navarra

I would like to acknowledge the encouragement and understanding provided by my loving wife, Jill; brother, Dr. Kenneth Lipkowitz; children, Kara and Michael Lipkowitz; and especially my mother, Rena; also the following individuals for their support over the years: fellow pharmacists and friends Stephen V. Lane, Robert B. Alpert, Kenneth Dubrovsky, Russell Hecht, Kenneth Treidel, Edward Camp, John Rimondi, Albert Lee, the late Max H. Siegel, Harry Pillion, Lewis Lippin, James Gluth, Irving and Solomon Wineberg, and the former Dean of the Duquesne University School of Pharmacy, Dr. John Adams, for not giving up on me, and four very special friends who guided me through my first years of practice in Uniontown, Pennsylvania: physicians Phillip Reilly, Cataldo "Doc" Corrado, Donald Franklin and Lydia Noche. Thanks also to the following for allowing me to tap their extensive knowledge of clinical nutrition: Laura Tadesco, R.D., C.D.E., Christine Rives, R.D., and Carolan Amirrata, and to Kimball Medical Center staff secretary Joanne Schwobel and Jere Grisham for their assistance in obtaining needed literature. And special thanks to Derek Burke, assistant editor at Facts On File.

—Myron Lipkowitz

FOREWORD

Approximately 3 million worried Americans wrote to members of Congress during 1993. Their letters attempted to head off governmental regulations that many feared might deprive the public of easy access to vitamins and other dietary supplements. The public was accustomed to buying any number of products they believed to be helpful—vitamin C tablets to ward off colds, garlic pills to lower blood pressure, calcium and magnesium for calming the nerves and strengthening bones.

The thought of putting restrictions on such products created a stir. Thanks to consumers who educated themselves on the often-controversial issues of dietary supplementation, over-the-counter supplement sales have been mounting for the past 10 years. According to the Council for Responsible Nutrition, a vitamins-and-minerals industry trade group based in Washington, D.C., supplements earned $4.1 billion in 1993, an 11-percent boost over the previous year. The passion for supplements expanded from preventive measures related to nutrition to treatments for various health problems.

In 1991, a new federal law, the Nutrition Labeling and Education Act, had given the Food and Drug Administration (FDA) the authority to allow distributors to make disease-related claims for foods and dietary supplements if the claims were supported by sufficient scientific evidence. The fear was that, in deciding which claims to allow, the FDA would be too restrictive. In effect, it may have deprived the public of the free flow of not only the supplements themselves but of the infor-mation the public had been enjoying. In turn, restricting the information distributors could pass on would thwart their ability to market their products, which might then be removed from store shelves.

One might attribute this outpouring of public sentiment in part to a media campaign launched by distributors who exaggerated the threat to dietary supplements. One television commercial produced by the Health Freedom Task Force, an industry group, even portrayed a fictional FDA raid on the home of a man (played by Mel Gibson) in the act of taking "illegal" vitamin C.

What, you may wonder, could be "illegal" vitamin C? Perhaps vitamin C bought on the "black market" without a prescription or in a dose larger than that allowed by imaginary FDA regulations. One thing is clear from the outcry that ensued: The issue captured the hearts and minds of so many Americans that it grew to major political proportions.

The federal Department of Health and Human Services responded to consumer inquiries by assuring that dietary supplements would remain available in the same manner as they had been, and that regulations adopted by the FDA did not require a doctor's prescription to purchase dietary supplements. The stated goal of the FDA was to ensure that the public would have access to *safe* products, and that health claims on the label or contained in promotional literature would be scientifically valid.[1]

Taken at face value, this goal is objectively an admirable one and within the responsibility of the

FDA. After all, the FDA had already approved health claims for the following disease conditions which they found to be nutrient-linked: ". . . dietary calcium and a reduced risk of osteoporosis; dietary sodium and an increased risk of hypertension; dietary saturated fat and cholesterol and an increased risk of coronary heart disease; dietary fat and an increased risk of cancer; consumption of fiber-containing grain products, fruit, and vegetables and a reduced risk of cancer and heart disease, and dietary folic acid and a reduced risk of neural tube defects."[2]

The FDA gave further assurance that it would continue to review research that could serve as the basis for other health claims. If the claims were scientifically justified, they would be authorized to appear on the labels. However, skeptics warned that demonstrating the required scientific proof for a typical health claim could take many years and cost many millions of dollars before satisfying the FDA. In addition, such scrutiny was not necessary because there were so few adverse effects associated with dietary supplements, unlike many drugs that already had been approved.[3]

The FDA nevertheless sought to educate and alert the public to illnesses and injuries connected with the use of certain dietary supplements.[4] The dangers known and unknown were viewed by the FDA to be more ominous in the absence of a systematic process for evaluating the safety of supplements.

An FDA publication suggested that dietary supplements as marketed are too diverse to be placed in one regulatory category and treated the same.[5] Vitamins and minerals have not only been marketed as supplements, but high-potency amino acids, botanicals, enzymes, animal extracts and bioflavonoids have been marketed the same way as well.

FDA responses did not prove reassuring enough to stop the progress of new legislative bills that had been introduced into Congress explicitly to protect public access to dietary supplements and to information about them. When the new law was enacted as the Dietary Supplement Health and Eduction Act of 1994 (DSHEA), Public Law 103-417 (see Appendix 7), there were more than 200 members of Congress who felt so strongly in support that they declared themselves sponsors of the legislation.

The basis for the congressional action is clear from the facts stated in section 2 of DSHEA.[6] The section affirms improving the health status of United States citizens as a national priority and acknowledges the importance of nutrition—and specifically the benefits of dietary supplements—for health and disease prevention.

The act also invokes sound economics. Healthy diets may reduce the need for expensive medical procedures, such as coronary bypass surgery. Also, it is advisable to make all reasonable efforts to decrease the enormous amount of money being spent on health care, more than $1 trillion in 1994, which amounted to about 12 percent of the nation's gross national product (GNP).

Another economic aspect noted in the act is that annual sales of dietary supplements amount to about $4 billion per year and that the industry consistently projects a positive trade balance. It is big business indeed. It serves almost half the country's citizens as customers who want to improve their health.

The DSHEA gives consumers the reassurance that ". . . the Federal Government should not take any actions to impose unreasonable regulatory barriers limiting or slowing the flow of safe products and accurate information . . ."[7] although swift action should be taken against unsafe or adulterated products.

To that end, the act calls for "a rational Federal framework" to supersede the patchwork regulatory policy that existed before its passage.[8] Accordingly, the act begins with a broad definition of the term dietary supplement, which includes vitamins, minerals, botanicals such as herbs, amino acids, dietary substances for use by humans to supplement the diet by increasing dietary intake and concentrates and combinations of these.

Furthermore, dietary supplements are expressly excluded from the definition of food additives so that laws applying to those products will not be applied to supplements.[9] The DSHEA also addresses a major concern of those who feared the loss of free access to safe products by providing that the supplements are presumed safe until proof to the contrary is provided by the FDA. This is in keeping with the congressional finding in the act that the supplements are "safe within a broad range of intake," and that safety problems are relatively rare.[10]

The act also strikes a blow for freedom of speech as set forth in the First Amendment to the United States Constitution. Proponents of the act had warned that unduly broad labeling regulations would hinder the free flow of information about products. For example, some feared that statements by retailers and general promotional articles made available by them to their customers might be found to constitute labeling of specific products. Imagine the burden on distributors if they were charged with mislabeling their products because of actions taken by retailers. How could they realistically defend themselves?

To address that concern, the DSHEA provides that publications, including promotional items and excerpts from books—if they are not false or misleading, they do not promote a particular brand and they are physically separate from the supplements in the store—would not be considered labeling when used in connection with the sale of supplements.

The act further tips the scales to encourage the free flow of information by providing that the government will have the burden of proving that a publication is false or misleading.[11] If that burden were the manufacturer's, a manufacturer would have to prove the contents of the publication to be true and not misleading. That could be an onerous, if not impossible, task.

Labeling statements about supplements claiming benefits related to a disease caused by a nutrient deficiency may be made if certain conditions are met. The statement must disclose the prevalence of such a disease in the United States, describe the role of the nutrient and the documented mechanism by which it works. Statements describing general well-being resulting from consumption of nutrients may also be made. Manufacturers must have substantiation that any statements they do make are truthful and not misleading. Any statement must also include the following language in boldface type:

"This statement has not been evaluated by the Food and Drug Administration. This product is not intended to diagnose, treat, cure, or prevent any disease."[12]

Products intended to diagnose, treat, cure or prevent any disease would be classified and regulated as drugs rather than as supplements under the law. Any manufacturer making a claim of benefit in the labeling of a supplement must notify the FDA within 30 days of beginning to market it with such a statement.

As for labeling, the act requires that names and quantities of ingredients be listed. The supplement will be considered misbranded if it misrepresents the quality, purity, strength or composition it truly contains.

A new ingredient—that is, one that was not marketed before October 15, 1994—contained in a supplement must meet certain requirements. For example, the presence of a new ingredient will be allowed if there is a history of safe use and if supporting documentation of that use is supplied to the FDA 75 days before the product is transported interstate.

The DSHEA also provides that a federal Commission on Dietary Supplement Labels be established. Its seven members are to be appointed by the president. The commission will study and make recommendations for the regulation and evaluation of label claims, including literature used in connection with the sale of a supplement. The commission is directed to consider how consumers should be provided with the accurate and scientifically valid information they need to make intelligent health-care choices. The commission is empowered to gather information and hold hearings. By October 1996, the commission is to submit a final report to the president and Congress. As part of its report, the commission will submit recommendations for any necessary regulations and even new legislation it may find advisable.

So we see, as we might have expected, the law pertaining to supplements purports to remain dynamic. Issues of health will remain scientifically complex, as will cherished freedoms we want to enjoy and see protected: freedom to make-nformed choices from among available health-care alternatives, freedom of speech, freedom of the marketplace. We know that all our freedoms must be limited to the extent that we try to respect the rights of others and provide for the general health and welfare of the public. Our society and its institutions—not unlike a tightrope-walker—face the difficult challenge of achieving a fair balance.

Those of us who have become impatient with the FDA at times should recall that its history and purpose have stressed its role in protecting the public from harmful substances and misinformation rather than maximizing freedom in the marketplace. Those who want to have access to a substance may feel victimized by regulations that hamper or completely deprive them of that access. On the other hand, someone who is harmed by a substance that proves hazardous may well decry the lack of regulation or lack of vigorous enforcement of regulations that might have protected her or him.

In the interest of speeding the process of scientific evaluation, the DSHEA provides for the creation of an Office of Dietary Supplements within the National Institutes of Health. The office is to explore the extent to which dietary supplements can play a more significant role in our health care. In that effort, the office is to collect and compile research and on that basis is to advise the director of the National Institutes of Health, the director of the centers for Disease Control and Prevention,

and the commissioner of Food and Drugs regarding dietary supplements.

We are a long way from the times of *caveat emptor* in many respects. This is not to say that all consumers are adequately protected. As a legal rule, "let the buyer beware" was more suitably applied in our early economic history when commerce primarily consisted of neighbor selling to neighbor commodities they both understood. In the 20th century, technology increasingly produces complex items to be sold to people who cannot know how they were made and handled or how they work. Consumers need adequate, even detailed information, especially on a topic such as supplements that have an effect on personal well-being, and in light of the frequently baffling myriad products from which to choose. The FDA is not going to make the choice for anyone. And people who are just going to pop pills don't need this book. But the authors have supplied to a willing eye and open mind a volume of both practical and interesting information on a great many supplements. The final benefits of supplements, of course, lie with the reader and his or her own state of body and mind.

—John G. Navarra, Jr., J.D.
Howell, New Jersey
February 1995

NOTES

1. From a letter from Carol R. Scheman, deputy commissioner for external affairs, Department of Health and Human Services, Public Health Service, Food and Drug Administration, Rockville, Md., June 10, 1994.
2. Ibid.
3. Rosman, Lisa, and Allan Cass. *The Supplement Wars: How the FDA and Congress Are Fighting Over Your Right to Choose Vitamins, Minerals and Dietary Supplements.* New Jersey Naturally, 1994 Winter/Spring, City Spirit Publications, Brooklyn, N.Y., p. 16.
4. *Illness and Injuries Associated with the Use of Selected Dietary Supplements,* Food and

Drug Administration Public Service Information, Appendix 9.

5. Ibid.
6. Public Law 103-417 [S.784] October 25, 1994: Dietary Supplement Health and Education Act of 1994, Section 2.

7. Ibid., Section 2 (13).
8. Ibid., Section 2 (15B).
9. Ibid., Section 3 (b).
10. Ibid., Section 2 (14).
11. Ibid., Section 5 (c).
12. Ibid., Section 6.

INTRODUCTION

Man's mind stretched to a new idea never goes
back to its original dimension.
—Oliver Wendell Holmes

Long before former president George Bush declared he hated broccoli and dubbed carrots "orange broccoli," people seemed to be in constant skirmishes over what foods are necessary for overall good nutrition. The American culture's affection for junk food and gourmet fare often manifests as meats, vegetables, fruits and starches that are hollandaised, glazed, grilled, creamed, sautéed, flambéed, candied, topped and glopped. Plain, wholesome food may represent "eating to live"—as in the painting *The Potato Eaters* by Van Gogh—rather than "living to eat."

In short, we have become nutritionally challenged, a society living on pizza, burgers and fries and wondering why *Time* magazine would run a cover story billed as "Girth of a Nation."[1]

The problem is not only obesity; it's also mindset. People sport either a laissez-faire attitude, as in, "Let them eat chips," or a general ignorance of nutrients. There is little in between, except possibly for registered dietitians (and not even all of them), health-food "nuts" and some conscientious types who prefer to eat sensibly.

Knowing what to eat involves recognizing, at least to a certain extent, that some foods are more nutritious than others. Furthermore, nutrition is an individual matter, especially for people with diabetes, heart disease, irritable bowel syndrome or an uncooperative gallbladder, for example. Nutritionists working with cancer patients may champion the intake of huge portions of ice cream with hot fudge and real whipped cream, or extra dollops of mayonnaise on a bologna sandwich—all hideous in terms of "good" nutrition. The rationale? Many of these patients have lost the desire to eat at all, so whatever appeals to them and offers the greatest number of calories may help keep up their energy and weight. The same principle applies to stubborn or fussy children whose parents allow them to live on cocktail wieners, if that's what they want, just to ensure they will eat *something*.

As if the daily routine of eating well weren't enough of a battle, the concept of food supplements compounds the confusion. Never mind the cost, but to take, or not to take?

The major studies conducted so far indicate mostly controversial results. A recent study in Finland, done under the auspices of the National Cancer Institute (NCI), tested beta-carotene supplements' effect on approximately 29,000 male smokers. Earlier studies suggested that people who regularly ate foods containing large amounts of beta-carotene were at low risk of developing lung cancer. But the Finnish study gave a startling result. The incidence of lung cancer in the Finnish men who took the supplement was 18 percent higher than in those who did not.

Also in the Finnish study, vitamin E was implicated as a possible troublemaker. It lowered the risk of prostate cancer as expected, but increased the death rate from hemorrhagic strokes.[2] On the other hand, studies have shown that calcium supplements (even in the form of Tums and other antacid tablets) do help prevent osteoporosis, vitamin C does lessen the wrath of many infections, vitamin A helps improve night vision and many other nutrients are tried and true in a variety of situations.

In general, people favor taking some form of supplement to their diets; vitamins, minerals, herbs and other substances and combinations are ingested to give us what our diets may not, even though vitamin and mineral supplements do not necessarily substitute for eating a healthful variety of foods (see Appendix 1, USDA Food Pyramid). Popping a stress-formula B-vitamin capsule, a garlic pill or a vitamin C tablet hooks directly into our cultural taste for things instant, easy, painless and, it is hoped, efficient.

In the 1950s, jars of "One-A-Day" multiple vitamins were snapped up by young moms eager to provide their families with a "magic bullet" that would compensate for any unwitting nutritional lack. It was a postwar era characterized by children who, despite Popeye's prowess-in-a-can, refused to eat spinach and turned up their noses at liver, rutabaga and brussels sprouts as well.

Moreover, food-processing and the supermarket emerged as enormously successful industries during that time. The "corner grocer" with his fresh produce became less popular as housing developments in suburban areas blossomed. The American family grew more interested in the modern conveniences of large freezers and processed foods. The Wonder Bread advertising campaign of 40 years ago comes to mind as an example: "Wonder Bread helps build strong bodies 12 ways." Nutritionists

and home economics teachers tried to tell us then that "enrichment" with 12 nutrients was necessary because the grain's original nutrients had been processed out of the product that ended up in our lunch boxes.

Youngsters following the example of older siblings and media role models promptly spurned whole-wheat bread—or any grainy kind that was good for you—because white bread somehow tasted better than brown bread. (White bread was also soft, and the taste blended with the flavor of whatever was on it or between two slices of it.) I remember Miss Sharp, my fifth-grade home economics teacher, who said, "Put a white slice on top of the sandwich and a brown one on the bottom, and when you eat, hold the white side toward you." One must admire her gift for compromise.

Miss Sharp also made each girl in her home-economics class (the boys took woodshop) eat a teaspoonful of wheat germ during a decade when the unappetizing key word was "germ." Grimaces shot around the room. I was the only girl who liked it, and I still eat it to this day. That experience in the 1950s influenced me to thrive on a merry assortment of both health and junk foods. I must also admit that, although I am not a disciplined supplement-taker, I believe in the nutritive and healing potential of vitamins, minerals and herbs and have experienced a fair amount of personal success in their use. Cranberry pills and marshmallow-root capsules from the health-food store, for instance, ended years of taking ineffective prescription medications for chronic bladder and urethral infections that had become the bane of my existence.

No doubt Miss Sharp would approve were she still around. Today, her baby-boomer pupils are middle-aged and may be junk-food junkies and the parents of finicky eaters. And conflicting ideas about the requirements of "good" nutrition struggle on. So many people became enamored of fast foods that nutritionists conducted scientific analyses of the nutrients (and dietary disadvantages) offered by the Whopper, the Big Mac, and other fast-food offerings.

Among the thornier questions are: How will the issue and study of nutrition become more significant in the future? Will the government's new Food Pyramid (see Appendix 1) truly guide a nation that embraces as great a gastronomic diversity as ours? Is there a spirituality of nutrition evolving, a philosophy of mind-body connection that may encourage people to become more vegetarian and take supplements with educated discretion?

Perhaps the only answerable question is the last, because the concept of mind-body connection has finally engaged itself as part of our health-care infrastructure. According to recent surveys in women's and other consumer magazines, people generally believe that one's way of thinking affects his or her physical state. That the media repeatedly call the increasing interest in vitamins, minerals and supplements "the vitamin craze" (see Bibliography for the *Time* magazine April 1994 article of that name) indicates the overall American disposition toward better nutrition, despite an appetite for empty calories, fats, sweets and poor sources of nutrients.

There are and always will be skeptics, however, including some who may have worthy points of view. In the *New York Times Magazine,* Nicholas Wade wrote:

> Nature doesn't yield its secrets easily. As with the oracle at Delphi, its answers may conceal a dangerous ambiguity. . . . It's tempting to infer that vitamins are the cause of better health. . . . But beneath that beguiling message, all that these observational studies really tell us is that there is an association between vitamins and health benefits. For a biologist, that's the statement of the puzzle, not its solution.
>
> Scientific trials will in time provide the verdict on vitamin supplements. For all who assumed the answer was already known, the Finnish trial offers two lessons. One is that science can't be rushed. The

other is not to put all your bets on those convenient little bottles: back to broccoli and bicycles.[3]

While Wade suggests the benefit of the doubt, Dr. Victor Herbert, a professor of medicine at New York City's Mount Sinai Medical School, set forth an uncompromisingly negative stance. He said taking supplementary nutrients creates nothing more than "expensive urine."[4] Many physicians, not trained in nutrition (or mind-body connection, for that matter), would agree. They tell their clients the food they eat supplies them with all the nutrients they need, which could possibly be true if people dutifully ate their carrots, broccoli, wheat germ and such.

But it isn't true, because people insist on eating what they like. They are not complying with basic nutritional information, and they are frequently baffled by conflicting reports on supplements. *Consumer Reports* (September 1994) says, "The ups and downs of nutrition advice have come to seem as capricious as the fluctuations of the stock market."[5] The article continues with evidence in favor of antioxidants—vitamin C, vitamin E and beta-carotene—that help protect us from the potentially destructive activities of the body's naturally produced molecules called free radicals. The article also discusses evidence that for certain people the taking of certain supplements may be harmful.

Because most scientists and health professionals have established that we must obtain vitamins from outside sources to maintain good health, there is a clear need for extensive research and controlled clinical studies that take a multitude of factors into account, such as:

(a) understanding what a balanced daily diet is, given an individual's ethnicity, age, circumstances and history;

(b) understanding emotional and spiritual aspects, known to some as "psychic vitamins," in our lives that may affect the individual metabolism of nutrients; and

(c) studying nutrients, including herbal sources, as substances that prevent and treat disease.

The broccoli study is one example. Broccoli and other cruciferous vegetables, including cabbage, cauliflower and brussels sprouts, contain the chemical compound sulforaphane. According to the findings of Dr. Paul Talalay, Dr. Gary H. Posner and other research scientists at Johns Hopkins University in Baltimore, Maryland, sulforaphane blocks the growth of cancerous tumors in rats and stimulates the production of anticancer enzymes in mouse cells. These intriguing results were published in the March 1992 issue of *The Proceedings of the National Academy of Sciences*.[6]

From this, scientists speculate that broccoli may provide a key to preventing colorectal cancer in humans. Sulforaphane in the *Brassica* genus of vegetables, whose most potent star is broccoli, is being tested at Fox Chase Cancer Center in Philadelphia, Pennsylvania, under the auspices of Dr. Paul F. Engstrom, senior vice president for population science, and Dr. Margie Clapper, who holds a Ph.D. in molecular and cell biology. The clinical trial with human participants seeks to determine the role of broccoli in preventing colorectal cancer.

"We're looking at individuals who are at high risk for colorectal cancer," Dr. Clapper said. "The criteria are those undergoing routine colonoscopy, those with a history of colorectal cancer who completed treatment at least two years ago, those with a history of colon polyps, and people with a family history of colorectal cancer."

Individuals with active colorectal cancer, colitis or radiation enteritis are among those not eligible for the broccoli trial. A sulforaphane treatment for active cancer may take years to emerge, if ever. The big questions for the clinical study are how much broccoli must a participant eat, and will it help if he or she actually likes broccoli.

Owing much to the techniques of pharmacy, participants do not eat any broccoli whether they like it or not. They take as a dietary supplement six broccoli tablets per day, two with each meal. Yes, broccoli tablets, made from real broccoli by a well-known supplement manufacturer. Available over the counter, they are green, malodorous and equivalent to approximately 30 grams of the vegetable, a typical restaurant serving of cooked broccoli. The cumulative dosage for participants is three grams a day.

Dr. Clapper said Fox Chase seeks 50 participants. At this writing, 31 have been recruited. In addition to taking the broccoli tablets, participants agree to undergo two flexible sigmoidoscopies, during which physicians can obtain colon tissue for biopsy, and give two blood samples before and after the study.[7]

Slowly but surely, the Fox Chase research exemplifies, skeptics are beginning to agree with those who believe in eating the most beneficial foods and food supplements. As nutrition takes center stage, the proverbial "food fight" over supplements will revert to a foolishness of the past.

Ironically, we may need first to step back in time and follow the culinary example of our biblical ancestors. The Bible is replete with references to the cultivation, preparation, consumption and significance of food, such as: ". . . A land of wheat, and barley, and vines, and fig trees, and pomegranates; a land of oil olive, and honey; A land wherein thou shalt eat bread without scarceness, thou shalt not lack any thing in it . . ." (Deuteronomy 8:8).

Basic food came from the earth, the sea and the animals. If one favored St. Benedict's philosophy of moderation in all things, basic foods taken in moderation (including meat, to the dismay of vegans) would constitute the next step toward a revitalized view of modern nutrition.

Furthermore, the Bible advocates using plants not only as food but as agents of healing:

"Along both banks of the river, fruit trees of every kind shall grow; their leaves shall not fade, nor their fruit fail. Every month they shall bear fresh fruit, for they shall be watered by the flow from the sanctuary. Their fruit shall serve for food, and their leaves for medicine" (Ezekiel 47:12).

If familiar vitamins and minerals have wrought havoc in the supplement wars, lesser-known herbal supplements, also to be used as remedies for illness, increase the confusion about what to take or not to take. As swiftly as "One-A-Day" multiple vitamins were accepted, many people now run to the health-food store to purchase any number of "foreign" products. "Biochavan," for example, is an Ayurvedic (traditional Hindu) herbal supplement designed to nourish, promote longevity and cater specifically to the needs and/or deficits of the various body types upon which the practice of Ayurvedic medicine is based.

It is sobering to know that people from the time of the Ancient Egyptians (and possibly before recorded history) used aloe, poppy, caraway seeds, garlic and hundreds of other herbs as both food and medicine. In the last few years, Americans have been leaning, if cautiously, toward tapping into the rewards of good nutrition as they were experienced by our ancestors. We are looking more carefully at natural instead of processed foods. Holistic concepts and practices now in the American mainstream—yoga, among others—teach us about the body's innate power and desire to resist damaging invaders and heal itself. While it is advisable to investigate products before ingesting them, such as powders made of deer antler and shark cartilage sold as treatments for certain maladies, it is also advisable to keep an open mind to foods and other substances that have actually been part of our culinary and pharmaceutical heritage for thousands of years.

Fears pertaining to nutrition still loom large: world hunger and malnutrition; the future effects of managed care on preventive and alternative health-care options; certain herbal teas making headlines as killers; dietary or health-food backlash; supplement quackery; the cruelty of animal-testing; and other dilemmas. But we might as well seek as intelligently as we can the opportunity to fortify our bodies without sacrificing the pleasures of food and drink—whether a sumptuous prime rib or a plain broiled flounder, an artichoke parmigiana or a portobello mushroom, a calming cup of warm milk with nutmeg or a goblet of wine. In the presence of these, "One-A-Days" risk being forgotten in the "fridge," and memories of Miss Sharp's home-economics class endure only as a rudimentary connection between nutrition and tastebuds.

—Tova Navarra

NOTES

1. Elmer-Dewitt, Philip. "Fat Times." *Time,* January 16, 1995, pp. 58–65.
2. "Taking Vitamins: Can They Prevent Disease?" *Consumer Reports,* September 1994, pp. 561–567.
3. Wade, Nicholas. "Method and Madness: Believing in Vitamins." *New York Times Magazine,* May 22, 1994, p. 20.
4. Toufexis, Anastasia. "The New Scoop on Vitamins." *Time,* April 6, 1992, p. 54.
5. "Taking Vitamins: Can They Prevent Disease?" *Consumer Reports,* p. 561.
6. Prochaska, Hans J., Annette B. Santamaria, and Paul Talalay. "Rapid Detection of Inducers of Enzymes That Protect Against Carcinogens." *The Proceedings of the National Academy of Sciences,* vol. 89, March 1992, pp. 2394–2398.
7. The two-year study, funded by the National Cancer Institute, was completed in April 1995.

VITAMINS, MINERALS AND SUPPLEMENTS A–Z

A

A, vitamin

A fat-soluble vitamin essential for growth and bone development in children, for vision (especially in low light), for healthy skin and mucous membrane surfaces, for reproduction and the integrity of the immune system. Vitamin A consists of several active compounds, including alpha-carotene, beta-carotene, retinal (retinaldehyde), retinol (vitamin A_1), retinoic acid and the carotenoids. Natural sources of vitamin A are egg yolks, fish-liver oils, liver, cream, butter, green leafy and yellow vegetables, pineapples, prunes, cantaloupes, oranges and limes. The richest sources include cod-liver oil, butter, butterfat in milk and egg yolk. Vitamin A can also be synthetically produced.

Documented reports of "night blindness" more than 3,500 years ago indicate a positive response to foods rich in vitamin A. In Ancient Egypt, there was evidence that juice prepared from cooked animal livers was placed in the eyes of those with poor night vision. This practice has persisted to modern times in some societies. Later, in the third and fourth centuries B.C., Hippocrates prescribed eating beef liver for the treatment of night blindness.

Early in the 20th century, Englishman Frederick Gowland Hopkins discovered a growth-stimulating substance in milk. Later, a German researcher named Stepp identified a substance he had labeled "minimal qualitative factors" as a lipid. In 1913, E. V. McCollum and Marguerite David demonstrated an essential growth factor for rats in butter and egg yolk, which they called "fat soluble A."

Simultaneously, Osborn and Mendel, working in New Haven, Connecticut, found a similar fat-soluble substance in cod-liver oil and butter.

Moore, an English scientist, demonstrated that beta-carotene obtained as a colored substance from plants was transformed in the human body to a colorless form of vitamin A, which was then stored in the liver. It was not until 1930 that Karrer and his group in Switzerland determined the chemical structures of vitamin A and beta-carotene. In 1935, Wald defined a biochemical in the retina that he termed retinene, later renamed retinal.

Beta-carotene

A provitamin, precursor chemical or building block that the human body converts to vitamin A, beta-carotene is one of many pigments called carotenoids that give the deep coloring found in orange or green vegetables and fruits. Although there are more than 500 naturally occurring carotenoids, only about 50 have provitamin A activity, or the ability to be converted to retinol.

Beta-carotene is the only carotenoid that can be converted to significant amounts of vitamin A, and only about one-sixth is converted in humans. Dietary fat is required for the adequate absorption of carotene. The deeper the orange coloring of a carrot, the higher the concentration of beta-carotene.

In an Arizona study, 26 of 49 patients with oral leukoplakia, a premalignant lesion, were given 60 milligrams daily of beta-carotene for six months, resulting in a significant reduction in the size of their lesions. However, excessive ingestion of beta-carotene and other carotenoids from dietary sources or supplements may cause a yellowing of the skin. Fortunately, the skin pigmentation is reversible with reduction in the quantity of beta-carotene consumed. There is no evidence that natural sources of beta-carotene are more effective than synthetic sources. (See also CANTHAXANTHIN.)

Retinol

The major vitamin A compound is found naturally in eggs, dairy products, liver and fish-liver oil. The compounds require proteins for their absorption from the intestines. Etretinate, a synthetic retinoid, appears to be effective in the treatment of psoriasis. Half of 32 patients being treated for advanced cervical cancer had a 50 percent regression in the size of their tumors when treated with oral 13-cis-retinoic acid and alpha interferon.

Vitamin A Deficiencies

The most common vitamin A deficiencies are caused by disorders of impaired fat absorption. These conditions include: (1) preschool-age children with cystic fibrosis, malabsorption syndromes or obstruction in the biliary system; (2) impaired storage or transport of the vitamin in cirrhosis and abetalipoproteinemia (an inherited metabolic disorder involving the synthesis of low-density cholesterol); and (3) increased metabolic demands during infancy, pregnancy and breastfeeding or with hyperthyroidism. Dietary deficiency of only vitamin A is rare and is usually combined with other vitamin deficiencies.

Nyctalopia, or night blindness, is the initial indication of inadequate vitamin A. With continued vitamin insufficiency, xerophthalmia (dryness of the conjunctiva and cornea) and keratomalacia (softness of the cornea) occur with perforation and ultimately cause blindness. This is especially common in the children of underdeveloped countries, where vitamin-A deficiency may be responsible for an estimated 250,000 cases of blindness annually. Although most symptoms of vitamin A deficiency improve with vitamin-A supplementation, there may be a permanent stunting of growth if the epiphyseal, or growth, plates close prematurely in bones.

Data collected from the 50,828 women enrolled in the Nurses' Health Study by researchers at the Brigham and Women's Hospital in Boston suggest that consuming foods high in vitamins A and C may reduce the incidence of cataracts. Antioxidant-rich vegetables such as spinach, sweet potatoes and squash appear to protect the eyes by preventing oxidation of proteins in the lens that lead to the formation of cataracts.

Measles seems to have a poorer prognosis in children who are vitamin A deficient. Children with severe measles infections should be given vitamin supplementation (see also MEASLES AND VITAMIN A DEFICIENCY).

One study of AIDS patients demonstrated that individuals with vitamin A deficiency died sooner than those with normal levels of the vitamin (see also AIDS AND VITAMIN DEFICIENCY).

Toxicity

Vitamin A excess can be toxic to a developing fetus. More than 15 mg of beta-carotene per day may impair fertility. Liver damage may result in a child from as little as the adult Recommended Daily Allowance (RDA) for a certain number of years and in adults from as little as five times the RDA for seven to 10 years. Chronic toxicity in infants and children causes pseudotumor cerebri (increased pressure in the brain that acts like a brain tumor), tinnitus (ringing in the ears), bulging fontanelles (swelling of the soft spot in the infant skull), increased cerebrospinal fluid, bone pain, lethargy, pruritus (itching), scaly rashes, cracks in the corners of the mouth, hyperostosis and metaphyseal cupping (abnormal bone growth) and paronychia (infections in the nail edges). Eye changes include diplopia (double vision), papilledema (swelling of the optic nerve), optic atrophy (wasting of the optic nerve) and eventually blindness.

In adults, chronic toxicity of vitamin A may cause vomiting, skin changes, irritability, headache, diminished menstrual bleeding, weakness and psychiatric disorders. Depression and symptoms suggestive of schizophrenia can be so severe that individuals have been placed in mental hospitals. Liver and spleen enlargement have been seen along with elevated levels of calcium in the blood. Chronic vitamin-A toxicity causes drying of the skin and mucous membranes, hair loss, brittle nails, loss of appetite and muscle, bone and joint and abdominal pains. Enlarged spleens and anemia may also result. Fatal anaphylactic shock (the most severe form of allergic reaction) and death have been reported following intravenous administration of vitamin A.

It has been estimated that almost 5 percent of vitamin A-supplement users in the United States exceed the 800 to 1,000 mcg recommended dietary allowance (RDA) of retinol approved by the Food and Nutrition Board of the National Research Council in 1980.

Teratogenicity (Birth Defects)

Doses greater than the RDA of 6,000 international units (I.U.) or 1,800 retinol equivalents of vitamin A should never be taken by pregnant or lactating women. Serious birth defects have been reported in infants born to mothers who took as little as 25,000 I.U. of vitamin A daily during conception and the first trimester of pregnancy. The Food and Drug Administration considers this vitamin in Pregnancy Category X, or having the potential for serious birth defects if taken in excess during pregnancy (see also PREGNANCY VITAMIN AND MINERAL REQUIREMENTS).

Dosage

The liver stores several months' supply of vitamin A in well-nourished individuals. Protein and possibly zinc may be involved in the utilization of the liver stores. Healthy breast-feeding infants, children and adults generally do not require vitamin A supplementation. Rarely should adult doses exceeding 25,000 I.U. daily be taken unless a deficiency is especially severe. See Table 2 for U.S. RDA for vitamin A.

Although breast milk normally supplies adequate vitamin A, infants of poorly nourished mothers should receive 1,400 I.U. of vitamin A daily for the first six months. Although milk is labeled as fortified with vitamins A and D, studies by the Boston University School of Medicine found wide variance in vitamin content of milk tested in both regular containers of whole milk and infant formulas. Investigators identified vitamin D toxicity in eight children and fear that incorrect amounts of these vitamins in the milk may result in vitamin

deficiencies or cases of toxicity. Only a third of milk samples tested had a vitamin content within 20 percent of the amount stated on the label. Seven of 10 samples had more than twice the amount stated.

The International Center for the Prevention and Treatment of Major Childhood Diseases reported that a single large dose of vitamin A (50,000 to 200,000 I.U. each) reduced death by 26 percent in a group of 3,700 malnourished children in India and Nepal.

Water-soluble vitamin A is six times more readily absorbed than an oily preparation and also more toxic to the same degree.

Drug Interactions

Cholestyramine, the cholesterol-lowering drug, and mineral oil may reduce absorption of vitamin A. Oral contraceptives (birth control pills) significantly increase blood levels of vitamin A.

Table 1 DOSAGE REQUIREMENTS FOR VITAMIN A DEFICIENCY STATUS	
Severe deficiency with xerophthalmia (see above)	Age > 8 500,000 I.U./ day for 3 days then by 50,000 I.U./day for 2 weeks
without xerophthalmia	Age > 8 100,000 I.U./ day for 3 days then 50,000 I.U./day for 2 weeks then 10,000 to 20,000 I.U./day for 2 months
	1 to 8 years 5,000 to 10,000 I.U./day orally for 2 months or 17,500 to 35,000 I.U./day intramuscularly for 10 days
	Infants 7,500 to 15,000 I.U./day intramuscularly for 10 days

Table 2
U.S. RDA FOR DIETARY VITAMIN A
SUPPLEMENTATION

Age	Daily Requirement	
	Retinol Units (RE)	International Units (IU)*
Birth to 1 year	375	1875
1 to 3 years	400	2000
4 to 6 years	500	2500
7 to 10 years	700	3300
Adolescent and adult males	1000	5000
Adolescent and adult females	800	4000
Special circumstances		
Elderly	no changes required	
Pregnant females	no additional requirement	
Lactation, initial		
6 months	1300	6500
after 6 months	1200	6000

[RE = Retinol equivalents: 1 RE = 3.33 IU of vitamin A or 10 IU of beta-carotene]

*The Recommended Dietary Allowances (RDAs) assumes more than half of the vitamin A intake will come from beta carotene, thus the values given are based on 1 RE = 5 IU.

(Sources: National Research Council Recommended Dietary Allowances 10th edition and The Essential Guide to Vitamins and Minerals by Elizabeth Somer, M.A., R.D.)

abrus

(rosary pea, love pea, Indian licorice, wild licorice vine, prayer-beads, weather plant or vine, coral-bead plant, red-bead vine, crab's eye, precatory bean)

A plant of the family Leguminosae, *Abrus precatorius,* whose whole seeds are used to treat fever, malaria, headache, dropsy and intestinal worms. *Abrus* is the Greek word meaning delicate, which describes the leaves of the plant; the other names refer to the seeds. As long as the seeds are completely intact, they are harmless or considered by herbologists to be therapeutic. However, the ingestion of a cracked seed, or even the absorption through the skin of the contents of cracked seeds used for necklaces and the like, may be fatal. Abrus is used in traditional Chinese medicine.

absorption

The process by which nutrients enter the circulatory system from the gastrointestinal tract. In order for vitamins and minerals to reach the bloodstream, they must dissolve in the stomach or intestines and diffuse across the membranes lining the digestive tract. Nutrients that fail to be absorbed may pass through the digestive tract and be excreted in the feces and therefore provide no nutritional value. The *U.S. Pharmacopoeia* (USP) establishes standards for the composition of drugs. Products that meet its rigid requirements assure the consumer that water-soluble products will dissolve within 30 minutes if uncoated or 45 minutes if coated. However, some products are designed for a prolonged release in order to reduce adverse effects. Evidence is lacking that chelated or bioflavonoid forms of vitamins work faster or are better absorbed than less expensive forms.

A dissolution test measures how soon a supplement dissolves in liquid and is more stringent than a disintegration test, which measures how long it takes for a product to break into tiny pieces.

acanthopanax

(spiny panax)

The plant of the family Araliaceae used in traditional Chinese medicine. From the Greek words *akantha,* or thorn, *pan,* or all, and *akes,* or remedy, acanthopanax is also known as thorny panax (panacea). *Acanthopanax gracilistylus* root bark is considered a tonic for weakness and for the treatment of rheumatism, impotence, lumbago and syphilis. The entire *Acanthopanax davidii* plant is used to treat mechanical injury, and the leaves of the *Acanthopanax trifoliatus* are used in preparations to treat tuberculosis, partial paralysis and bleeding in the lungs.

acidophilus

(Lactobacillus acidophilus)

A bacterium occurring naturally in the intestines that assists in the digestion of proteins, reduces blood cholesterol levels, fights fungal infections and augments nutrient absorption and distribution. Acidophilus also helps the body combat the effects of harmful substances by reinforcing the intestines' balance of what are called "friendly" bacteria or "good flora." For example, a *Candida* (yeast) infection is the result of an excess of coliform, instead of lactobacillus, bacteria that provided an accommodating climate in which *Candida* flourished. An acidophilus supplement has an antibacterial effect, thus defeating the coliform bacterial environment and restoring intestinal health.

Acidophilus is also found in yogurt, kefir, cheese, buttermilk and other "soured milk" or fermented-milk products. Non-dairy acidophilus include DDS Acidophilus, Neo-Flora, Kyo-Dophilus and Primadophilus and are available in powdered, tablet or capsule form in health-food stores and pharmacies. When a food containing the "good bacteria" of yogurt cultures is heated, the bacteria are destroyed. Frozen yogurt products do not contain the beneficial *lactobacillus acidophilus* culture. (See YOGURT.)

acne

Inflammation of the sebaceous glands and hair follicles that causes pustules and other skin eruptions, especially during adolescence. Pitting and scarring of the skin may result. Vitamin A has been used to treat acne for many years. However, oral forms can be toxic in the high doses required for significant improvement. Isotretinoin (13-cis-retinoic acid), or Accutane (trade name), is a very potent synthetic derivative of vitamin A. Unfortunately the drug has a great many adverse effects and is teratogenic (causes birth defects) if taken early in pregnancy. Tetinoin (all-trans-retinoic acid) or Retin-A, is another vitamin A derivative that is useful in treating acne when applied topi-

cally. Beta-carotene, which is converted to vitamin A in the body, is nontoxic and may also improve acne.

Selenium and vitamin E in one study showed significant improvement in acne and also seborrheic dermatitis (a form of severe dandruff). Pyridoxine (vitamin B_6) may also have value for severe acne, but large doses may cause toxicity to the central nervous system and must be used cautiously.

(See also A, VITAMIN.)

aconite

(aconitum, monkshood, fu tzu)

A north-temperate herb, of the family Ranunculaceae, with thick roots and flowers that resemble the garb of Benedictine monks. Monkshood was known to the Greeks in mythology and ancient times as containing a poisonous juice of various uses, including for poisoning the wells and other water supply of encroaching enemies, for criminals to drink as a death penalty and on one Greek island as a euthanasia method for the ill elderly.

In folklore, a concoction of monkshood and deadly nightshade was believed to enable witches to fly. Some herbologists believe the concoction may induce a sensation of flight, which fostered the fables.

Used in China for more than 2,000 years, aconite, including *Aconitum carmichaelii, chinensis* and *transectum,* has many benefits when the plant parts have been dried. Among them are treatment for pain, colds, chills, vomiting, rheumatoid arthritis, loss of appetite and kidney inflammation. Aconite is also considered a stimulant, heart tonic, narcotic, mild laxative and local anesthetic.

acorn

The oak tree nut encapsulated in a woody covering with indurated bracts, like tiny "jewelry settings," from which the acorn had grown. Of the *Quercus* species, shelled and ground acorns are made into a meal that can be used as a food or drink. Herbalists claim that acorns are nutritive, containing flavonoids, sugar, starch, albumin (a protein) and fats, to individuals with wasting diseases including tuberculosis and AIDS, as well as medicinal for those with diarrhea.

acrodermatitis enteropathica

An inherited disease resulting in an inability to absorb zinc. Infants with this disorder have poor appetite, severe diarrhea, impaired night vision, hair loss, skin rashes, depressed immunity and bizarre neurological and psychological disturbances. These children fail to thrive and if untreated may die. Family members share a tendency to have diminished zinc levels as well.

Zinc is poorly absorbed from cow's milk, and manifestations of acrodermatitis enteropathica were initially recognized when symptoms of zinc deficiency appeared in infants fed cow's milk. These infants improved when switched to more easily digested breastmilk.

(See also ZINC.)

adder's tongue

(lamb's tongue, snake leaf, rattlesnake violet, erythonium, dog-tooth violet, serpent's tongue, yellow snowdrop)

A perennial, flowering herb, *Erythonium americanum,* that grows in rich soil all over the United States, whose bulbs and leaves are used as an emetic (to induce vomiting) and as a poultice for scrofula and other skin conditions.

additives

Chemicals or substances added to foods, medications or supplements as coloring or flavoring agents, preservatives, sweeteners or to improve consistency. Adverse reactions are rare from the approximately 2,800 substances approved by the Food and Drug Administration (FDA). An esti-mated 12,000 other chemicals enter the food supply unintentionally.

One important and potentially life-threatening reaction can occur in persons susceptible to the preservatives known as sulfiting agents. These additives can cause asthma or life-threatening anaphylaxis (allergic shock), with symptoms including a flushed feeling, drop in blood pressure and tingling sensations.

Dyes approved in the Food, Drug and Cosmetic Act (FD&C) of 1938 are derivatives of coal tar. Tartrazine or FD&C yellow dye number 5 is frequently implicated as a cause of hyperactivity in children and asthma. However, less than 10 percent of individuals suspected of having adverse reactions to these additives reacted when challenged in a controlled study. Asthmatics who are allergic to aspirin may also react when exposed to the dye tartrazine.

Butylated hydroxanisol (BHA) and butylated hydroxytoluene (BHT) are used in low doses as antioxidants (see ANTIOXIDANTS) in grain products, including breakfast cereals, and have not been shown to cause any allergic problems. However, since antioxidants are thought by some to prevent cancer and herpes infections and to retard aging, they are often used in megadoses in various health-food preparations that may be toxic.

The azo dye amaranth (FD&C red number 5) was banned by the United States in 1975 because of suspected carcinogenicity. Aspartame (Nutra-sweet) is often blamed for adverse effects, but except for a few cases of urticaria (hives), there is no scientific proof of ill effects. Tartrazine is also frequently implicated in causing hives. However, well-controlled studies such as those at the Scripps Clinic and Research Foundation have rarely confirmed these suspicions. The dyes do play a role as sensitizers, or allergens, in allergic dermatitis. They are often suspected of inducing adverse effects both in the skin and when ingested. Skin reactions are relatively common; when dyes are used in foods and supplements, they are rarely proven to be the source of the adverse effect.

agastache
(huo xiang, wrinkled giant hyssop)
The herb *Agastache rugosa* of the family Labiatae, native to China, Japan, northern Vietnam and Laos, that is used in traditional Chinese medicine for treating fever, headache, nausea and vomiting, diarrhea, gas, colds and cholera. *Agastache* is Greek for many-spiked, which describes the plant's flowering spikes.

agave
(American agave, spiked aloe, American century, century plant, flowering aloe)
A perennial plant, *Agave americana,* of the tropical regions of America and in some parts of Europe, considered to be an antiseptic, diuretic and laxative. It has been used in the treatment of liver disease and pulmonary tuberculosis.

aging
See NUTRITION AND AGING.

agrimony
(xian he cao, sticklewort, cocklebur, burr marigold)
A fruit-bearing, yellow-flowered herb with toothed leaves, of the genus *Agrimonia* of the rose family. Available in powdered or capsule form, agrimony is thought to relieve gastrointestinal disorders and to strengthen the liver, gallbladder and kidneys. Agrimony, which contains vitamins B and K and other nutrients, is also said to inhibit any type of bleeding. In Chinese traditional medicine, agrimony, especially *Agrimonia eupatoria* and *pilosa,* is used to treat dysentery, stomach pain, and vomiting of blood, bleeding in the uterus, blood in the urine and stool and exhaustion.

AIDS (acquired immunodeficiency syndrome) and vitamin deficiency
Some individuals with AIDS, in addition to many other health deficits, seem to lack the ability to absorb nutrients including vitamins and minerals that leads to malnutrition. Studies conducted by researchers at Johns Hopkins University, Baltimore, Maryland have found lower levels of vitamin A in individuals who test positive for HIV. Those with AIDS and vitamin A deficiency died up to six times more rapidly than those who had normal vitamin A levels.

(See also A, VITAMIN.)

ailanthus
(tree-of-heaven, varnish tree, copal tree)
The tree *Ailanthus altissima,* of the family Simaroubaceae, indigenous to China, whose root bark and fruit are used in Chinese traditional medicine to treat dysentery, piles, bloody stools, vaginal discharge, premature ejaculation and tapeworm, and to increase menstrual flow.

akebia
(mu tong, five-leaf akebia, chocolate vine)
The vine *Akebia quinata* or *trifoliata,* of the family Lardizabalaceae, whose stem, fruit stalk and root are used in Chinese traditional medicine. Native to China, Japan and Korea, akebia is thought to relieve fever and inflammation of the skin, induce the secretion of breast milk for a new mother, induce perspiration and increase menstrual flow. The fruit stalk is used as a purgative.

albizia
(mimosa tree, silk tree)
An ornamental tree, *Albizia julibrissin,* of the family Leguminosae, grown from Iran to Japan and cultivated in other countries, whose bark and flowers are considered medicinal by traditional Chinese practitioners. The bark is said to tranquilize, relieve pain, improve circulation and treat insomnia, bleeding, fractures and lung cancer. The flowers are used as a general tonic.

alcoholism

The excessive, debilitating intake of alcoholic beverages, accompanied by a decreased desire for food. The substitution of alcohol for food causes multiple nutritional deficiencies and interferes with the absorption of nutrients when they are ingested. Beriberi, Korsakoff's syndrome and Wernicke's disease, all disorders of thiamine deficiency, are prevalent in alcoholism. Riboflavin, vitamin B_{12}, magnesium, potassium and selenium are other vitamins and minerals that are frequently deficient in alcoholics.

Women who drink more than two alcoholic drinks daily have a 25- to 50-percent increased risk of hip fractures. A group of white men between the ages of 49 and 61 years with a history of alcohol abuse for at least 10 years were found to have spinal bone densities averaging 58 percent of the normal density. The cause for these findings has not been determined.

alder

(holly, winterberry, feverbush, black alder, brook alder, striped alder)
A deciduous shrub, *Ilex verticillata,* common to swamplands of northeastern America and England, whose bark and fruit are used in the preparation of infusions or decoctions to treat worms and dyspepsia. An excessive quantity of the berries may be poisonous.

alehoof

(ground ivy, cat's foot, gill-go-by-ground, turn hoof, hay maids, alehoof, gill-creep-by-ground, creeping Charlie, gillrun, hedge maids, turnhoof)
A flowering perennial herb, *Nepeta hederacea,* found in the eastern states, on the Pacific coast and in Europe, whose leaves and flowering herb are used an an appetizer, astringent, digestive, diuretic, stimulant and tonic. Ground ivy is commonly thought to relieve diarrhea, colds, sore throat, bronchitis, headache, hypoacidity, neurasthenia and liver problems. Large quantities of ground ivy can be poisonous.

aleurites

(tung: oil tree, China wood-oil tree)
A tree indigenous to central Asia and cultivated elsewhere, *Aleurites fordii,* of the family Euphorbiaceae, known to have insecticidal properties. The oil, used in the manufacture of India ink, is also claimed to treat boils, burns and other topical anomaly, according to traditional Chinese medicine. The immature fruits are used to treat anemic conditions and the absence of menses.

alfalfa

An edible herb grass, succulent perennial and legume, *Medicago sativa,* containing calcium, magnesium, phosphorus, potassium, iron, essential enzymes, choline, sodium and vitamins A, B_6, D, K and P, cited for its beneficial effects against arthritis, intestinal ulcers, liver disorders, eczema, asthma, anemia, bleeding gums, gastritis, hemorrhoids, burns, fungal infections, cancer and hypertension, among other problems. In Arabic, alfalfa means father, and as herbalist, acupuncturist and author Michael Tierra, of California, says, perhaps this refers to alfalfa's "patriarchal" function as a highly esteemed restorative tonic. The chlorophyll content of alfalfa is thought to contribute to its potency. While alfalfa sprouts may be purchased at most supermarkets and eaten raw in salad, alfalfa is also available as a liquid, especially recommended to be taken during a fasting period.

Known as Mu-Su in Chinese medicine, alfalfa is effective as a raw green food, powder or tea. Its vitamin P (rutin) is reported to build the strength of capillaries and reduce inflammation of the stomach lining, thus an antiulcer treatment. Alfalfa is said to increase the flow of mother's milk and relieve low back pain. Alfalfa tea contributes to the digestive process for sugars, fats, starches and protein. Native Americans, who introduced the plant as a fresh green after it was brought from Europe to the United States in the mid-1800s, also ground alfalfa seeds into flour and added it to breads, gruel and other foods. People of the Great Plains region of America often referred to alfalfa as buffalo grass.

According to Ayurvedic medicine (*ayu* means life and *veda* means knowing in Sanskrit, the classical language of India and Hinduism), alfalfa is used as an anti-inflammatory, a natural pain reliever (for sciatica, for example) and as an agent that cleanses the large intestine of toxins.

algae

The Latin word for seaweed. Algae belongs to a group of aquatic plants—subphylum Algae of the phylum Thallophyta, the lowest division of the animal kingdom—including pond scums, stoneworts and seaweeds that contain chlorophyll. Ranging in size from microscopic to massive and found in salt or fresh water or moist places such as swamps, algae have no roots, stems or leaves. Kelp and Irish moss are forms of algae. (See IRISH MOSS; KELP.)

Blue-green algae, which grows in brackish water, has not been approved for sale in the United States. However, harvested wild, it is marketed as an organic food containing vitamins and all the amino acids and as beneficial in the daily diet. Some marketers and distributors of blue-green algae claim that algae increases energy; alleviates stress, anxiety and depression; relieves hypoglycemia, fatigue, constipation and allergies; and improves digestion, memory and immune functions.

According to the late nutritionist and author Adelle Davis, whose best-selling books of the 1950s to the 1970s influenced the public view and study of nutrition, algae in the form of kelp constitutes a treatment for an inadequate supply of iodine to the thyroid gland, which regulates metabolism, especially in areas affected by fallout from bomb testing. Kelp and other seaweeds contain iodine that is necessary for healthy thyroid functioning and protection against radioactive material easily absorbed by, and thus damaging to, the thyroid.

alisma

(ze xie, water plantain, mad-dog weed)

The North American and East Asian herb *Alisma plantago-aquatica,* of the family Alismataceae, considered to have anticancer properties and the ability to lower blood sugar in animals. In traditional Chinese medicine, the underground stem is used to treat hypertension, diabetes, kidney inflammation, venereal diseases, vertigo, lumbago and painful urination.

allergy to foods

See FOOD ALLERGY.

allium

(garlic)

The plant *Allium sativum,* of the family Amaryllidaceae, of European origin and cultivated all over the world. The garlic bulb, divided into cloves, is popular as both a food flavoring and medicinal/nutritive agent. Eastern and Western medical disciplines recognize the value of garlic as a natural antibiotic for colds, sore throat, phlegm in the respiratory tract, asthma, bronchitis, abscesses and tuberculosis. Garlic is also known to reduce high blood pressure and cholesterol.

The Ancient Egyptians used garlic to cure headaches, tumors, heart disorders and intestinal worms. Ancient Olympic athletes ate garlic to increase their energy. In the first century A.D., garlic was prescribed by Dioscorides, chief physician to the Roman army, as an anthelmintic (intestinal worm-killer) agent. Garlic may also have anticarcinogenic properties and is used as an antidote against various toxins. First known to be used in Chinese medicine during the reign of Emperor Huang Di, garlic has been gaining popularity and credibility by researchers as an agent that promotes immune-system support and fights viruses.

allspice

An aromatic spice, *Pimenta officinalis,* prepared from the berries of the West Indian tree *Pimenta dioica* (the allspice tree), of the myrtle family. According to herbalists, allspice has medicinal properties similar to those of cloves: it warms the body, increases circulation, promotes digestive health, and treats nausea, vomiting and intestinal gas.

(See also CLOVE.)

aloe

A member of the Lily family, *Aloe vera,* also known as "the burn plant," and whose name in Sanskrit, *kumari,* means goddess. Indigenous to East and South Africa, the succulent aloe is grown in the West Indies, tropical areas, some Mediterranean countries and in the southwestern and southeastern United States. While the aloe plant's gel has long been used as a topical remedy for minor burns, sunburn and abrasions, insect bites, diaper and heat rashes and rashes from poison ivy, oak or sumac, aloe may also be taken internally. Herbalists and nutritionists often use chrystallized aloe in extract form as a laxative and "cleanser" for the liver, kidneys and spleen.

In Ayurvedic (Indian/Hindu) medicine, aloe is considered a general liver tonic, a pain reliever of muscle spasms associated with menstruation, a mild laxative, a blood purifier and therefore beneficial to the liver, gallbladder and stomach, and a balancer of *vata, pitta* and *kapha*—the Ayurvedic aspects of human constitution, or body types.

However, the internal use of aloe, which contains a substance called anthraquinone, has come under question because it has been known to cause gastrointestinal cramping.

The National Aloe Science Council, a trade association created in 1972 by 30 manufacturers of aloe products, plans to establish scientific studies, ethics and standards for the production of aloe, including as juices and drinks, to satisfy the requirements of the Food and Drug Administration (FDA).

alum root

(American sanicle, crane's bill)

The root of an herb of the genus *Sanicula* (of the carrot family) used in folk medicine as an astringent for sore throats or canker sores or as an anodyne (pain-reliever) and anti-inflammatory for diarrhea, hemorrhoids, ulcers and excessive menstruation.

aluminum

A mineral with no known nutritional benefit and which may be harmful to bone or the brain tissues. High levels of aluminum in the diet may interfere with the absorption or utilization of other essential minerals, including calcium, phosphorus, magnesium, selenium and fluoride. Muscle pain and weakness and bone deterioration are signs of aluminum toxicity. Studies in rats suggest that aluminum accumulation in the brain may be a cause of Alzheimer's disease. Sources of dietary aluminum include food additives, acidic foods cooked in aluminum pans that absorb or leach the mineral and some antacids.

(See also ALZHEIMER'S DISEASE.)

Alzheimer's disease

Progressive and irreversible disorder, characterized mainly by loss of memory, named for the German neurologist Alois Alzheimer (1864–1915). As the dementia worsens, it results in loss of the control of body functions and eventual death.

Although the cause of Alzheimer's disease is unknown, scientists have implicated both aluminum and zinc deposits in the brain as possible causes. Failing appetite in Alzheimer's patients may result in severe vitamin deficiencies, and they should be given supplements.

amalaki
An Ayurvedic herb thought to rejuvenate tissue, relieve gastrointestinal irritation and stabilize blood sugar-related problems.

amaranth
(love lies bleeding, red cockscomb, pile wort, prince's feather, velvet flower)
A common weed, *Amaranthus hybridus,* of the family Amaranthaceae (also listed as *Amaranthus hypochondriacus* of the family Americanceae), whose seeds and greens (called pigweed in the West because it is fed to pigs) are used as food and other parts as medicinal preparations for the treatment of throat, stomach and intestinal ulcers, dysentery, diarrhea and bleeding. Amaranth greens are said to taste like spinach and contain iron, other minerals and vitamins A and C. The greens are also considered valuable as an acid neutralizer to a diet high in acid-producing grains, beans, meat and milk products.

American Cancer Society guidelines on diet and nutrition
To help people make educated choices about nutrition, the Society publishes nutritional guidelines to advise the public on dietary practices that may reduce the risk of cancer. The guidelines are meant to be practiced as a whole, creating a total dietary pattern to follow for lowered cancer risk. (1) maintain a dersirable body weight; (2) eat a varied diet; (3) include a variety of vegetables and fruits in the daily diet; eat more high-fiber foods such as whole grain cereals, legumes, vegetables and fruits; (4) cut down on total fat intake; (5) limit consumption of alcoholic beverages, if you drink at all; limit consumption of salt-cured, smoked and nitrite-preserved foods. (Used with permission, American Cancer Society, Inc.)

American Dietetic Association position statements
The philosophy and requirements set forth by the American Dietetic Association pertaining to public policy on nutrition, including:

(1) It is the position of the American Dietetic Association that the U.S. government establish a national policy on enrichment and fortification of the food supply that protects against nutrient insufficiencies and toxicities.
(2) To assure the American public safe, nontoxic dietary supplements, it is the position of The American Dietetic Association that dietary supplements be regulated like foods and that all associated health claims be based on significant scientific agreement.

See Appendix 6 for complete text.

amino acids
A group of organic compounds considered the "building blocks" of proteins. Of the nearly 80 amino acids found in nature, about 20 are required for human growth and metabolism. Essential amino acids are those provided by foods; nonessential amino acids are produced naturally by the body and therefore not required through food intake. The essential amino acids are histidine, isoleucine, leucine, lysine, methionine, cysteine, phenylalanine, tyrosine, threomine, tryptophan and valine. The nonessentials are alanine, aspartic acid, arginine (nonessential in adults but essential in infants because infants' bodies cannot produce enough of the compound in time to meet the metabolic demand), citrulline, glutamic acid, glycine, hydroxyglutamic acid, hydroxyproline, norleucine, proline and serine.

Examples of complete proteins, that is, those containing all the essential amino acids, are milk, milk products, eggs and meat. Vegetables, grains and gelatin are incomplete proteins. In a normal

Table 3
20 AMINO ACIDS SPECIFIED BY THE GENETIC CODE

Alanine	*Leucine
Arginine	*Lysine
Asparagine	*Methionine
Aspartic acid	*Phenylalanine
Cysteine	Proline
Glutamic acid	Serine
Glutamine	*Threonine
Glycine	*Tryptophan
*Histadine	Tyrosine
*Isoleucine	*Valine

* = Essential amino acids

adult maintaining a constant weight, the recommended daily protein intake is about 0.8 grams per kilogram of body weight, or about 46 grams of protein per day for women and 56 grams per day for men.

During digestion, amino acids transfer from the walls of the intestine and the portal vein into the blood. From the blood they move through the liver into the bloodstream, and are then distributed to the tissues as required so the tissues can produce their own protein. Amino acids not needed by the body for the building and repair of tissue are broken down into ammonia, carbon dioxide and water, producing heat and energy. They may also become the end products of digestion, such as urea, which is eliminated by the body.

One component of all proteins is the gas nitrogen, found in compounds including ammonia, nitrites and nitrates and essential to plant and animal life as a tissue-builder. The physical state of nitrogen balance refers to an equal amount of nitrogen ingested and excreted daily by the body. The Western diet, tends to foster a negative nitrogen balance. However, the body can withstand a negative nitrogen balance for a certain period because body proteins and other compounds containing nitrogen are continuously being synthesized and degraded as amino acids and re-utilized to satisfy any needs.

Inadequate intake of proteins, responsible for the growth and repair of cells, may lead to nutritional disorders including kwashiorkor and marasmus, commonly seen in African and Asian countries. Anorexia nervosa, an eating disorder characterized by extreme slenderness and malnourishment because of a lack of protein and calories, is often the result of compulsive dieting. Lack of protein may also result in anemia, a reduced number of red blood cells, and therefore reduced oxygen circulation, stemming from defective nucleoprotein synthesis, iron deficiency and other causes.

Ovolactovegetarians, who eat eggs, milk and cheese, can obtain sufficient amounts of essential amino acids, but vegans, who eat only vegetables and grains, may be at risk of protein deficiency.

Requirements
Allowances are expressed as protein but reflect requirements for amino acids. Proteins and other compounds containing nitrogen are continuously being synthesized and degraded as amino acids are reutilized. However, some amino acids are lost in a process called oxidative catabolism. Metabolic breakdown products of amino acids such as urea, creatinine and uric acid are excreted in the urine. Nitrogen is also lost in hair and nails and as skin sloughs. Therefore, a continuous supply of amino acids is required. During the metabolic processes the keto acid portion of the compounds are utilized for energy or converted to carbohydrate or fat.

Deficiencies
Inadequate nutrition is the major cause of protein and therefore amino acid deficiency, a cause seldom seen in the United States.

Supplementation
Many unproven claims have been attributed to amino acid supplements, either in balanced formulations or as individual products. Allegations range from strengthening the immune system to reducing dependency on drugs. Additionally, there may be

as yet unrecognized risks associated with these supplements, and they should not be used except under the supervision of a physician or university-trained nutritionist.

High-protein intake or unbalanced diets seem to suppress the appetite. A combination of phenylalanine, valine, methionine and tryptophan taken by a group of obese persons one half-hour before lunch reduced their food intake by almost 25 percent. In a group of normal weight individuals, tryptophan alone suppressed the appetite.

Phenylalanine and tyrosine may be low in persons suffering from depression. These amino acids are involved in the manufacture of the neurotransmitters dopamine, norepinephrine and epinephrine (adrenaline). Trytophan is converted to another important neurotransmitter serotonin. Interestingly, antidepressant drugs such as fluoxetine (Prozac) exert their effect by blocking the utilization of serotonin. Amitriptyline (Elavil) and other tricyclic type antidepressants act similarly by blocking the action of both norepinephrine and serotonin at the level of the neurons. As the compounds appear to terminate the activity of these nerves, depression is counteracted.

Caution must be used in taking individual amino acid supplements because the risks have not been adequately defined at this time.

Toxicity
There is no strong evidence that ingestion of excessive amino acids is harmful in persons with normal kidney function.

amino acid chelates
A method of combining amino acids with a metal such as iron. Advocates for the use of chelated minerals claim that they improve absorption of poorly absorbed minerals three to five times over the absorption of unchelated minerals. Detractors of these compounds feel they are not worth the extra expense. In addition, when minerals are taken with meals, they are naturally chelated by the digestive system.

amomum
(sha ren, round cardamom)
An herb native to Java, *Amomum compactum* and *illosum,* of the family Zingiberaceae, whose seeds are used as an aromatic spice. In Asian medicinal practices, the cardamom fruit are used to expel gas, prevent vomiting and stimulate stomach secretions.

amorphophallus
(devil's tongue, snake palm)
The tropical herb *Amorphophallus riveri,* of the family Araceae, whose stem is used in Chinese medicine to treat poisonous snake bites and whose flowering stalk is used to reduce fever.

ampelopsis
A deciduous plant native to China and Japan, *Ampelopsis japonica,* of the family Vitaceae, whose roots are considered by Chinese traditional practitioners to be an anticonvulsant, purgative, cooling and anti-inflammatory. The roots are also used to expel phlegm.

amygdalin
(also known as laetrile or "vitamin B_{17}")
A potentially toxic substance extracted from the pits of apricots and falsely reputed to cure cancer. This substance is not a vitamin and has no nutritional value. Initially promoted by Ernst Krebs, a biochemist, in 1952, the drug was found worthless in clinical trials by the National Cancer Institute and other scientific organizations. Since there is no known need for this substance, it does not meet the criteria to be classified a vitamin (see VITAMIN). In addition, the product contains 6 percent cyanide and has caused chronic cyanide poisoning and death. Despite this, many cancer sufferers desperate to find a cure turned to illegal or foreign sources of the drug. Perhaps the greatest tragedy

was that many individuals with potentially treatable cancers delayed conventional therapy until it was too late.

androgràphis
(creat)

The Asian herb, also considered a weed, *Andrographis paniculata,* of the family Acanthaceae, used in Chinese medicine to treat flu, pneumonia, bronchitis, whooping cough, hypertension, bites, burns and infection of the gallbladder.

anemarrhena
(zhi mu)

A native northern Chinese plant, *Anemarrhena asphodeloides,* of the family Lilliaceae, best known in Chinese medicine for its extract, which yields steroidal saponins, anti-inflammatory agents effective against lumbago. The underground stem is used for preparations to treat congestion and thirst as a result of fever, excessive perspiration, pneumonia, chronic cough, measles, vertigo, nausea and vomiting related to pregnancy, and premature ejaculation. Large doses of the medicinal underground stem of the plant are toxic and may inhibit cardiac function.

anemia

Diminished number of erythrocytes, or red blood cells, or in the quantity of hemoglobin caused by decreased production or blood loss.

(See also ANEMIA, MACROCYTIC; ANEMIA, MICROCYTIC.)

anemia, macrocytic

A type of anemia characterized by below-normal numbers of red blood cells that are larger than normal size. The red blood cells, or erythrocytes, are recognized by their increased mean corpuscular volume (MCV) and mean corpuscular hemoglobin (MCHC). Pernicious anemia, a vitamin B_{12} deficiency, and folate deficiencies are types of macrocytic anemia. (See B_{12}, VITAMIN; FOLIC ACID.)

anemia, microcytic

A type of anemia characterized by below-normal numbers of red blood cells that are smaller than normal size. The red blood cells, or erythrocytes, are recognized by a diminished mean corpuscular volume (MCV) and mean corpuscular hemoglobin (MCHC). Iron deficiency is the most common cause of this type of anemia.

(See also IRON; PYRIDOXINE.)

anemone

Temperate herb of the family Ranunculaceae containing glycoside ranunculin, a poison. The sap of the anemone causes skin irritation and blisters and, when taken internally, may cause various problems ranging from severe gastrointestinal and kidney inflammation to respiratory failure. The *Anemone hupehensis* (Japanese anemone) is used in Chinese medicine, however, to treat ringworm and lymphatic tuberculosis, and the roots of the *Anemone cernua* are used to treat sore throat, toothache, stomachache and bone fractures and pain. *Anemone chinensis* roots are used to treat diarrhea.

angelica
(dang gui, holy ghost plant, root of the holy ghost, archangel, masterwort, purple angelica, alexanders)

The genus *Angelica atropurpurea* of herbs of the Ammiaceae family used as a flavoring oil. In powdered form or capsules, angelica is touted by nutritionists (though not proven by scientists) to be an effective heart-strengthener and for use against heart and lung disease. It is also claimed to remedy gastrointestinal problems, including indigestion and gas, and to have the ability to create a distaste for alcoholic beverages. In addition, angelica is said to be effective against menstrual irregularity, colds and coldness.

anise
The herb *Pimpinella anisum,* a member of the Umbellifer family, whose leaves, stalks and seeds are used as a licoricelike flavoring and as a salad ingredient. Cultivated by the Ancient Egyptians, Greeks and Romans and touted by Chinese, Japanese and other herbalists, anise is said to have a therapeutic effect on intestinal gas, indigestion, bad breath, coughing and congestion, and a property that increases breast milk. Anise is also known as a mild diuretic.

antacids as calcium supplements
Agents that neutralize excessive acid in the stomach and intestines. TUMS and Rolaids, among the over-the-counter antacids, contain calcium carbonate and are widely promoted as calcium supplements.

antibiotics and vitamin interactions
See Appendix 4 Drug and Nutrient Interactions.

anticarcinogens
See CANCER PREVENTION; CANCER TREATMENT WITH VITAMINS.

anticonvulsants and vitamin interactions
Drugs used in the treatment of seizure disorders, including phenytoin (Dilantin), carbamazepine (Tegretol), phenobarbital and primidone, that interfere with the absorption or action of certain vitamins. Phenytoin, phenobarbital and primidone compete with the absorption of folic acid, thus long-term use may cause a folate deficiency. However, the consumption of large doses of folic acid may block the effectiveness of phenytoin, increasing the likelihood of seizures.

Calcium-containing antacids may interfere with the absorption of anticonvulsants, and the doses should be staggered to prevent this. Osteomalacia (the increased softness of bones as a cause of deformities, such as the adult form of rickets) has been associated with phenytoin and is thought to be due to the drug's interference with vitamin D metabolism.

antioxidants
Substances, including vitamins A, C and E and the trace elements selenium, manganese and zinc, thought to protect the cells from destructive oxidation by free radicals. Free radicals are compounds naturally produced in the body. They contain one or more unpaired electrons, or "electrical charges," and are therefore unstable. To achieve stability, free radicals "borrow" or "steal" electrons from stable compounds. This process allows formerly stable compounds to become reactive and cause the oxidation that may interfere with normal cell function and possibly mutate cells.

Peroxides are among the free radicals that are byproducts formed when fat molecules react with oxygen. Free radicals are also formed by radiation and are present in air pollution, ozone and cigarette smoke. Other examples of oxidation are the rusting of iron and the browning of apples and lettuce left exposed to the air. Oxidation also occurs when cooking fats become rancid.

Fatty cell membranes are choice targets for attack by free radicals. These substances alter cell functions by interfering with the transport of nutrients, oxygen and water into the cell and the removal of waste materials. Free radicals may also assault nucleic acids and the genetic code in each cell. The resulting cell damage may disrupt growth or repair of damaged or aging tissues. Some researchers implicate free radicals as a cause of premature aging.

In a six-month study at the Washington University School of Medicine, 11 young men were given supplemental antioxidants consisting of 600

International Units (IU) of vitamin E, 1,000 milligrams of vitamin C, and 30 milligrams (50,000 IU) of beta-carotene daily. A nine-man control group was given a placebo (an inactive look-alike) supplement. After running for 35 minutes on a treadmill at the beginning and end of the study, free-radical production was measured in each group. The vitamin-users produced 17 to 36 percent fewer free radicals than the control group.

Antioxidants have been promoted as cancer-preventing agents. Unfortunately, this has yet to be proven. In one study involving more than 850 people, mostly men, known to have had at least one benign polyp in the colon, subjects were given antioxidant supplements for four years. There was no difference in the recurrence of polyps among the group that took beta-carotene, vitamins C and E, all three vitamins or a placebo. Colon polyps begin as benign growths, but some have the potential to become malignant if they are not removed.

Preliminary evidence from a Harvard University study looks promising for vitamin E's ability to modify the incidence of heart disease. However, vitamins A, C and E may be more appropriately considered redox agents. Although antioxident in the physiologic quantities present in food, they are pro-oxidant in the larger quantities found in some supplements. Therefore, more research is needed to determine if there is any benefit from taking large doses of these vitamins.

(See also ASCORBIC ACID; BETA-CAROTENE; CARDIOVASCULAR DISEASE PREVENTION AND ANTIOXIDANT VITAMINS; E, VITAMIN; EYE DISEASES.)

antithiamine factors
(ATF)
Substances in the diet that diminish the bioavailability (the ability of body tissues to utilize a substance present in the diet) of thiamine in the diet. Inadequate thiamine causes beriberi, a potentially fatal vitamin-deficiency disease. There are two types of ATF: thermolabile (destroyed by heat) and thermostabile (ability to withstand heat). Thiaminase I is found in the viscera of freshwater fish, some saltwater fish, shellfish, in ferns and some plants and some bacteria. Thiaminase II is found in some bacteria and fungi. These substances break down the thiamine during food preparation, storage or as the vitamin passes through the gastrointestinal tract. Frequent ingestion of raw freshwater fish and shellfish may cause thiamine deficiency. However, cooking prevents this process.

Thermostabile ATF are found in ferns, tea, betel nut, some other plants, vegetables and animal tissues. Ascorbic acid, or vitamin C, prevalent in citrus fruits improves thiamine status in those who habitually chew tea leaves or betel nut.

(See also BERIBERI; THIAMINE.)

anxiety and stress
Illness as well as physical and emotional stress that may deplete the body of some vitamin storage. Many advocate the use of megadoses of supplements, especially niacin and the other B-complex vitamins, for conditions ranging from minor anxiety and depression to schizophrenia and major depression. The large doses recommended by some are not only of unproven benefit, but may actually be toxic. (See MEGAVITAMINS.)

apple
A tree of the *Malus* species, cultivated throughout the world and whose fruit, flowers, buds, leaves, twigs and bark are used as a food, beverage, and medicine. Apple seeds are toxic and are not recommended for consumption. Herbalists and naturopaths (practitioners of natural treatments) claim that apples, which contain malic and tartaric acids and potassium, sodium, magnesium and iron salts, help dissolve kidney or gallbladder stones. Chinese practitioners also claim that apple cider and other preparations are effective against diabetes, hypoglycemia, nausea and vomiting, fever and influenza. French herbalist Maurice Méssegué, author of *Of Men and Plants: Autobiography of the World's Most Famous Plant Healer* (MacMillan,

1973), used an apple blossom infusion as a treatment for sore throats and colds.

apricot seed
(ku xing ren)
The seed of the fruit of the tree *Prunus armeniaca,* of the Rosaceae family, whose kernel is said to provide a lung tonic, according to Chinese traditional medicine, but is also thought of as a source of laetrile, or "vitamin B_{17}," not considered a true vitamin, or amygdalin. Once praised as an anticancer agent, laetrile is not considered therapeutic or nutritive, and it contains cyanide, which in large doses may be lethal. (See AMYGDALIN.)

aquilaria
(chen xiang, eagle-wood tree)
A tropical tree, *Aquilaria agallocha,* of the family Thymelaeaceae, whose wood is grated and used in the preparation of Chinese medicines for rheumatism, smallpox and illness related to childbirth.

arbutus, trailing
(gravel plant, winter pink, mountain pink, wild May flower, gravel laurel)
A small evergreen plant, *Epigaea repens,* of the Ericaceae family, considered by Native American herbalists to be effective in the treatment of debilitated bladder, diarrhea and bloody or infected urine.

arctium
(cuckold, great burdock, edible burdock)
Derived from the Greek word *arctos,* meaning bear, a flowering, fruit-bearing weed, *Arctium lappa,* of the family Compositaea, found in Asia and Europe. American Indians and Europeans used the plant as an antibacterial agent. In the Middle Ages, it was considered a remedy for gallstones and kidney stones. In Chinese medicine, arctium leaves are used for dizziness and rheumatism, and

the fruit and seeds are used for colds, sore throat, pneumonia, scarlet fever, smallpox, mumps, measles in the early stage and skin eruptions such as pimples and St. Anthony's fire. The roots are a mild laxative and can induce sweating and urinary flow.

areca
(da fu pi, pinang, catechu, betel nut, betel palm)
A flowering, fruit-bearing palm tree, *Areca catechu,* of the family Palmae, whose ripe seeds are used in Chinese medicine to treat diarrhea, indigestion, lumbago and urinary tract problems. The seeds also increase menstrual flow and expel tapeworms and roundworms. The areca kernel is flavored and chewed by people throughout the Old World tropics as a narcotic. It turns their saliva bright red.

arginine
A nonessential amino acid produced by the breakdown of proteins and used to treat elevated ammonia levels in liver failure. Arginine supplementation seems to play a role in treating chronic inflammatory conditions. Following major surgery, it has been shown to reduce the patient's need to stay in the hospital. Arginine is necessary for the synthesis of polyamine and nucleic acid and can stimulate the secretion of the hormones prolactin, insulin, growth and glucagon.

Arginine is promoted by some as a way to increase sperm count, muscle tone and physical stamina and alertness. It should be avoided in growing children because it could cause joint and bone deformities. Excessive doses of supplements may cause thickening of the skin.

arnica
(leopard's bane)
A flowering plant, *Arnica montana,* of the family Compositae, prescribed in minute doses as an internal tonic by herbalists and homeopaths. Ar-

nica oil and liniment are used freely, however, for bruises and other injuries such as aches, strains and painful skin problems in which the skin has not been broken.

arsenic
Non-metallic element with a garlicky odor. Although it has been used in some medicinal preparations in the past, it is rarely used today. Although no human deficiency has been identified, some scientists feel arsenic and other trace minerals (see TRACE ELEMENTS) may play a role in human enzyme systems. Arsenic has been proven to be essential for normal growth and reproduction in rats, minipigs, chicken and goats. An estimated 0.4 mg to 0.9 mg daily intake of arsenic is far below amounts known to be toxic.

arsesmart
(walter pepper, peach-wort, dead arssmare)
An American plant, *Polygonum hydropiper,* of the family Polygonaceae, used in Native American medicine as a stimulant, diuretic and diaphoretic (to induce sweating). Homeopaths prescribe arsesmart for amenorrhea, colic, cough, diarrhea, dysentery, eczema, epilepsy, gonorrhea, gravel, hemorrhoids, cardiac problems, hysteria, laryngitis, ulcers and splenic ailments.

In Russian medical and herbal literature, polygonum is recognized as an effective herbal treatment for various problems.

Polygonum contains oil, several minerals and rutin and vitamins C and K. Folk-medicine practitioners believe it also stops bleeding.

arthritis
Inflammatory disorder of the joints. The deformities common to severe rheumatoid arthritis can be crippling, and medical treatment is often inadequate for the relief of pain and does little if anything to prevent worsening of the disease. In addition, medical treatment may have many serious adverse effects. The antioxidant vitamins, omega-6 fatty acids (fish oil) and other supplements are promoted as "cures" for arthritis, but remain unproven. Double-blind clinical trials with these products are difficult because the pain of arthritis waxes and wanes even if no treatment is given.

(See also ANTIOXIDANTS; GERMANIUM; OMEGA-3 FATTY ACIDS; OMEGA-6 FATTY ACIDS.)

artichoke
(blessed thistle, garden artichoke, globe artichoke)
A perennial plant, *Cynara scolymus,* of the thistle family, whose flower heads are eaten as a vegetable and whose leaves and root are considered medicinal by herbalists. Extracts from these parts are said to have healing properties in cases of arteriosclerosis, liver dysfunction, postoperative anemia, chronic protein in the urine and indigestion.

arum
(cocky baby, dragon root, starchwort, gaglee, Portland arrowroot, ladysmock)
A perennial plant, *Arum maculatum,* whose arrowhead-shaped leaves are poisonous when eaten, but whose rootstock is considered a diaphoretic and expectorant.

asafoetida
(devil's dung, gum asafetida)
The plant *Ferula assafoetida,* of the Umbelliferae family, whose gum resin is often used in place of garlic in parts of Asia because it does not leave an offensive odor on the breath as garlic does. An ingredient in Worcestershire sauce, asafoetida is said to be effective in the treatment of coldness, respiratory distress including coughs, mood

swings, hysteria, weak digestion, intestinal gas, yeast (*Candida albicans*) overgrowth, hypoglycemia and food allergies.

In Ayurvedic medicine, a pinch of asafoetida cooked with lentils is said to aid digestion. It also is thought to relieve gas in the intestines, relieve pain and remove toxins.

asarum

(hazelwort, public house plant, asarabacca, wild nard)

A European perennial plant, *Asarum europaeum,* whose rootstock and leaves are considered medicinal, mainly as an emetic (to induce vomiting).

ascorbic acid, or vitamin C

A water-soluble compound that acts as a coenzyme, a reducing agent and antioxidant. The word ascorbic is derived from the Latin, meaning "without scurvy." Humans, other primates, guinea pigs and some birds lack the enzyme (L-glu-conolactone) that forms ascorbic acid in the body. The inability to manufacture ascorbic acid is due to an inborn mutation in carbohydrate metabolism. In most other animals, the vitamin is synthesized from glucose. Inadequate dietary supply of the vitamin causes scurvy.

History of Vitamin C

Scurvy is the oldest recognized nutritional-deficiency disease. Symptoms include loss of energy; pain in legs and joints; anemia; spongy, bleeding gums; bad breath; loosening of teeth; subcutaneous hemorrhages and bleeding from mucous membranes; and muscle pain. It is also characterized by abnormal formation of bones and teeth. Scurvy can be cured by vitamin C.

From the 16th through 18th centuries, scurvy was responsible for the death of one-half to two-thirds of the crew on prolonged ocean voyages during which the diet consisted only of cereals and meat. In 1747 British naval surgeon and physician James Lind recommended that limes and lemons

be included on board ships of the British navy. Although the navy initially ignored Lind's recommendation, it finally complied, and British sailors became known as "limeys."

Actions

Vitamin C supplies electrons to enzymes that require metal ions. It also acts with the substances prolyl and lysyl hydroxylases in the manufacture of collagen. Collagen is the proteinaceous, fibrous material—or "body cement"—found in the connective tissues of the body, including skin, bone, ligaments, cartilage and dentin of teeth and comprising approximately 30 percent of body protein.

Some scientists feel that vitamin C (and vitamin E) may protect against carcinogens such as nitrosamine. This chemical is formed in the body from nitrates and nitrites found in processed meat products such as lunch meats and hot dogs.

Data from the Prospective Basel [Switzerland] Study published in 1984 and other studies seem to support the premise that the antioxidant properties of vitamin C and other nutrients may prevent some cancers. However, there is no conclusive evidence that they are curative.

Deficiency

Signs and symptoms of scurvy occur after about three to 12 months of a severe lack of dietary vitamin C. As the deficiency worsens, splinter hemorrhages develop near the tips of nails, gums become swollen, purple and bleed. Wounds fail to heal, bleeding may occur spontaneously from any part of the body, ankle and leg edema occurs, and there is diminished urinary output. A classic sign of scurvy is the formation of thick hair follicles with surrounding redness or bleeding.

Some authors on nutrition claim that vitamin C increases sperm count, motility and viability. Lack of vitamin C may have some deleterious effect on sperm, particularly in the case of severe deficiency.

Vitamin D deficiency results in imperfect formation of or inability to form the calcified lattice, or framework, of bone tissue. This poor bone structure is also characteristic of scurvy. In the presence of coexisting vitamin C and D deficiencies, important symptoms and X-ray findings of scurvy may be masked or modified causing confusion in the diagnosis.

Possible but Unproven Benefits

English researchers have found that 1,000 milligrams per day of vitamin C given to healthy persons inhibit a destructive process in proteins known as glycosylation. Since this process is thought to cause diabetic complications, investigators speculate that complications may be delayed or prevented by vitamin C.

Vitamin C, along with folic acid, carotenoids and fiber, has been linked to a reduced incidence of breast cancer in a study of 626 patients in New York State. However, high-fiber intake rather than vitamin C and beta-carotene seemed to reduce colorectal cancer risk in a Canadian study.

Boston researchers found that vitamin C and A supplements taken for many years appeared to reduce the incidence of cataracts (see A, VITAMIN). Many nutritionists recognize that a balanced intake of multiple fruits and vegetables is probably a much better approach to reducing cancer risks than the use of any supplement, because different cancers seem to be protected by different vitamins or other factors.

Dosage and RDA

The U.S. recommended dietary allowances (RDA) for vitamin C are 35 mg daily from birth through one year of age, 40 mg from one to four years, and 60 mg over age four, including pregnant and lactating women. Scurvy usually responds to doses of 250 mg daily until signs of the disorder have begun to disappear. Then 100 mg daily prevents recurrence. Requirements increase up to 500 percent during periods of environmental stresses, such as exposure to extremes in temperature, burns, trauma and surgery. Cigarette smokers have a 50-percent increased need for vitamin C to maintain normal blood levels. Women taking oral contraceptives also have an increased need for the vitamin.

There is probably no significant benefit from taking natural rather than synthetic vitamin C (see NATURAL VITAMINS). Timed-release vitamin C may be less effective in raising vitamin C levels than regular, less expensive tablets.

There is evidence that doses of vitamin C need to be taken every 12 hours rather than once daily, because the body eliminates large doses in that time and timed-release formulas in about 16 hours.

Citrus fruits, tomatoes, potatoes and leafy vegetables are good sources of vitamin C. Much of the natural vitamin C in foods, however, is lost during storage and certain cooking processes, or is present in forms not bioavailable.

The Vitamin C Controversy and Dr. Linus Pauling

Nobel Prize–winning scientist Dr. Linus Pauling (1901–1994) believed there are wide variations in the vitamin requirements of animals and man. Dr. Pauling and others have claimed large amounts of vitamin C are not only beneficial, but strengthen the immune system. Unfortunately, proof is lacking that vitamin C supplementation prevents or cures colds or cures cancer. However, the popularity of the vitamin indicates a discernible success rate in prevention or treatment of colds and other infections. There may be some cancer-protective properties of vitamin C.

A virtual war over vitamin C has existed for years between "establishment" scientists (including many physicians) and nutritionists. The scientists demand proof that megadoses, which can approach 10 grams of vitamin C per day, have any benefits. In addition, scientists believe megadoses may be harmful. (See toxicity section below). To counter unsubstantiated claims by Dr. Pauling, the Mayo Clinic ran scientifically controlled studies that failed to prove any lasting benefits of vitamin C in a group of cancer patients.

New, more optimistic studies include an analysis of carotenoid and vitamin A, C and E intake for the prevention of age-related macular degeneration (AMD), conducted by Dr. Johanna M. Seddon of the Department of Ophthalmology of the Massachusetts Eye and Ear Infirmary, Harvard Medical School, Boston, Massachusetts, and colleagues.

Another study, conducted from 1993 to 1994 by the University of Medicine and Dentistry of New Jersey-Medical School, in Newark, New Jersey, indicated that elderly people who eat well and take daily multivitamins generally have stronger T-lymphocytes, the white blood cells that fight infection.

Furthermore, luminaries such as Kenneth Cooper, M.D., of the Cooper Aerobics Center in Dallas, Texas; Bruce Ames, Ph.D., professor of biochemistry at the University of California; William Castelli, M.D., director of the Framingham Heart Study; Dean Ornish, M.D., director of the Preventive Medicine Research Institute in Sausalito, California; Walter C. Millett, M.D., Dr. P. H., epidemiologist at the Harvard School of Public Health, and Margo N. Woods, D.Sc., director of the nutrition unit at Tufts University School of Medicine, report that they take vitamin C in doses ranging from 50 to 3,000 mg per day.

Toxicity and Other Adverse Effects
Vitamin C increases the absorption of iron. Elevated iron levels can be dangerous in some individuals and may even increase the risk of cardiovascular disease (see IRON). Even if large doses of vitamin C are not toxic to most persons, the process in which the body eliminates the excess vitamin may be. Theoretically, with doses of 1,000 to 10,000 mg per day, great quantities of urine are produced to eliminate the 99 percent of vitamin C not utilized. If insufficient fluids are not replaced, the vitamin C may crystallize and damage the kidneys. In order for vitamin C to be eliminated by the kidneys, this acidic substance must be neutralized. Calcium salts may be required in the process, possibly causing the formation of kidney stones. Large doses of the vitamin may cause water to be pulled into the colon from the circulatory system, thus causing diarrhea.

Vitamin C reacts to tests for diabetes and may give a false impression that blood sugar is too high, causing patients to increase insulin doses. This increased dose may result in insulin shock. The acidity of chewable vitamin C tablets, if used regularly and in large quantities, can dissolve tooth enamel.

Persons taking large doses of vitamin C should not suddenly stop taking it, but gradually taper the dose. Advocates of megadoses of vitamin C claim that the deep yellow color of urine indicates saturation of the body tissues, assuring adequate vitamin supply. However, the skeptics rebut this theory by saying the excess is at best a waste of money and at worst, actually harmful.

ash tree
(weeping ash, European ash, American white ash)
A tree, *Fraxinus excelsior,* of the Oleaceae family, of the north temperate zone and extending into southern regions including Mexico and Java, whose bark and leaves are used by herbalists in the treatment of gout, arthritis, rheumatic pain, obesity, dropsy and fevers. Homeopathic application of ash includes the treatment of uterine problems. In Russia, Manchuria and China, ash leaves and bark are made into a tea thought to stimulate circulation in the extremities.

ashwagandha
("Indian ginseng")
An Ayurvedic preparation of the roots and leaves of the *Withania somnifera* plant, with its active constituents known as *withanolides.* The standardized measure of withanolides is 4.5 mg per tablet. Ashwagandha has been widely used as an "adaptogen," a term coined by advocates and manufacturers of natural dietary supplements that refers to an agent that helps the body adapt to physical, emotional and environmental stresses for optimal well-being.

asparagus
(sparrowgrass)
A popular spring vegetable, *Asparagus officinalis,* of the Liliaceae family, whose shoots are eaten

and whose root is said to provide a respected "Yin tonic," which, in Chinese traditional medicine, refers to its healing properties for tuberculosis, AIDS, female hormonal and reproductive problems, dryness of the lungs and throat, and to promote love and compassion (possibly attributable to its steroidal glycosides). Asparagus shoots are considered useful for bladder infections. As a general body tonic, asparagus root is said to fight fatigue, various forms of "burnout" or exhaustion and knee, joint and back aches.

asthma and vitamin supplements

Ascorbic acid (vitamin C) and other vitamins promoted for the treatment of asthma and allergic rhinitis (hay fever). Some studies have actually demonstrated improvement in spirometry (lung function tests), the standard for measuring response to asthma treatment. However, results are inconsistent, and benefits have not been seen in all studies.

astragalus
(huang qi)
An herb, *Astragalus membranaceus,* or *cochinchinensis,* of the family Lilliaceae, whose roots contain betaine, B-sitosterol, choline, dimethoxy-isoflavane, glucoronic acid, kumatakenin and sucrose, thought to be of use in the treatment of chronic lung weakness. In Chinese medicine, astragalus in tonic form is used to protect the immune system, as a diuretic to reduce edema (excessive tissue fluids), and as an anhidrotic, an agent that inhibits perspiration. The herb is also used to promote healing and adrenal gland function, to increase metabolism and fight fatigue.

atherosclerosis
See CARDIOVASCULAR DISEASE PREVENTION AND ANTIOXIDANT VITAMINS.

athletes' needs
See EXERCISE AND SUPPLEMENTS.

atractylis
(bai zhu, atractylodes)
An herb of Manchuria, Korea, northern and eastern China and Japan, *Atractylis ovata* (also *macrocephala*), of the Compositae family, whose roots are used in Chinese medicine to treat indigestion, skin problems, fever, nervousness, loss of appetite, chronic bronchitis, cough, night blindness, diarrhea and anemia associated with pregnancy.

aurantium
(zhi ke)
The fruit of the plant *Citrus aurantium,* used in Chinese medicine to tonify and disperse the body's energy, called *Qi* (pronounced "chee"), especially in counteracting spasms and symptoms including poor digestion, muscle weakness, a feeling of heaviness and water retention.

averrhoa
Originally a Malayan plant, *Averrhoa carambola,* of the Oxalidaceae family, whose fruit, commonly known as starfruit, is used in Chinese medicine to increase the flow of urine, treat wounds and stop bleeding. The starfruit was named for the Arabian physician Averrhoes (1149–1217).

avidin
A protein in egg white that binds to biotin (of the Vitamin B complex) and prevents its absorption. A biotin deficiency may result if large amounts of raw egg white are ingested.

B

B₁, vitamin
See THIAMINE.

B₂, vitamin
See RIBOFLAVIN.

B₃, vitamin
See NIACIN.

B₅, vitamin
See PANTOTHENIC ACID.

B₆ vitamin group
See PYRIDOXINE.

B₁₂, vitamin
(colbalamin, cyanocobalamin, hydroxocobalamin)
A component of the vitamin B complex essential to the growth and repair of all body cells. Vitamin B_{12} is a generic term for several cobalt-containing compounds, of which cyanocobalamin is the most stable form. Synthetic vitamin B_{12} contains a cyanide group not found naturally.

This water-soluble vitamin is derived from certain microorganisms. In the stomach, hydrochloric acid and pepsin release cyanocobalamin from dietary protein to which it is tightly bound. Parietal cells in the gastric mucosa (stomach lining) secrete a substance called intrinsic factor. The vitamin then binds to salivary R proteins and, after passing into the small intestine, is altered by pancreatic enzymes at the level of the jejunum. For simplifi-cation, the small intestine, or bowel, is a long tube, approximately 22 feet in length. The upper two-fifths is called the jejunum and the remaining three-fifths the ileum. In the jejunum, cyanocobalamin binds to a substance called intrinsic factor. The resulting intrinsic factor-cyanocobalamin complex formed is resistant to proteolysis (further breakdown by digestive enzymes) and passes unchanged until it adheres to special receptors on mucosal cells lining the distal ileum (the lower end of the bowel). It is at this level that vitamin B_{12} is absorbed.

Discovery
In the early 1800s, the name pernicious (meaning deadly or fatal) anemia was first used to describe a serious disease affecting older adults. Death usually occurred within two to five years. The 1926 discovery by George Richards Minot that nutrients in liver cured pernicious anemia led to the isolation of the vitamin (later termed B-12), for which Minot, William Parry Murphy and George Whipple received a Nobel Prize in 1934. Others, including Edwin Cohn and William Castle, were also involved in this important medical advancement.

The initial treatment for pernicious anemia was one pound of raw liver daily. The researchers reasoned that there must be extrinsic, or external, and intrinsic, or internal, factors involved in this anemia. These factors turned out to be vitamin B_{12} and intrinsic factor, respectively (see above).

Uses of Vitamin B₁₂
In addition to its growth and repair abilities, the vitamin is essential for the formation of mature red blood cells and central nervous system function. It interacts with folic acid coenzymes and is involved in the synthesis of DNA and methionine, an essential amino acid.

Experiments with laboratory mice suggest that vitamin B$_{12}$, when combined with vitamin C, may inhibit the formation of cancerous tumors in mice. Mice given either of the vitamins alone were not protected from developing tumors. Early studies suggested that vitamin C supplements might destroy vitamin B$_{12}$ in the body. However, later better designed studies showed that the presence of vitamin C actually promotes the absorption of cyanocobalamin. The hydroxo-cobalamin form of B$_{12}$ may be preferred for the treatment of vitamin B$_{12}$ deficiency, since optic neuropathies (disorders of the optic nerve) may worsen with the use of the cyanocobalamin compound.

Dietary Sources

Vitamin B$_{12}$ is produced only by bacteria and must be obtained from animal products or fermented foods such as miso from fermented soybeans. The average American diet supplies an estimated 5 to 15 mcg daily. However, this amount of the vitamin B$_{12}$ is sufficient only if intrinsic factor (see above) is available and adequate calcium is present.

Deficiencies

Dietary deficiencies are rare except in strict vegetarians. Whether from inadequate dietary intake or from inadequate secretion of intrinsic factor (required for the absorption of B$_{12}$ from the small intestine) by the stomach, anemia occurs from insufficient vitamin B$_{12}$. The classical type of anemia that results from a lack of intrinsic factor is termed "pernicious." This anemia is caused by improper replication of the genetic code. Anemia is recognized by decreased numbers of larger-than-normal red blood cells called macrocytic cells. Less frequently white blood cells and platelets are diminished, which increases susceptibility to colds, other infections, poor blood clotting and bruising.

Manifestations of anemia include fatigue, a feeling of weakness, dizziness (lightheadedness or vertigo) and tinnitus (ringing in the ears). In severe cases there may be palpitations, angina (chest pain) and congestive heart failure (shortness of breath). Due to its slow and gradual onset, anemia may be quite advanced before the individual becomes pale,

has a rapid pulse, slight fever and appears to have mild jaundice (yellowing of the skin and the whites of the eyes). In late stages, the heart, liver and spleen may become enlarged.

Faulty formation of epithelial cells lining the gastrointestinal tract causes nausea, vomiting, diarrhea, anorexia (poor appetite) and poor absorption of food, possibly resulting in malnutrition. There may be skin rashes and a sore tongue that appears smooth, beefy and red.

Most troublesome, however, may be the irreversible neurologic disorders caused by vitamin B$_{12}$ deficiency before characteristic anemia occurs. Nerve damage is characterized by disorientation, numbness, tingling, confusion, agitation, irritability, dimmed vision, dizziness, delusions or hallucinations. B$_{12}$ is essential to the production of myelin, the substance that covers and protects our nerves. Destruction of this sheath, called demyelination, is the first step in a process that, if uninterrupted, may result eventually in the death of the involved nerves. Peripheral, spinal nerves or the brain itself may become involved. Unfortunately, irreparable damage may occur before the cause is recognized.

Hypochlorhydria or achlorhydria are states in which there is a deficiency or total absence of hydrochloric acid in the stomach. When this occurs, the cyanocobalamin bound to proteins in food may not be released in sufficient amounts to combine with R protein and intrinsic factor. This condition eventually results in B$_{12}$ deficiency. In addition, the acid-deficient environment in the stomach allows an overgrowth of gastric bacteria, which in turn produces compounds called analogs that are physically similar but not identical to vitamin B$_{12}$. These vitaminlike compounds compete with the vitamin for absorption, causing a deficiency of the vitamin. The ulcer drug omeprazole (Prilosec) may cause a vitamin B$_{12}$ deficiency because of its effectiveness in reducing the secretion of acid in the stomach.

Smokers were found to have lower levels of B$_{12}$ and folic acid in a study published in the *Journal*

| Table 4 | Table 5 |

Table 4
CAUSES OF VITAMIN B$_{12}$ DEFICIENCY

Dietary:

Total vegans (vegetarian) diet

Infants breastfed by vegan mothers

Rarely alcoholism (folate deficiency is more common)

Dietary faddism, ignorance, religious beliefs, poverty

Inadequate absorption of vitamin B$_{12}$

Deficiency of intrinsic factor secretion in the stomach (total or diminished), including pernicious anemia, destruction of the gastric mucosa or surgical resection of the stomach

Inhibition of intrinsic factor by immune factors

Disorders of the small intestine such as celiac disease, sprue, bacterial overgrowth, fish tapeworm infestation, malignancy, surgical removal of portions of the intestine

Drugs including para-aminosalicylic acid (PAS), colchicine, neomycin, alcohol, possibly oral contraceptives and omeprazol (Prilosec)

Table 5
CONDITIONS THAT MAY REQUIRE VITAMIN B$_{12}$ SUPPLEMENTATION

Alcoholism

Anemia, hemolytic (a condition in which anemia is caused by destruction of red blood cells)

Cancer of the bowel or pancreas

Fever, prolonged or chronic

Fish tapeworm infestation

Gastrectomy (surgical removal of all or part of the stomach)

Gastritis, atrophic with achlorhydria (a condition in which the stomach lining wastes away and loses the ability to secrete acid)

Metabolic disorders:

(1) homocystinuria, usually a genetic disorder causing failure to thrive, can also be caused by inadequate vitamin B$_{12}$ or folate deficiency.

(2) methylmalonic aciduria, an inherited disorder involved in the metabolism of vitamin B$_{12}$.

Hyperthyroidism

Infection, prolonged or chronic

Kidney disease

Liver disorders

Malabsorption disorders associated with diarrhea

Stress, prolonged

---

of the American Medical Association in 1988. In the study, precancerous changes in bronchial cells of the lungs were noticed in smokers. Supplementation of those vitamins seemed to modify the abnormal cells, suggesting a potential protective effect.

Prolonged exposure to extremely high doses of nitrous oxide, or "laughing gas," may lead to vitamin B$_{12}$ deficiency.

Anemia may result when there is a vast overgrowth of bacteria in the intestines that compete for available vitamin B$_{12}$ with the host. This condition occurs following surgical removal, or resection, of portions of the small intestine.

Dosage

Supplementation of vitamin B$_{12}$ may be necessary during pregnancy and breast-feeding in vegetarians. For infant formulas 0.15 mcg/kcal (micrograms per kilocalories of B$_{12}$) is required for each 1000 calories of formula consumed. Multivitamins with folic acid should also contain vitamin B$_{12}$.

People with pernicious anemia require injections of vitamin B$_{12}$, because the lack of intrinsic factor in these individuals prevents absorption of dietary or oral supplements in the intestine.

Toxicity

Although synthetic vitamin B$_{12}$ contains a cyanide molecule, there is no known toxicity. However, doses greater than 10,000 times the RDA may rarely cause allergic reactions with the formation of antivitamin antibodies. This is more likely to occur with the hydroxocobalamin form of B$_{12}$. There may also be acnelike rashes. A suspicion also exists that extreme excesses (doses exceeding 10,000 mcg per day) of the vitamin enhances the spread of some cancers.

B$_{15}$**, vitamin**
See PANGAMIC ACID.

B$_{17}$**, vitamin**
See AMYGDALIN.

baeckea
An evergreen tree originating in Australia, *Baeckea frutescens,* of the Myrtaceae family, whose leaves are used by Chinese practitioners to treat sunstroke and fever.

bala
In Ayurvedic medicine, the Sanskrit name for country mallow. (See MALLOW.)

balamcanda
(black-berry lily, leopard flower)
An herb native to China and Japan, *Belamcanda chinensis,* of the Iridaceae family, whose underground stem is used by Chinese practitioners to treat tonsillitis, laryngitis, gonorrhea, breast cancer, dysuria (painful urination), asthma, cough, swollen liver and spleen and malaria.

balm
(balm mint, blue balm, melissa, sweet balm, dropsy plant, garden balm, bee balm)
An herb common to the Mediterranean area and the Near East and cultivated in other regions including the United States, *Melissa officinalis.* The herb and leaves, which smell like lemon when bruised, are used by herbalists as a calmative and antispasmodic, and to treat migraine, bronchial cough, toothache, melancholy, cramps, dyspepsia, flatulence, some forms of asthma and female reproductive disorders. Balm tea also has diaphoretic properties.

Balm of Gilead
(quaking aspen, white poplar)
The *Populus balsamifera,* or *balsamifera candicans,* and *Populus tremula* trees' buds used in the making of cough syrups and expectorants. Poplar bark is said to relieve fever and aches and pains. Quaking aspen bark is said to reduce fever and headaches and relieve aches and pains.

balmony
(snake head, turtle head, salt rheum weed, bitter herb)
A perennial herb, *Chelone glabra,* of the Scrophulariaceae family, found in the United States, whose leaves are considered medicinal, especially for improving the appetite. A tea made of the leaves is thought to stimulate the stomach and flow of liver fluids and relieve jaundice, malarial problems and gastrointestinal disturbances. Balmony is also used to expel worms from the body.

balsam fir
(Christmas tree)
One of the nine species of fir trees in the United States, *Terebinthine canadensis,* of the Coniferae family, whose bark and twigs are considered medicinal for the treatment of rheumatism, kidney dysfunctions, gleet, cystitis, typhoid fever and capillary bronchitis, among other ailments. As a stimulant and expectorant, balsam fir yields products similar in effect to Balm of Gilead. (See BALM OF GILEAD.)

bambusa
(giant thorny bamboo)
A native Indian plant cultivated in other regions (bamboo is the Malay name), *Bambusa arundinacea,* of the Gramineae family, whose stem, sap and unfolded leaves are used in Chinese medicine to treat fever and rheumatism. Bamboo shavings,

known as *zhu ru,* of the *Phyllostachys nigra* species, are used for lung problems.

baptisia
(wild indigo)

A leguminous, flowering plant of the genus *Baptisia tinctoria,* of the family Leguminosae, whose name derives from the Greek word *baptisis,* which means dipping. The roots and leaves are used in herbal medicine as a treatment for blood poisoning, ulcerations, typhoid dysentery, typhoid pneumonia, meningitis, diphtheria, sore throat and severe inflammatory disorders. Considered a strong anti-inflammatory and antibiotic, baptisia is also used for swollen glands and infections characterized by putrid discharges. It is also thought to have antiviral properties.

barberry
(pipperidge bush)

A deciduous shrub of the genus *Berberis* and the family *Berberiaceae,* whose bark is powdered and made into capsules. Homeopaths claim that tincture of the bark of the barberry root promotes the secretion of bile and is effective against bad breath, indigestion, rheumatism, skin conditions, bladder infections, sore throat, menstrual pain, fistula, calculus, herpes, ophthalmia, jaundice and other liver disorders, knee pain, lumbago, tumors and problems of the spleen. Barberry has been called an "old woman's medicine," which refers to its use as a stomach and liver tonic. The Native Americans used barberry-root tea as a blood tonic, cough medicine and remedy for rheumatism, ulcers, heartburn and even tuberculosis. Herbalists also allege barberry's effectiveness against cholera, ringworm and bronchitis. Barberries and barberry juice are prescribed for fever, diarrhea and other symptoms of typhus.

The official Pharmacopoeia of Russia has cited two barberry species, Amur barberry and Barberry common, as therapeutic treatment for high blood pressure and problems of the female genital organs. Russian folklore has it that barberry treats inflammation, excessive menses, and gallbladder problems, and has a general ability to stop bleeding.

In Ayurvedic medicine, barberry is known by the Sanskrit name *daruharidra.*

barley
(prelate)

A cereal grass of the genus *Hordeum,* including *Hordeum vulgare,* whose seed is used in malt beverages, breakfast cereals, animal feed and to make barley water for the treatment of fever, diarrhea and intestinal irritation.

Found in tombs in Asia Minor around 3500 B.C., barley seeds had been the most favored grain for bread-making in Europe until wheat and rye became more popular. Today, barley is also grown in the United States, especially California, North and South Dakota and Minnesota, and in Canada.

When introduced to Native Americans by early settlers in North America, barley was recognized to be a generally beneficial nutrient. It contains proteins, sugars, starch, fats and B vitamins. Barley is thought to be effective in the treatment of arthritis and rheumatism. Barley water, made by boiling pearl barley in water and strained, is used for fevers, diarrhea in children, bowel and stomach inflammation and as an addition to any diet to promote healthy intestinal bacterial conditions. In Chinese traditional medicine, barley is considered an anti-inflammatory diuretic and a treatment for tumors, gallbladder disorders and jaundice.

basil

An annual herb, *Ocimum basilicum,* thought to relieve nausea, headaches, intestinal gas in infants, anxiety, infections and lack of menstruation. Basil, which grows wild in India, parts of Africa, Japan,

Iran and Malaysia, among other countries, is also a popular flavoring in European and Mediterranean dishes. There is varied folklore pertaining to basil. To the French, basil has been dubbed the *herbe royale* (royal herb); Jewish lore holds that basil offers strength during fasting. To the Italians, basil symbolizes love, and to the Greeks, hate, although the Greek word for king, *basileus,* may be the reason for basil's having been known as the king of herbs. Basil, possibly derived from *basilicus,* meaning serpent, may also have been an ancient antidote for poisonous insect bites. English herbalist Nicholas Culpeper added to basil's folklore by calling it "an herb of Mars and under the Scorpion . . . it is no marvel if it carry a virulent quality with it." Contemporary herbalists believe basil to yield gentle yet reliable therapeutic effects.

In Ayurvedic medicine, *tulsi* is the Sanskrit name for "holy basil."

basswood

The linden tree, *Tilia americana,* or *Tilia europaea,* native to Europe and the eastern United States, whose flowers are used medicinally for nervousness, indigestion, cramps, insomnia and initial symptoms of a cold. Linden-flower tea is considered by European herbalists to be therapeutic, while linden-flower baths are thought to relieve hyperactivity, insomnia and anxiety. The linden tree also yields linden-flower honey, inner bark that is prepared to treat burns as well as to make rope, and wood especially appealing to woodcarvers.

bay

A tree native to Mediterranean shores, *Laurus nobilis,* also known as sweet bay or bay laurel, whose leaves are used chiefly as a flavoring in foods but also as a gastrointestinal tonic and to relieve gas. Cultivated in groves near the healing temples in Ancient Greece, the bay tree was considered sacred to Apollo, Greek god of the sun, and its branches were fashioned into wreaths to be worn by exalted luminaries such as heroes and great artists.

bayberry

A shrub of the Myricaceae family, also known as American bayberries, wax myrtle, wax berry, tallow shrub, candle berry and American vegetable wax. Bayberry grows in sandy swamps and other wet woodland areas in the West Indies, along the east coast of the United States from southern New Jersey to Florida, and west to Arkansas and Texas. Besides its berries yielding an aromatic wax used to make candles, bayberry is said to have medicinal properties in its root bark. Herbalists claim that bayberry, or *myrica cerifera,* provides treatment for bronchitis and other bronchopulmonary diseases, cholera, scarlet fever, goiter, typhoid, diseases of the intestinal tract, and uterine, stomach, lung or bowel hemorrhage, among other ailments. The ancient physician Galen noted that bayberries helped relieve colds. Herbalists also prescribe bayberry for sore throats (as a gargle solution) and to improve the circulation of blood throughout the body. Because of the alleged astringent and narcotic properties of the wax, bayberry has also been used as a topical bath for skin irritations including boils and carbuncles.

The Sanskrit name for bayberry in Ayruvedic medicine is *katphala.*

bearberry
See UVA URSI.

bear's foot

A perennial flower, *Polymnia uvedalia,* member of the astor family, shaped like a bear's foot. Also known as leafcup, balsam resin, yellow leafcup and uvedalia, the bear's foot is found in North America. Its root is claimed to have both internal and external therapeutic effects. When boiled in water, the root allegedly provides relief of mammitis (nonmalignant inflammation of the breast), enlarged cervical nodules, enlarged spleen, scrofula, chronic rheumatism and certain malarial conditions. Made into a salve, bear's foot is applied to swollen areas and used as a hair tonic when massaged into the scalp.

beech
A tree, *Fagus grandifolia* and *Fagus sylvatica,* known for its beechnuts and medicinal leaves that thrives in North America and Europe. According to English herbalist John Gerard, in the 16th century leaves were used in topical treatments of swelling, blisters, excoriations, skin rashes including poison ivy, frostbite and burns. When chewed, the leaves were thought to relieve chapped lips and painful gums. Gerard also claims that beechnuts ease kidney pain, and beechwater (found in the hollow of the tree) washes can cure assorted problems such as scabs on people, horses, sheep and cows.

beechdrop
Cancer root, a parasite of the Orabanchaceae, or broom-rape, family. This wiry plant has a scaly root and bears flowers in late summer. The tops, stems and root are considered medicinal, having an astringent effect on the body. They are used in the form of tinctures and extracts by homeopaths to treat cancer, asthma, palpitations, gonorrhea, headaches, mouth and stomach ulcers and diarrhea. Externally, beechdrop is said to be effective against all forms of dermatitis.

bee pollen
The dusty bloom on the body of the bee. Pollen, a mass of microspores resembling a fine flour found in seed plants, is collected by "pollen baskets" on each hind tibia of the bee. Many nutrition-ists and herbalists consider bee pollen a 100-percent nutritionally balanced food because it contains enzymes, amino acids, vitamins, hormones and other substances required for healing and rejuvenation of bodily functions. Some of the indications for using bee pollen are aging, allergies, indigestion, prostate disease, sore throat, acne, sexual problems and fatigue, according to some nutritionists, homeopaths and herbalists.

belladonna
(poison black cherry, deadly nightshade, dwale)
A perennial plant, *Atropa belladonna,* found in the eastern United States and in Europe, whose leaves, tops (any growth above the leaves or from leaves) and berries are used as a narcotic, anticholinergic, antispasmodic, calmative, diaphoretic and diuretic. A well-known poison, belladonna (meaning "beautiful lady" in Italian) is the source of various alkaloids, including atropine and scopolamine, used to treat gastrointestinal spasms and diarrhea, according to the United States Pharmacopoeia (USP).

benincasa
(dong gua pi, white gourd, wax gourd, Chinese preserving melon)
An annual plant native to southeast Asia, *Benincasa hispida,* of the Cucurbitaceae family, eaten as a vegetable and used for making pickles, whose seeds, rind and fruits are used by Chinese practitioners to treat fever, piles, diabetes, urinary tract diseases, gonorrhea and intestinal inflammation.

benzoin
A balsamic resin derived from the tree *Styrax benzoin* or *Styrax paralleloneuris,* used internally as a stimulant expectorant and an inhalant for the treatment of laryngitis and bronchitis, according to the United States Pharmacopoeia (USP).

bergamot

A mint of the genus *Monarda,* or an essential oil derived from the rind of the orange *Citrus bergamia,* used in the making of perfume. Bergamot is a popular, aromatic tea that may offer some of the soothing effects of other mints. (See MINT.)

beriberi

A disease affecting the neurological, cerebral and cardiovascular systems that is caused by a severe lack of thiamine, or vitamin B_1, in the diet. *Beri* is the Singhalese word meaning weakness, one of the symptoms of beriberi. Other symptoms include abdominal discomfort, poor memory, numbness in the legs, palpitations and increased heart rate, calf-muscle tenderness, sleep disturbances, constipation, anorexia and pain in the heart and chest area.

Symptoms including edema, or swelling, of the legs, face, trunk and serous cavities, high blood pressure, decreased urine output, distended neck veins and muscle tension are characteristic of "wet beriberi."

Symptoms of the form of beriberi known as "dry beriberi" include difficulty walking, loss of memory and disorientation, a staggering gait, jerky eye movements and other signs of the Wernicke-Korsakoff syndrome, which is identified by encephalopathy, or any dysfunction of the brain. Wernicke-Korsakoff syndrome is usually seen in alcoholics, although it can occur in others with malnutrition.

Beriberi, also known as dietetic neuritis, has been endemic in Asia, particularly Burma, Thailand and Vietnam, the Philippines and other Pacific islands, and formerly in regions of the United States in which rice is grown. People who rely on milled rice as their chief food are at risk of developing beriberi. When the grain was hulled and pounded at home, it retained its thiamine content in the bran left on the kernel of rice. But when rice is highly polished during a commercial milling process, it loses its valuable thiamine content. Prevention of beriberi has been implemented by manufacturers of flour and cereals: Thiamine is added to the products, called "enriched," to reduce the incidence of thiamine deficiency.

Secondary conditions may also result from inadequate or impaired absorption or impaired bodily utilization of thiamine. Alcoholics are at risk of a neuritis nearly identical to beriberi, because the consistent consumption of alcoholic beverages suppresses the desire for food and depletes the body of nutrients.

Thiamine may be administered orally or by injection as treatment for the disease. Dietary sources of thiamine include whole and enriched grains, legumes and other vegetables, lean pork, eggs, liver and milk. Infants with beriberi may be treated by administering thiamine to the breast-feeding mother and the infant.

(See also ANTITHIAMINE FACTORS; THIAMINE.)

beta-carotene

A provitamin, precursor chemical or building block that is converted to vitamin A in humans. (See A, VITAMIN.)

beth root

(birth root, wake robin, Indian balm, American ground lily)

A flowering herb of temperate North America and eastern Asia, *Trillium pendulum,* wild, or *edectum,* of the Liliaceae family, whose root was used by Native Americans as a pain reliever, especially during childbirth. Beth root is also considered a tonic for bleeding and female reproductive disorders including profuse menstruation and leukorrhea. It is also used in the treatment of lung conditions and, in homeopathic medicine, for writer's cramp, fainting, dysentery and diabetes.

bharngi

The Sanskrit name, in Ayurvedic medicine, for the herb *Clerodendrum serratum,* of the family Verbenaceae.

bhringaraj

The Sanskrit name, in Ayurvedic medicine, for the herb *Eclipta,* of the Compositae family, used as tonic, alterative, nervine and hemostatic. (See ECLIPTA.)

bhumyamalaki

The Sanskrit name, in Ayurvedic medicine, for the herb *Phyllanthus nururi.*

bibhitaki

The Sanskrit name for Beleric myrobalan, used in Ayruvedic herbal medicine as a strong laxative and antidote for *kapha,* a *dosha,* or body type, characterized generally by sluggishness. From the species *Terminalia belerica* of the family Combretaceae. Used as tonic, astringent, expectorant and laxative.

bilberry

(huckleberry, whortleberry, hurtleberry)
An herb, *Vaccinium myrtillus,* of the Ericaceae family, that is thought to strengthen capillaries of the eye muscles, thereby reducing eyestrain and increasing night vision.

bilva

An Ayruvedic herbal medicine (*bilva* in Sanskrit translated as "bel").

bioflavonoids ("vitamin P")

A group of naturally occurring compounds containing a common structure, widely distributed in plants with biological activity in animals including humans. Citrus bioflavonoids are derived from the rind of green citrus fruits, rose hips and black currants. Although plentiful in the diet, these substances are broken down in the intestine and little if any are absorbed intact. It was theorized in the 1930s that bioflavonoids were useful to treat individuals with fragile or damaged blood vessels. Originally called vitamin P, this substance was renamed when researchers realized they could not prove the group of bioflavonoids to be either essential nutrients or have any value as drugs. Some researchers claim that bioflavonoids boost the effects of vitamin C.

biota

(bai zi ren)
A Chinese medicinal herb, *Biota orientalis,* whose seeds are used in the treatment of heart problems.

biotin

A coenzyme manufactured by bacteria normally found in the human intestinal tract and essential in the metabolism of both fats and carbohydrates. Because it is manufactured in humans, it is not a true vitamin. (See VITAMIN.)

Raw egg white contains the antivitamin substance avidin, which, if ingested in high and prolonged quantity, results in a rash and glossitis (inflammation of the tongue) caused by biotin deficiency. Long-term total parenteral nutrition (TPN), an intravenous method of nourishing people who are extremely ill and/or incapable of eating, may also cause biotin deficiency.

Infants may exhibit the rash seborrheic dermatitis and hair loss due to a lack of biotin, but hair

FOOD SOURCES OF BIOTIN

Chicken	Yeast	Rice bran
Lamb	Soybeans	Eggs (must
Pork	Milk	be cooked[1])
Beef	Cheese	
Veal	Saltwater fish	
Liver	Whole wheat flour	

[1] Avidin, a substance in raw egg white, antagonizes the action of biotin but is destroyed by cooking.

loss only responds to supplementation in a true deficiency of the substance.

There are reports that some individuals may exhibit such Alzheimer-like signs and symptoms as disorientation, speech disorders, loss of memory, restless legs, tremors and unsteady gait that are actually caused by biotin deficiency. Biotin deficiencies are rare except for some genetically impaired groups of individuals and body-builders who eat large quantities of raw eggs (see table). Also, persons treated with antibiotics for a prolonged time might have impaired bacterial synthesis of biotin because of the destruction of normal bacterial flora in the gut.

Although there is no recommended daily allowance (RDA) for biotin, a dosage of 150 to 300 mcg daily promptly improves biotin deficiency.

Biotin is found in many B-complex and multivitamin supplements and is also available as d-biotin tablets. Biotin is thought to be without toxic or other adverse effects.

birch

A tree whose leaves are used in the making of tea that is claimed to help alleviate urinary problems, intestinal worms and rheumatism.

bird's nest

(ice plant, ova-ova, fit plant, Indian pipe)
A flowering plant, *Monotropa uniflora,* found in North America from Maine to the Carolinas and in regions toward Missouri, considered an antispasmodic, tonic and sedative, especially for use in St. Vitus' dance (chorea, including Huntington's disease, among other types) and seizures in children.

birth control pills and vitamin deficiency

See CONTRACEPTIVES, ORAL.

birth defects and vitamin deficiency

See FOLIC ACID.

bistort

(dragonwort, adderwort, snakeweed)
The plant *Polygonum bistorta,* of the family Polygonaceae, whose root is considered by herbalists to be an astringent to treat bleeding and diarrhea. External uses include toothpowder said to be effective against gum disease and a douche to eliminate vaginal discharge.

bitter root

(dog bane, milk weed, westernwall)
A perennial, flowering plant of North America, *Apocynum androsaemifolium,* of the family Apocynaceae, whose root is considered medicinal, especially in the treatment of venereal diseases, Bright's disease, rheumatic gout, worms, diabetes, heart diseases, dropsy, facial neuralgia, nausea and vomiting. Used externally, bitter-root milk is said to remove warts.

blackberry

The bush *Rubus fruticosus,* of the family Rosaceae, whose berries are nutritionally beneficial, especially to anemic individuals, and whose leaves and root bark are used as treatment for sore throat, fever, colds, diarrhea, bleeding and dysentery. Blackberries contain sugars, vitamins C and A and other nutrients, and, in Chinese traditional medicine, are thought to provide a cooling "Yin tonic" for nourishing the blood.

black cohosh

(bugbane, black snakeroot, rattleroot)
An herb containing natural estrogen with none of the carcinogenic properties found in synthetic estrogen. Black cohosh is claimed to be effective for the treatment of menstrual cramps and to regulate menses.

black haw

(stagbush, American sloe)
The *Viburnum prunifolium,* of the family Caprifo-

liaceae, whose stem and root bark are used in herbal medicine as a uterine tonic to prevent miscarriage, relieve menstrual pain and help relieve menopausal distress such as hot flashes and night sweats, and as an antispasmodic for treating diarrhea, asthma, palpitations and other cardiac problems, nervousness and mood swings.

bladderwrack
See SEAWRACK.

black pepper
(*maricha,* in Sanskrit)
A pungent, hot spice used throughout the world mainly to improve the taste of foods, from the East Indian plant of the Piperaceae family. Pepper is used in Ayurvedic medicine to relieve swelling, hives (external use), intestinal worms, dry hemorrhoids, constipation, flatulence and loss of appetite.

blessed thistle
(holy thistle, St. Benedict thistle)
An annual plant native to southern Europe or western Asia cultivated elsewhere, that is thought to be a tonic to stimulate circulation to the heart, stomach and liver. Many herbalists believe blessed thistle, *Cnicus benedictus* of the family Compositae, increases the flow of oxygen to the brain and boosts memory capabilities. It is also said to reduce fever, stop bleeding and resolve blood clots and treat hepatitis. Artichoke leaves, a member of the thistle family and usually eaten as a vegetable, are also used for a tea thought to restore normal liver functioning. Milk thistle is considered a healing and protective liver tonic. (See ARTICHOKE.)

bletilla
A ground orchid of China and Japan, *Bletilla striata,* of the Orchidaceae family, whose stem is used in Chinese medicine to treat tuberculosis,

chest pain, bloody sputum or vomitus, coughs, abscesses and swellings.

blindness and vitamin deficiency
See EYE DISEASES.

blood coagulation
See K, VITAMIN.

blood levels of vitamins
Laboratory tests available to determine adequacy or deficiencies of vitamins or minerals. Only a few tests are frequently used, including vitamin B_{12}, folic acid and iron levels to assist in the diagnosis of anemia. Minerals can be measured also, but most often these tests are run to detect toxicity.

TESTS AVAILABLE

	Use
Calcium (blood)	Elevated calcium levels occur in hyperparathyroidism, some kidney disorders, some cancers, especially tumors of lung, kidney, pancreas and ovary or metastatic cancer. Also hypervitaminosis A or D, myeloma, sarcoidosis, milk-alkali syndrome (excessive use of calcium-containing drugs), hyperthyroidism, acromegaly, Addison's disease, drugs including diuretics and estrogens. Causes of low calcium levels: low levels of albumin and total protein, hyperparathyroidism, osteomalacia, vitamin D deficiency, rickets, kidney disorders, malabsorption or malnutrition, neonatal tetany, Milkman's syndrome, pan-

TESTS AVAILABLE

	Use
	cratitis, high phosphorus, IV fluids, drugs including anticonvulsants and barbiturates.
(urine)	Elevated in some bone disorders, kidney stones and other kidney disorders, rickets, vitamin D toxicity, hyperparathyroidism. Decreased when taking oral contraceptives, vitamin deficiency, some kidney disorders, vitamin D-resistant rickets, hypoparathyroidism.
Carotene (blood)	Elevated in pregnancy and excessive intake of carrots. Depressed in malabsorption, some metabolic disorders, heat stroke and liver necrosis.
Ferritin (blood)	Evaluation of microcytic anemia, iron storage disorders, iron metabolism.
Folates (folic acid) (blood)	Anemia evaluation.
Iron (blood)	Anemia evaluation.
Vitamin A	Hypervitaminosis A. Vitamin A deficiency.
Vitamin B_1	Deficiency.
Vitamin B_2	Deficiency.
Vitamin B_6	Deficiency.
Vitamin B_{12}	Deficiency. Anemia evaluation.
Vitamin C	Evaluation of scurvy.
Vitamin D	Evaluation of parathyroid and kidney disorders.
Vitamin E	Deficiency in hemolytic disease in premature infants, neuromuscular disease in infants and adults with cholestasis.

bloodroot

(redroot, red Indian paint, tetterwort)
An herb, *Sanguinaria canadensis,* of the Papaveraceae family, thought to be a treatment for coughs and colds and a stimulant to the heart and digestive system. In herbal medicine, bloodroot is used as an expectorant for asthma, productive coughing, croup, sinus congestion and laryngitis. External uses include tinctures or powders to treat athlete's foot, skin rashes and cancer and gum disease.

blue cohosh

(papooseroot, squawroot)
An herb, *Caulophyllum thalictroides,* of the Berberidaceae family, similar in effect to black cohosh. The rhizome, or root stem, is used in herbal medicine to relive labor pain and various difficulties related to menses, such as lack of menses, irregularities and menstrual pain. It is also used for the treatment of worms and genitourinary disorders. (See BLACK COHOSH.)

blue flag

(flag lily, poison flag, liver lily, fleur-de-lis, wild iris)
An herb, *Iris versicolor,* of the family Iridaceae, whose rhizome, or root stem, is used in extract form, thought to be effective in the treatment of cancer, skin diseases, blood dyscrasias, constipation, rheumatism and liver ailments. In herbal medicine, blue flag is also used as an appetite suppressant for obese individuals.

blue vervain

The herb *Verbena officinalis,* of the family Verbenaceae, whose aerial portions or tops, are used in herbal medicine in the treatment of liver disorders, menstrual pain, nervousness, ascites, mastitis, influenza, colds and fever. Vervain is also thought to increase the flow of breast milk.

blue violet

A flowering herb claimed to relieve headache, head congestion and internal ulcers.

bone growth and structure
See CALCIUM; OSTEOPOROSIS; RICKETS.

bone meal
Ground or crushed bone used as feed, fertilizer and a source of easily absorbed calcium. Bone meal is also high in phosphorus.

boneset
(feverwort, thoroughwort)
An herb, *Eupatorium perfoliatum,* of the family Compositae, prepared as an infusion to treat colds, influenza and constipation. Boneset is also thought to relax muscles, stomach, intestines, uterus and gall ducts.

borage
(burrage)
A flowering European herb, *Borago officinalis,* of the family Boraginaceae, thought to reduce fever and irritation of skin and mucous membranes, including the mucous membranes of the lung. Borage, whose seeds are a rich source of gamma linolenic oil, is also said to increase breast milk.

boron
A nonmetallic element found as a compound in such substances as boric acid or borax and in plant and animal tissues. Along with arsenic and aluminum, boron, or bromine, is considered a nonessential trace element of no known function or need in the human diet. There is some evidence that postmenopausal women on low-boron diets may be at increased risk for osteoporosis, and a diet high in fruits and vegetables may prevent calcium loss and bone demineralization.

boswellic acid
One of four triterpene acids found in the herb *Boswellia serrata* that has been standardized in amount and used in Ayurvedic herbal treatments for various problems. Boswellia and vitamin E are combined in a topical preparation for arthritic pain relief.

brahmi
In Ayurvedic medicine, Sanskrit for gotu kola. (See GOTU KOLA.)

bran
The cracked outer coating of the seed of a cereal grain such as oats or wheat that has been separated from the milled product, i.e., flour or meal, through the process of sifting (bolting). Added to the diet, bran is used to prevent and treat constipation because of its indigestible cellulose content, which introduces bulk into the intestines. Any edible product containing digestion-resistant cellulose, hemicellulose, lignin, gums, mucilages and pectin is considered helpful to the elimination function of the body. Studies have been made on the effectiveness of added fiber to the diets of individuals with high blood pressure, diabetes, colon cancer, gallstones, irritable bowel syndrome, colon polyps and other problems. Oat bran became extremely fashionable during the early 1990s when some researchers proclaimed it a cancer-preventing agent. The studies have not yet proven all the claims, but it is accepted that foods rich in fiber, including whole-grain products, bran flakes, beans, fruits, leafy vegetables, nuts, root vegetables and prunes, are beneficial in the prevention of constipation.

brand name products
See GENERIC PRODUCTS.

brassica
(mustard)
The cabbage plant, *Brassica juncea, cernua, napiformis, oleracea* or *gongylodes,* of the Cruciferae

family, whose seeds and leaves are used by Chinese herbalists to treat various disorders, including colds, lumbago, rheumatism, ulcers, cystitis, stomach problems, diabetes, pneumonia, arthritis and neuralgia.

breast disease and vitamins

The controversial results from several studies designed to determine if antioxidant vitamins protect against breast or other cancers. In 1984, British investigators measured frozen blood from more than 5,000 women and determined that those with breast cancer had significantly lower beta-carotene than healthy women. The same observers found that those with low vitamin E levels were five times more likely to develop breast cancer.

In 1990, researchers at the University of Toronto analyzed data from a number of studies and concluded that large amounts of vitamin C seemed to protect women against breast cancer. However, participants in the Harvard Medical School's Nurses Health Study, who consumed more than 1,300 mg vitamin C or 600 I.U. of vitamin E daily, had no apparent protection against breast cancer when compared to those not taking the antioxidants.

brewer's yeast

Species of yeast suitable for use in brewing. One such yeast is *Saccaromyces cerevisiae,* a low-potency source of the B-complex vitamins.

(See also YEAST, BREWER'S.)

brindal berry

The English name of *amlavetasa,* the Sanskrit name of an Ayurvedic herb.

brucea

A shrub native to the Malay Archipelago, East Indies and China, *Brucea javanica,* of the Sima-

roubaceae family, whose seeds are used by Chinese herbalists to treat both constipation and diarrhea, amoebic and chronic dysentery and piles.

buchu

The plant *Agathosma betulina,* of the family Rutaceae, whose leaves have been touted for their effectiveness as a diuretic, an agent that helps rid the body of excess water, and urinary pain-reliever. Buchu leaves were used by the Hottentots of South Africa.

buckthorn

A tree, *Rhamnus cathartica,* whose bark is said to promote regular bowels and alleviate appendicitis, worms and warts. Buckthorn berries are made into a syrup with honey, allspice and ginger that is considered as a laxative for children.

buddleia

(butterfly bush)

A flowering shrub of China, *Buddleia officinialis,* of the family Loganiaceae, named for English botanist Adam Buddle (1660–1715). The shrub's flower buds contain buddlein, an alkaloid, and the flowers and leaves are used in Chinese medicine to treat night blindness, eyestrain and cataracts. The roots of the poisonous *Buddleia lindleyana* are used for stunning fish, killing insects and treating asthma and bloody, productive cough.

buffered vitamins

Modification of vitamins that are acidic, such as ascorbic acid (vitamin C), so that megadoses can be taken without irritating the stomach. Sodium ascorbate, a buffered form of vitamin C, should be avoided by people with hypertension and others on low-sodium diets.

bupleurum
(ch'ai hu)

An herb, *Bupleurum chinese,* of the family Umbelliferae, whose root is considered in Chinese herbal medicine to be a liver detoxicant and an agent against nausea, anxiety, dizziness, pain and fever. Bupleurum is also thought to strengthen the eyes and limbs.

burdock
(lappa, beggar's buttons, bardane)

An herb, *Arctium lappa,* of the family Compositae, whose root, seeds, and leaves are claimed to purify the blood by removing toxins and treat severe skin problems and arthritis. In Japan, burdock root, called *gobo,* is eaten like carrots.

burns and nutrition

The effects of dietary factors in people with severe burns. Burns cause a loss of fluids and electrolytes, which may be life-threatening. Since burn patients may require total bedrest, serum calcium may fall to levels that precipitate bone loss. This condition can be minimized by calcium supplementation and starting exercise as soon as possible. In addition, zinc levels fall, impairing wound healing and causing loss of appetite.

butcher's-broom
(kneeholy, sweet broom, pettier)

The herb *Ruscus aculeatus,* of the family Liliaceae, used in herbal medicine as a vascular anti-inflammatory and a pain-reliever in arthritis and rheumatism. Hemorrhoid pain and swelling are treated with an ointment made from butcher's-broom.

butternut

An American oily-nut tree, *Juglans cinerea,* of the walnut family, whose bark is thought to strengthen the intestines and relieve constipation, fever and colds.

C

C, vitamin
See ASCORBIC ACID.

cabbage
A common leafy vegetable originating in Europe, *Brassica oleracea,* that was given high praise by the Ancient Greeks and Romans, particularly Hippocrates, Pythagorus and Cato the Elder, as a medicinal plant. In *Herbal,* a 17th-century writing by Nicholas Culpeper, cabbage (earlier known as colewort) was credited with healing all manner of ills, including kidney stones and shortness of breath. Dubbed "the poor man's medicine" in Europe, cabbage is considered effective in cleansing the liver (because of its sulfur content) and keeping the intestines healthy (because of its vitamin C, bulk, water and fermentation bacteria). Cabbage has also been used in the treatment of worms, anxiety and depression.

(See BRASSICA.)

cadmium
A metal similar in appearance and properties to tin. Elemental cadmium and its salts are toxic. It is unknown if traces of this mineral are essential in human nutrition. If required, it is sufficiently plentiful in food, water and air to satisfy human needs.

caesalpinia
(sappan tree, brazilwood)
A tree, *Caesalpinia sappan,* of the Leguminosae family, native to the Malay Peninsula and India, that yields heartwood, from which synthetic aniline dyes are made. In Chinese medicine, heartwood also can be made into a decoction for the treatment of bleeding during and after childbirth, excessive menstrual flow, coughing blood and bruises, among other similar uses.

cajunput
(cajeput, white tea tree, tea tree)
The tree *Melaleuca leucadendron,* of the family Myrtaceae, whose oil is distilled and used in herbal medicine preparations to treat colds, flu and yeast (*Candida albicans*) infections. Internal use of cajunput is restricted, however. External uses include treatment of arthritis pain, fungal infections, pimples, cradle cap, plantar warts, cuts, bruises and various topical injuries, itching and scalp irritation. Inhalation of the oil vapors may be effective for congested sinuses.

calamus
(sweet flag, haulm, sweet sedge)
The plant *Acorus calamus,* of the family Aracae, named from the Greek word *kalamos,* meaning reed, whose aromatic rhizome, or root stem, contains a carcinogenic essential oil, B-asarone. (The American, as opposed to the European, calamus is reported to lack this oil.) In herbal medicine, calamus has been used for treating liver, stomach and intestinal ailments. It is also said to help overcome the desire for tobacco. Native Americans chew the calamus root to boost their stamina and endurance. The Chinese consider the calamus root therapeutic for hypertension, coughs, constricted veins, irregular heart rhythms, lung congestion and bacterial infection. Asian Indians use calamus root as a cooking spice and for nervousness, particularly in

40

Ayurvedic medicine, which maintains that calamus root increases concentration. Ayurvedic practitioners also believe that calamus root's anti-anxiety properties aid in helping individuals with a marijuana habit. Both in marijuana and tobacco cessation therapies, calamus is said to create a slight nausea when taken in conjunction with either substance.

calciferol
See D, VITAMIN.

calcium
The most abundant mineral and the fifth most-plentiful substance in the body. The average adult contains from 2 to 3 pounds of calcium, of which 99 percent is found in the bones and teeth. The remaining 1 percent is found in the circulatory system and aids in regulating various body functions. The newborn's skeleton contains about 30 grams of calcium, most of which is deposited during the third trimester of pregnancy.

Calcium, which is absorbed from the small intestine, requires the presence of vitamin D.

Uses

Essential for healthy bone composition, calcium alone cannot increase bone mass after the age of 20. Although calcium supplements probably do little to reduce the incidence of hip fractures in the elderly, there is little downside to supplements. A French study in elderly women given 800 International Units of vitamin D_3 (see D, VITAMIN) and 1.2 grams of calcium daily demonstrated more than a 40-percent reduction in hip fractures.

Results have been mixed in studies designed to see if high calcium intake lowers blood pressure. While animal studies seem to indicate that high calcium intake may protect against colon cancer, proof in humans is lacking.

Deficiency

Osteoporosis is the most common and serious complication of inadequate calcium intake or absorption. As calcium intake diminishes, calcium is resorbed from bones, especially the spine and jaw, the first bones to show evidence of osteoporosis. Vitamin D is essential for the utilization of calcium, and it may be prudent for women at highest risk, such as those older than 65 who are housebound, reside in nursing homes or live in areas where winters are long with minimal sun exposure, to take 200–400 I.U. of vitamin D daily.

It has been found in several studies that women taking thiazide diuretics for the treatment of hypertension had a reduction in the number of hip fractures as high as 30 percent. It is known that these drugs interfere with the excretion of calcium by the kidneys, and that the increased blood levels may result. However, other studies dispute the findings and report only a modest 10-percent increase in bone density for women on up to 10 years of thiazide therapy.

Regular weight-bearing, vigorous exercise seems to protect against osteoporosis because stressed bone stimulates new bone production via osteoblast cells. But any benefit is lost within one year of ceasing the exercise.

Low blood-calcium levels cause increased muscle sensitivity, resulting in muscle spasms, or tetany. Muscle cramps occur when blood-calcium levels are very low and are particularly more common during pregnancy. Infants fed undiluted cow's milk are at increased risk for tetany.

Recommended Daily Allowances

In 1994 The National Institutes of Health Consensus Development Panel made new recommendations for calcium intake (see TABLE 6). This expert group recommends a modest increase in calcium for most individuals that should not exceed 2,000 mg per day. Higher levels should be monitored carefully and may cause adverse effects. Peak bone mass is probably attained from ages 11 to 24 years. Women older than 50 who are on estrogen have a lower requirement equalivalent to premenopausal women. Since calcium absorption from cow's milk is less efficient than from human milk, formula-fed infants have an increased requirement.

Table 6
1994 RECOMMENDATIONS BY THE NATIONAL INSTITUTES OF HEALTH CONSENSUS DEVELOPMENT PANEL ON CALCIUM REQUIREMENTS

Infants up to 6 months	400 mg/day
Infants 6 to 12 months	600 mg/day
Children 1 to 5 years	800 mg/day
Children 6 to 10 years	800–1,200 mg/day
Adolescents and young adults (11 to 24 years)	1,200–1,500 mg/day
Men 25 to 65 years	1,000 mg/day
Men older than 65 years	1,500 mg/day
Women 25 to 50 years	1,000 mg/day
Women older than 50 years	1,000 mg/day with estrogen therapy 1,500 mg/day if not on estrogens
Pregnant or nursing women	1,200–1,500 mg/day

Supplements Available

Calcium supplements, generic or brand-name, are readily absorbed and best when taken with meals. Dietary sources such as cheese, milk and yogurt are much more expensive. Care must be taken to assure that sources of calcium used do not contain toxic amounts of lead. Seventy brands of calcium supplements were analyzed for lead content. Five categories of the supplements were identified: dolomite, bone meal, refined- and natural-source calcium carbonate and calcium chelates. Lead levels ranged from 0.03 mcg/gram to 8.83 mcg/gram. Twenty-five percent of the products supplied daily lead quantities exceeding the federal Food and Drug Administration's "provisional" total tolerable daily intake of lead for infants and children through age 6. Therefore, caution must be used to assure that calcium supplements, especially those given to children with milk intolerance, have lead contents as low or lower than the levels found in milk products.

Table 7
CALCIUM MYTHS

- **Myth:** The body can only utilize small quantities of calcium.
  Truth: Most adults can tolerate up to 2,500 mg of calcium per day.
- **Myth:** All foods containing calcium are absorbed equally.
  Truth: Soybeans, kale, bread and dairy products contain readily absorbable calcium, whereas calcium-rich spinach provides almost no available calcium.
- **Myth:** High fiber interferes with the absorption of calcium.
  Truth: While bran, spinach and rhubarb do inhibit calcium absorption, psyllium (Metamucil) does not.
- **Myth:** All calcium supplements are the same.
  Truth: Calcium citrate is the most easily absorbed but contains a lower concentration of calcium (24 percent) than calcium carbonate (40 percent). Calcium lactate contains only 13 percent and calcium gluconate 9 percent of calcium per tablet.
- **Myth:** Calcium intake must be reduced in persons with kidney stones.
  Truth: Low-calcium diet may actually increase the risk of calcium kidney stones.
- **Myth:** Calcium must be in the form of a soluble salt to be absorbed.
  Truth: With rare exceptions. Taking supplements with meals is the key to calcium absorption.
- **Myth:** Persons with achlorhydria (inadequate secretion of hydrochloric acid in the stomach) are unable to absorb calcium carbonate and require calcium citrate, a more expensive form of supplement.
  Truth: These individuals can absorb calcium carbonate if it is taken with meals.
- **Myth:** Persons taking calcium-channel blocking drugs such as verapamil (Calan, Isoptin, Veralan); diltiazem (Cardizem, Dilacor); nifedipine (Procardia, Adalat) and others used to treat hypertension, angina pectoris and heart arrhythmia (irregularities) should avoid calcium supplements.

Table 7 (cont.)
CALCIUM MYTHS

Truth: Calcium supplements can be taken by those individuals.

• Myth: All calcium supplements are equally safe.

Truth: Dolomite and bone meal have high concentrations of calcium, but may be contaminated by lead or other toxins.

In addition to the possibility of lead contamination, calcium in dolomite is very poorly absorbed. Although bone meal is easily absorbed, it also contains large amounts of phosphorus, which may be undesirable (see PHOSPHORUS).

Toxicity

Most adults can tolerate a calcium intake of up to 2,500 mg per day, but constipation and possibly increased incidence of kidney stones may occur with persistence of high ingestion. Very high levels of calcium may interfere with the absorption of iron, zinc and other minerals from the intestine. Renal function may deteriorate in the presence of continued excessive calcium intake. In any case of hypercalcemia (high calcium), hypomagnesemia (low magnesium) and hypokalemia (low potassium) should also be considered.

calcium-channel blocking drugs

Drugs used in the treatment of high blood pressure and heart disorders. They play no role in blood-calcium levels and do not interact with calcium supplements.

(See CALCIUM.)

calcium pantothenate

A form of pantothenic acid contained in supplements of the B-complex vitamin. (See PANTO-THENIC ACID.)

calendula

(pot marigold)

A flowering herb, *Calendula officinalis,* whose flower petals have been used as topical treatment of wounds, sores and wasp and bee stings. Infusions, or teas, made from the flowers have been used to treat toothache, conjunctivitis (inflammation of the lining membrane of the eye), ulcers and fever. Calendula petals also have the culinary advantage of being less expensive than saffron, an important spice in Asian Indian and Spanish cuisine.

calico

(sheep laurel, spoonwood, mountain laurel, lambkill)

The flowering, evergreen bush *Kalmia latifolia,* of the Ericaceae family, found in hilly, rocky regions of the United States, whose leaves have been used in folk medicine as an antisyphilitic, astringent and sedative. While herbalists claim that large doses of calico may be poisonous, they also use it in the treatment of fevers, jaundice, inflammation and neuralgia. In homeopathic practice, a tincture of calico leaves is thought to relieve angina pectoris (chest pain), Bright's disease, dropsy, painful menstruation, gout, headache, sun headaches, syphilitic sore throat, ill effects of tobacco, ringing in the ears, dizziness, vomiting, lumbago and other problems.

calorie-dense foods

Foods that contain minimal amounts of vitamins or minerals but relatively large amounts of calories. Calorie-dense foods include those high in fat and sugar such as bacon, hot dogs and cookies.

camellia

Flowering shrubs and small trees of the Theaceae family, named for the Moravian Jesuit George

Joseph Camellus of the 17th century. The flowers of *Camellia japonica,* indigenous to China and Japan, are used by Chinese practitioners to treat bleeding of the uterus and nose and coughing of blood. The tea plant, *Camellia sinensis,* yields caffeinated green tea and black tea from its leaves and is used as a tonic for the central nervous system, heart and flow of urine.

camomile

(chamomile, Hungarian camomile, single camomile)

A common European herb of the genus *Anthemis,* especially *A. nobilis,* and the related genus *Matricaria,* including *M. chamomilla* and *M. recutita,* of the Compositae family, whose leaves and flower heads contain medicinal properties. With its high calcium content, camomile tea is a popular remedy for indigestion, colds, flu, teething pain, back pain, diarrhea, menstrual cramps, anxiety and insomnia. German camomile is considered the most potent anti-inflammatory of all other varieties of camomile, which may account for its effectiveness against the pain of sciatica, gout and herniated vertebral disc.

campsis

(Chinese trumpet creeper, Chinese trumpet flower)

A flowering vine, *Campsis grandiflora,* of the family Bignoniaceae, whose flowers and roots are considered medicinal by Chinese practitioners. The Greek word for curve, *campsis* has curved stamens. The flowers are used to treat diabetes, itching, fever, rectal bleeding, painful menses, skin allergy and other problems. The roots are said to relieve rheumatoid arthritis and muscle paralysis.

canarium

(kenari-nut tree)

The tree *Canarium album,* of the family Burseraceae, native to Indochina and South China, that yields a fruit resembling an olive and containing an oily kernel used for candies and cooking. The fruit is also used in Chinese medicine for sore throat and diarrhea, and as an antidote for poisoning by contaminated or poisonous fish. The seeds are powdered and used as an anti-inflammatory.

cancer prevention

Relatively risk-free measures that may prevent or delay the onset of cancer, or malignancy. Cancer is a disease in which cells lose their normal structure, exhibit unlimited growth and spread by invasion of surrounding tissues or by the circulatory system in a process called metastasis to distant sites. The cancerous, or abnormal, cells interfere with the tissues' ability to function. Initially healthy cells or their genetic code is altered by exposure to a substance called a mutagen or carcinogen. A second phase called the promotion stage is necessary for cancer to occur. This phase may take many years to develop and may not be apparent for 20 to 30 years. For cancer to develop, the abnormal cell must be in contact with something that will stimulate its growth.

The National Academy of Sciences believes that up to 60 percent of cancer is caused by nutritional factors. Diets high in vitamin A and beta-carotene, the plant form of vitamin A that the body converts to vitamin A, appear to have cancer-protective properties. Those who have diets low in vitamin A and beta-carotene seem to have an increased risk of developing cancer. Both smokers and chewers of tobacco have low vitamin A levels and increased precancerous cells in the tissues of the mouth, throat and lungs. Smokers may also have low levels of vitamin B_{12} and folate. Vitamin A may also offer protection to persons exposed to "secondhand" smoke and pollution.

The antioxidant vitamin E has been promoted as a cancer preventive because of its apparent ability to stabilize cell membranes and reduce free radicals. So far, study results have been mixed and inconclusive.

Experiments with vitamin K suggest that it may block the growth of cancerous cells in some tumors.

Folic-acid deficiency may predispose some women to cervical cancer. Folate supplements appear to prevent damage to cervical cells. Vitamin C seems to block the conversion of nitrites in processed foods to nitrosamines, which are thought to be carcinogenic to the stomach, colon and bladder. Its antioxidant properties also may have protective properties similar to vitamin E. Individuals with colon cancer may consume diets low in calcium and vitamin D.

Selenium is another antioxidant. People who live in areas where the selenium content of soil is high have lower incidence of cancers. Similarly, patients with malignancies including Hodgkin's disease, breast, colon and bladder cancer and leukemia have low blood levels of selenium.

While diets rich in vitamins and minerals may be protective against malignancy, the safety of large doses, or megadoses, of vitamins is questionable. Some studies suggest that excessive amounts of vitamin C, iron and zinc may inhibit the immune response, thus increasing the risk for cancer, infections or other diseases.

(See also AMERICAN CANCER SOCIETY CANCER PREVENTION, DIETARY GUIDELINES; ANTIOXIDANTS.)

cancer treatment with vitamins

Alternative and highly controversial nutrient therapy for malignant disorders. Traditional treatment for cancer is often frustrating because it frequently fails to prevent pain and death, and nausea may be unbearable. Therefore, anything that promises to prevent, cure or at least slow the process is welcome. Unfortunately, some practitioners offer alternative cancer therapies that rely on unproven vitamin or mineral regimens that may be toxic as well as ineffective. Additionally, they may be substituted for traditional or experimental drug protocols that may be effective.

Even well-meaning scientists, such as Nobel Prize–recipient Dr. Linus Pauling, have been caught up in promoting vitamins, especially vitamin C, as a cancer treatment. A study published in the *Proceedings of the National Academy of Sciences* in 1976 by Linus Pauling and Scottish researcher Ewan Cameron reported that 100 terminally ill cancer patients who received large doses of vitamin C lived up to 20 times longer than those who did not receive supplements. However, the article sparked great controversy among scientists who doubted the validity of the study. Examination of study methods show that there may have been bias, unintentional or not, in favor of the group that received vitamin C. Other studies have also produced contradictory results. A properly controlled "double-blind" study at the Mayo Clinic found that those cancer patients receiving 10 grams of vitamin C daily appeared to do no better than the group receiving a placebo.

Pauling objected vigorously to the fact that patients in the Mayo study had previously received chemotherapy, thus influencing the outcome.

Multiple vitamin-mineral supplements that supply at least the recommended daily allowances (RDA) are frequently given to patients as part of their therapeutic regimen. Occasionally the use of other supplements appears to be beneficial. For instance, zinc improves the sensation of taste in some cancer patients, which therefore may improve appetite and nutritional status. Interestingly, the basis for the anticancer drug methotrexate's effect comes from its ability to fool cancer cells into thinking the drug is folic acid. Since folic acid stimulates the reproductive processes of cells, methotrexate effectively blocks the spread of cancer cells. Thus, folic acid supplementation may actually stimulate a tumor.

cannabis
See HEMP SEED.

canthaxanthin

A carotenoid, similar to beta-carotene, but, unlike beta-carotene, it is not converted to vitamin A in the body. Early research indicated this substance might have some cancer-protective properties.

capsicum

(cayenne, red pepper, bird pepper, African pepper, chili pepper)

The plants *Capsicum mimimum (Roxb), frutescens* and *annuum,* of the family Solanaceae, grown in America (mainly south of Tennessee), Asia and Africa, whose fruit is eaten as a vegetable and used in the making of the hot, pungent spice. Chinese and other herbalists use the fruit as a tonic to stimulate the heart and circulation and stomach activity, unfortunately linked also with stomach distress and intestinal gas. Cayenne, however, is thought to be effective against bleeding in the lungs, toothache (the leaves are the medicinal part for this), cramps and other ailments. Homeopathic medicine includes dried cayenne pods as treatment for mouth ulcers, diarrhea, delirium tremens, asthma, headache, motion sickness, obesity, gout, sciatica, sore throat and a number of other problems.

The Russians commonly use red pepper (Kayansky Peretz) in vodka as a home remedy for colds, stomach problems, rheumatism and lack of appetite.

capsule

A hard or soft enclosure suitable as a container for drugs. Capsules are usually made from gelatin and animal by-products. "Vegicaps" by Solgar are available from one manufacturer for vegetarians and those who adhere to a kosher diet.

(See also GELATIN.)

caraway

A flowering biennial or perennial plant, *Carum carvi,* of the Umbellifer family, whose aromatic seeds are used as seasoning in various ethnic cuisines and by Chinese practitioners and other herbalists to aid digestion; expel gas; calm the nerves; counteract spasms, colic in infants and uterine cramps; and promote the onset of menstruation and lactation. When cooked and eaten, the roots are thought to tonify the intestines. Caraway grows wild in the northern United States, Europe and Asia, and is cultivated in most parts of the world, particularly in England, the Netherlands and Morocco.

carbohydrate

A major class of chemical substances composed of carbon, hydrogen and oxygen, including sugars, dextrins, glycogen, starches and celluloses. As a fundamental source of energy, carbohydrates are stored in all the body's tissues as glycogen and are especially plentiful in the liver and muscles. Carbohydrates are dispatched from their storage sites when necessary.

The abundance of glucose and its polymers surpasses the quantity of all other organic chemical compounds found on earth, including fuel hydrocarbons just below the earth's crust.

Carbohydrates are absorbed by the body in the form of glucose, galactose and fructose—three sugars. Among the sources of carbohydrates are legumes, whole grains, vegetables, potatoes, fruits, honey and sugars. Because the calories obtained from sugars and candy lack essential amino acids, vitamins and minerals, they are considered "empty calories."

cardamom

(sha ren, bastard cardamom, Malabar cardamom, ela [Sanskrit])

A perennial native to southern and eastern India, *Elettaria cardamomum,* of the ginger family, used as a spice and in folk and Ayurvedic medicine as an appetite stimulant, antiflatulent (carminative) and stomachic (an agent that invigorates stomach function).

cardiomyopathy

A disease of the heart muscle in which the heart may become enlarged and lose its pumping efficiency, resulting in congestive heart failure. Selenium deficiency predisposes some individuals, primarily children, to a form of cardiomyopathy called Keshan's disease. (See SELENIUM.)

cardiovascular disease prevention and antioxidant vitamins

The presence of oxidized low-density, or LDL, cholesterol is thought to clog arteries by stimulating macrophages, cells in the immune system, to ingest LDL particles converting them to "foam cells." The oxidized LDL also damages the arterial walls, accumulating fats, cellular debris, platelets and the mineral calcium in the process. When the build-up becomes sufficient, the coronary arteries (blood vessels that supply life-sustaining blood to the heart muscle) become clogged, leading to angina pectoris (the pain of heart disease) and myocardial infarctions (heart attacks). Atherosclerosis also can occur in the carotid arteries and the extremities, often leading to strokes. Supplements of the antioxidant vitamin E seem to lower the risk of heart attacks by up to 37 percent, according to one of two Harvard University studies involving 39,910 male pharmacists and other health-care professionals followed for four years. Doses from 100 to 249 International Units (I.U.) of vitamin E daily were adequate with no extra benefit from higher doses. Since vitamin E also seems to reduce blood clotting similar to the effects of aspirin, the question of which mechanism, the influence of the vitamin on blood clotting or the antioxidant effects on LDL, is responsible for this risk reduction remains.

The second of the two Harvard studies followed 87,245 healthy female nurses for eight years and found that those taking 100 I.U. of vitamin E daily were 34 percent less likely to suffer a heart attack.

A comparison of a small group of men taking 800 I.U. of vitamin E daily suggests protection against the oxidation of LDL more effective than beta-carotene, vitamin C or placebo in a test tube. The study, conducted at the University of Texas, was reported in 1993. (See also ANTIOXIDANTS, E, VITAMIN.)

Conclusion

Studies suggest, but do not prove, that approximately 100 I.U. of vitamin E daily reduces the risk of heart disease. It is impossible to get 100 I.U. of vitamin E from a balanced diet, but there does not seem to be any harmful effect from taking that quantity of vitamin E in a supplement.

carica

(papay, pawpaw)

The plant *Carica papaya,* of the Caricaceae family, thought to have originated in Mexico and Costa Rica, whose dried fruit pulp, leaves and latex are used by Chinese practitioners. The pulp reduces foot distress, including swelling. The leaves are for the treatment of ulcerations, boils, wounds and swellings. The latex, a meat tenderizer and ingredient in the manufacture of chewing gum and cosmetic products, is dried and used to expel intestinal worms and treat splenomegaly (enlarged spleen), skin blemishes, warts and corns.

carotenoids

A group of yellow to deep red pigments, synthesized by plants, that concentrate in animal fat when ingested. An example is beta-carotene, which is converted to vitamin A in the body.

(See also A, VITAMIN.)

carrot

An herb, *Daucus carota,* of the family Umbelliferae, whose orange-colored root is edible. An average carrot is about 7 inches in length and provides roughly four times the Recommended Daily Allowance (RDA) of beta-carotene, which the human body converts to vitamin A. Although it contains only about 30 calories, a carrot will also provide fiber, vitamin C and potassium. Canned and frozen carrots lose about half their vitamin C but retain most of the beta-carotene and other nutrients. Excessive intake of carrots will result in a deep yellow or orange skin discoloration that can be reversed by eliminating carrots from the diet.

carthamus
(hong hua, false saffron, bastard saffron, safflower)
A flowering herb, *Carthamus tinctorius,* of the Compositae family, that may have originated in Eurasia and whose flowers are used in Chinese medicine to treat internal bleeding, painful menses and coughing blood. Other uses include to induce menstruation and stimulate the circulation. It is also prescribed for women after giving birth or carrying a dead fetus.

cascara sagrada
(Persian bark, sacred bark, chittem bark)
A flowering tree of the West Coast of the United States and in South America, *Rhamnus purshiana,* of the Rhamnaceae family, whose aged, dried bark extract is used as a cathartic, listed in the United States Pharmacopoeia (USP). Cascara was recognized by Native Americans as an effective laxative. In Russia, cascara sagrada is called Krushina or Joster, and is also used in homeopathic medicine for the treatment of rheumatism.

cassia
(sicklepod, sickle senna)
A flowering herb of the Philippines, Indonesia, India, Japan and China, *Cassia tora,* of the Leguminosae family, whose seeds are used in Chinese medicine to treat herpes, eye ailments such as conjunctivitis, vertigo, earache, constipation and skin diseases.

castor bean
(castor-oil plant, Palma Christi)
The plant *Ricinus communis,* of the Euphorbiaceae family, whose bean or seed yields an oil when pressed that is used internally as a cathartic (castor oil) and externally as an emollient. The oil contains glycerides of ricinoleic, isoricinoleic, stearic, linoleic and dihydroxystearic acids, which act as laxatives in the digestive tract. After the beans have been pressed to extract the oil, the poisonous substance ricin is left. In the past, castor oil was routinely given to children to keep their bowels regular. Its terrible taste often created indelible memories of childhood. Herbalists also prescribe castor oil as a treatment for food poisoning, and, administered along with anti-worm medications, to expel worms. Castor oil is recognized in the United States Pharmacopoeia (USP).

catalysis
A process in which a velocity of a chemical reaction is increased by the presence of a substance that is not consumed by the reaction. Enzymes, synthesized from amino acids, act in conjunction with B-complex vitamins as catalysts in the body.

catalyst
See CATALYSIS.

cataracts and vitamins
See EYE DISEASES.

catnip
(catmint)
A highly aromatic mint, *Nepeta cataria,* of the Labiatae family, commonly known for its attractiveness to cats. But a tea made from the leaves, according to herbalists, is used for relieving the accumulated effects of stress, including nervousness and insomnia. Catnip is also prescribed

as a treatment for diarrhea, fevers and colds, and hyperactivity in children. Catnip may be combined with camomile, spearmint and lemon balm as a remedy for insomnia.

celandine
(tetterwort, chelidonium)
An evergreen perennial of the United States and Europe, *Chelidonium majus,* of the Papaveraceae family, whose herb and root are used in herbal medicine as a diuretic, an expectorant and a laxative. Early use of celandine included the treatment of jaundice. In Russian folk medicine, celandine preparations are used for spasmatic conditions of the liver, kidney, bladder and gallbladder, stomach problems and swellings. Among the homeopathic applications of celandine are liver, spleen and skin disorders, cancer, chorea, gonorrhea, hemorrhoids, headache, nosebleed, whooping cough, jaundice, stomachache, diarrhea, pneumonia, rheumatism, gallstones and influenza. External uses include the treatment of metastatic skin conditions, warts and cuts. The celandine plant is poisonous to animals.

celery
(smallage)
A biennial or annual herb, *Apium graveolens,* of the Umbelliferae family, that originated in southern Europe, Asia and Africa, whose root and seeds are considered of medicinal use by herbalists as a tonic, nerve sedative and carminative. In India and Pakistan, celery (*ajmoda*) is used to treat numerous problems, such as bronchitis, asthma, liver and spleen ailments, rheumatism, hiccoughs, intestinal gas, hives, urinary retention and discharges, lack of menses, fever and cough. Homeopathic medicine uses celery-seed tincture for tension headache, heartburn, toothache, vomiting, hives and the retention of urine.

celiac disease
See MALABSORPTION.

celosia
(wood flower)
A weed of Asian origin, *Celosia argentea* and *cristata* (cockscomb), of the Amarantaceae family, named from the Greek word *kelos,* meaning burned, used in Chinese medicine for dysentery, various menstrual difficulties, bleeding in the intestines and lungs, cough, eye inflammations and abnormal sensitivity, headache and worms.

The plant was eaten by prisoners of war in Thailand during World War II to prevent nutritionally related diseases such as beriberi and pellagra, and it has been known also as an aphrodisiac and anticancer agent.

(See also BERIBERI; PELLAGRA.)

centaury
(bitter clover, rose pink)
A flowering plant, *Sabbatia angularis,* of the family Gentianaceae, grown in Europe and the United States, used in herbal medicine as a tonic, fever-reducer and diaphoretic, and for the treatment of dyspepsia, rheumatic and other joint pain, diarrhea, eye inflammations and homesickness (which may be a form of depression in this context). In Russian folk medicine, centaury tea with vodka is given for parasitic tapeworm, hypertension and liver and gallbladder maladies.

centella
(Asian pennywort, Indian pennywort)
A tropical weed, *Centella asiatica,* of the Umbelliferae family, sometimes eaten as a vegetable and, in Chinese medicine, used to stimulate the appetite, promote digestion and treat ulcers, skin problems and bowel complaints.

chaenomeles
(Japanese quince)
Deciduous shrub native to China and cultivated in Japan and elsewhere, *Chaenomeles speciosa,* of

the family Rosaceae, named from the Greek words *chaino* (split) and *meles* (apple), whose fruit is used in Chinese medicine for the relief of sunstroke, indigestion, colic, joint pain, cholera, muscle spasms and diarrhea.

chaga
(birch mushroom)
A North American and Canadian tree, *Inonotus obliquus,* of the family Polyporaceae, whose internal granulated parts (from the middle layer of a fungus, or mushroom-type growth sawn off the tree, as if removing a blackened wart) are used by Native Americans for medicinal purposes. In herbal folk medicine, chaga was given great credit for effectiveness against stomach pain, cancer, tuberculosis of the bone and other disorders. The Medical Academy of Science in Moscow touts chaga for malignancies and inoperable conditions, for purifying the blood and regenerating (or rejuvenating) organs.

chamomile
See CAMOMILE.

chaparral
(chaparro [Mexican], greasewood, creosote bush, gobonadora, dwarf evergreen oak)
The plant *Larrea divaricata,* of the family Zygophyllaceae, and plants of more than 100 botanical types of desert Artimesia, whose leaves and stems are considered in Native American medicine to be antiseptic, tonic and diuretic. "Chaparral tea" is an old Indian remedy for melanoma. Chaparral contains nordihydroguariaetic acid (NDGA), thought to be the substance that inhibits cancerous growth. It is also used by herbalists for the treatment of chronic backache, leukemia, prostate disorders, pulmonary ailments, kidney infection and arthritis, among others. It is considered an expectorant and weight-reducer.

chelation
A process in which metal complexes are formed. Chelating agents are used as treatments for metal poisoning. Although promoted by some as "better" supplements, there is no scientific basis for this.
  (See also CHELATED MINERAL SUPPLEMENTS.)

chelated mineral supplements
Minerals in which a natural or synthetic substance called the *chelator* is chemically combined and advocated as being better absorbed and therefore more available for utilization by the body. However, this claim may not be true, since the acidic nature of stomach juices breaks down the chelated product into its individual components. Therefore, there is probably no difference in absorption of chelated or nonchelated minerals. There are a few instances when chelated compounds such as iron or zinc may be less irritating to the stomach and therefore better tolerated. Chromium picolinate, another chelated mineral, may also be better absorbed.
  (See also AMINO ACID CHELATES.)

cherry bark
(choke cherry, wild black cherry bark)
A large North American fruit tree, *Prunus virginiana,* of the Rosaceae family, whose bark is used as a vehicle and flavoring in cough medicines. Homeopaths and Native American herbal-medicine practitioners use cherry bark, which contains hydrocyanic acid and malic acid, to prepare remedies for diarrhea (in children), bronchitis and dyspepsia.

chestnut
(Spanish chestnut, horse chestnut)
A North American, Asian and southern European tree, *Castanea dentata,* of the family Fagacaae, that produces nuts containing carbohydrates; minerals including phosphate of potash, magnesia,

sodium, and iron; and some protein. The leaves and inner bark are considered medicinal as a tonic, sedative and astringent. Herbalists use a tea of chestnut leaves for chronic cough, hiccoughs, fever and diarrhea. The horse chestnut is cultivated in Russia as Konsky cashtan, and, as in folk medicine, is used to treat arthritis, rheumatism, intestinal inflammation, gynecological problems and hemorrhoids.

chewable vitamins
Supplements that can be chewed to make them more palatable for children or those who have difficulty swallowing tablets or capsules. Young children must be observed for overdoses because these products may taste like candy. Chewable vitamin C may cause tooth decay because the acidic nature of the vitamin may wear away tooth enamel.

chickweed
(starwort, adder's mouth, tongue-grass, satin flower, stitchwort, starweed, winterweed)
An annual or biennial weed, *Stellaria media,* of the Caryophyllaceae family, found throughout the world and used in Native American and herbal medicine as a carminative, demulcent, expectorant and laxative. Also a vegetable, chickweed resembles spinach and can be eaten in salad. Homeopathic uses of chickweed include treatment of gout, inflammation of the liver, psoriasis and rheumatism.

chicory
(succory, endive)
An American and European perennial, *Cichorium intybus,* of the Compositae family, whose rootstock and flowering herb are used in folk, Native American and homeopathic medicine. Chicory tea is said to remove phlegm from the stomach, purify the liver and spleen and counteract gout, arthritis

and stiff joints. A tincture made of the dried root is used for amblyopia, constipation and headache. Chicory (Tzicory, in Russian folk medicine) is also used as a sedative of the heart and central nervous system.

chimonanthus
(wintersweet)
A Chinese flowering deciduous shrub, *Chimonanthus praecox,* of the Calycanthaceae family, whose flowers are used in Chinese medicine to treat sore throat and burns. *Chimonanthus* is the Greek word for winter flower.

chitrak
(plumbago)
An Ayurvedic herb thought to reduce hyperacidity and promote digestion.

chlerodendron
(glory-bower, tubeflower, Kashmir-bouquet)
Tropical shrubs or trees of the Verbenaceae family, named from the Greek words for chance and tree, whose leaves are used by Chinese practitioners to treat hypertension, beriberi, nosebleed, gonorrhea, intestinal bleeding, rheumatism and dermatitis.

Chlorella
The genus name of unicellular green algae. (See ALGAE.)

chloride
A salt of hydrochloric acid and principal inorganic anion in the extracellular fluid necessary to maintain a normal fluid and electrolyte balance in the body. Normal chloride occurs in concentrations of 96 to 106 milliequivalents per liter of plasma. Higher concentrations are present in the gastric juices and cerebrospinal fluid.

Chloride deficiency occurs only when there is also a loss of sodium caused by excessive sweating, chronic diarrhea or vomiting or some kidney disorders. These losses may result in metabolic alkalosis, a disorder of the body's pH, or acid-base balance, which may lead to coma or death.

Dietary intake is generally as sodium chloride (common table salt). Small amounts are available when potassium chloride supplements are used for the treatment of potassium deficiencies associated with diuretic use.

Toxicity
Only in the presence of severe dehydration is excessive dietary intake of chloride, as salt, of any significance. Hyperchloremia may cause high blood pressure.

(See also POTASSIUM; SODIUM.)

chlorophyll
The green color in plants in which photosynthesis takes place. (See ALGAE.)

cholesterol
See CARDIOVASCULAR DISEASE PREVENTION AND ANTIOXIDANT VITAMINS.

choline
A substance found throughout animal and plant tissues or made synthetically. Choline is not a vitamin despite claims by some that it is part of the B-complex. First discovered in hog bile in 1862, the amino acid methionine and folic acid are essential for its synthesis in humans.

Choline is important for the structure of all cell membranes, lipoproteins and surfactant for normal lung function. Choline may be vital in the production and transportation of fats from the liver and may prevent fatty liver. Investigators are trying to determine if alcoholic cirrhosis is caused by the toxic effects of alcohol alone or of that toxicity aggravated by nutritional deficiencies including choline.

Choline may also have important functions in the central nervous system as a component of sphinogomyelin in membranes and the neurotransmitter acetylcholine. Acetylcholine may be deficient in some neurological disorders of the elderly, and large dietary intake of choline was thought by some researchers to be of some possible benefit for memory loss. Unfortunately, this benefit has proved elusive in conditions such as Alzheimer's disease. There have been claims that chronic headache sufferers benefit from choline supplements.

Dietary Sources
The average diet contains 400 to 900 mg of choline found principally as lecithin in eggs, liver and other organ meats, lean meats, brewer's yeast, wheat germ, soybeans, peanuts and green peas. Lecithins are used as an emulsifier in chocolate and margarine, whereas vegetables such as cauliflower and lettuce contain free choline.

The American Academy of Pediatrics recommends that infant formula contain 7 mg of choline per 100 kilocalories equivalent to that found in human milk to assure adequate growth and development in newborns.

Toxicity
While large doses of choline produce liver and spleen damage and possibly alter the immune system in laboratory animals, this finding has not been demonstrated in humans. But an abnormal accumulation of sphinogomyelins in the nervous system results in the hereditary Niemann-Pick disease, characterized by enlargement of the liver and spleen, anemia and progressive physical and mental deterioration. With an onset in infancy, Niemann-Pick usually results in death before a child is three.

chromium
A trace mineral thought by some to be deficient in people with diabetes and having an influence on insulin and carbohydrate metabolism. Chromium, in association with insulin, may also play an important role in the synthesis of protein. Stud-

ies have not been completed to determine the validity of these claims.

(See also DIABETES MELLITUS.)

chronic fatigue syndrome (CFS)
(chronic mononucleosis, chronic Epstein-Barr virus infection, post-viral fatigue syndrome, myalgic encephalomyelitis)

A disorder characterized by overwhelming fatigue associated with a prolonged recovery period. Tasks that were formerly routine become difficult or impossible. The fatigue is accompanied by poor concentration and memory, depression, headaches, sleep disturbances, aches and pains.

The condition may begin insidiously without apparent cause, or following an acute infection, described as early as 1869 as "neurasthenia . . . a physical not a mental state" by the American neurologist George Beard. Clusters of cases have been blamed on mass hysteria since clinical findings are usually nonexistent.

Recently, several viruses have been proposed as causes, but so far this has not been scientifically documented. Epstein-Barr virus, enteroviruses, retroviruses, herpes virus type 6 and the T-cell lymphotropic virus type II have all been implicated as possible causes of CFS.

Alternative therapies including megavitamin formulas; royal jelly, a substance obtained from bees; and diets restricting yeasts and sugar have been prescribed for CFS. However, the Chronic Fatigue Syndrome Research Group at the Center for Disease Control in Atlanta warns that no dietary or vitamin therapy has proven effective in treating the condition.

An Australian study has demonstrated improvements in physical, psychological and functional symptoms following therapy with intravenous gamma globulin, suggesting that chronic fatigue syndrome, by whatever name, is an organic disease process and not a psychosomatic disorder.

(See also FATIGUE.)

chrysanthemum, Chinese
(chu hua or ju hua)

A flowering plant of the Compositae family, named from the Greek words *chyros* (golden) and *anthos* (flower). *Chrysanthemum morifolium* flowers are used in Chinese medicine as a tea in order to stimulate circulation and vision and treat menstrual, digestive, liver and potency problems, night blindness and nervous disorders. The flowers and stem of *Chrysanthemum indicum* are used to treat hypertension and skin infections.

cibotium
(Scythian lamb)

A Chinese and Malaysian forest fern, *Cibotium barometz,* of the Dicksoniaceae family, whose stem is used by Chinese practitioners as a liver and kidney tonic, and to treat infertility, lumbago, rheumatism and bone diseases.

cigarette smoking effects on vitamins and minerals

Smokers have lower bone density than nonsmokers, and calcium supplements may be helpful. Vitamin C is metabolized, or broken down, more quickly in smokers, who may require more than twice as much of the vitamin. The National Research Council recommends at least 100 mg of vitamin C daily. Vitamin E deficiency may also be more likely in smokers.

cimicifuga
(bugbane)

An herb, *Cimicifuga foetida,* of the Ranunculaceae family, of Europe, Siberia and China, named from the Latin words *cimicis* (bug) and *fugio* (to flee), and thought to have insecticidal properties. In Chinese medicine, bugbane root is used as a sedative, painkiller and treatment for measles, headache and diarrhea.

cinnamomum

(cinnamon, rou gui, gui zhi, twak [Sanskrit])
Evergreen trees and shrubs of the Lauraceae family, found from Southeast Asia to Australia. *Cinnamomum camphora* (camphor tree) of China, Taiwan and Japan yields wood and oil used externally to relieve pain and congestion. *Cinnamomum zeylanicum,* of India, Sri Lanka and the Malay Peninsula, is the source of cinnamon, the spice known throughout the world, as well as cinnamon oil, which, according to Chinese medicine, may be a narcotic poison when taken internally and a treatment for nausea and vomiting. The *zeylonicum* bark is used to treat rheumatism, tuberculosis and headache, and as a respiratory and circulatory stimulant.

The *Cinnamomum cassia* native to Burma yields cassia oil used in the making of chocolate and, from its bark, twigs and branches, medicinal preparations that relieve menstrual problems, indigestion, headache, fever, colds and joint and abdominal pain.

citrus

(chen pi, orange or tangerine peel)
Fruit-bearing, evergreen shrubs and trees of the Rutaceae family, originally of South and Southeast Asia and now cultivated throughout the world if the climate permits, whose leaves, roots, fruit and fruit peels are generally recognized as medicinal by most conventional practices of medicine and nutrition, including allopathic, Chinese traditional, Ayurvedic and Native American. Some of the fruits of the citrus shrubs and trees are oranges, lemons and grapefruits, rich in vitamin C.

In Chinese medicine, the leaves, root and fruit peel of citron, or *Citrus medica* native to India, are used to treat lumbago. Any citrus fruit offers vitamin C, which wards off scurvy (history has it that, to prevent scurvy, English sailors sucked limes to obtain the nutrient and therefore became known as "limeys"). Chinese practitioners also use both ripe and unripe fruits to relieve diarrhea, cramps, chest congestion and spleen and stomach problems.

(See also ASCORBIC ACID.)

cleavers

(goose grass, bedstraw, catchstraw, clivers)
A flowering herb, *Galium aparine,* of the Rubiaceae family, commonly found in Europe and the United States, especially along river banks, and used in Native American medicine as a tonic, diuretic and as a remedy for the occurrence of stones in bodily organs.

clematis

A climbing vine (in Greek, *klematis* means climbing plant) of the Ranunculaceae family. *Clematis chinensis* roots are used in Chinese medicine as a treatment for jaundice, constipation, irregular menses, lumbago, arthritis, backache, alcohol poisoning and scanty urine. The stem of *Clematis montana,* of the Himalayas, provides a remedy for excessive or painful urination and insomnia.

chlerodendron

(glory-bower, tubeflower, Kashmir-bouquet)
Tropical shrubs or trees of the Verbenaceae family, named from the Greek words for chance and tree, whose leaves are used by Chinese practitioners to treat hypertension, beriberi, nosebleed, gonorrhea, intestinal bleeding, rheumatism and dermatitis.

clove

(ding xiang, lavanga [Sanskrit])
A tropical evergreen tree, *Caryophyllus aromaticus, Eugenia caryophyllus* or *Syzygium aromaticum* of the myrtle family, used as a spice and a source of oil. Native to the Spice Islands and the Philippines, though cultivated in South America, Sumatra and the West Indies, clove oil relieves

toothaches and nausea. The oil is distilled from the dried flower buds.

cnidium
(chuanxiong, "Chinese lovage")
A Chinese, Siberian and eastern European herb, *Cnidium monnieri,* of the Umbelliferae family, whose seeds are used in Chinese medicine and are thought to be a stimulant (particularly for menstrual flow), aphrodisiac and sedative.

cobalamins
See B_{12}, VITAMIN.

cobolt
A metallic element that is an essential constituent of vitamin B_{12}. There is no evidence of human deficiency, and therefore no Recommended Daily Allowance (RDA) has been established.
(See also B_{12}, VITAMIN.)

cocaine abuse
See TYROSINE.

cod liver oil
A supplement rich in omega-3 fatty acids and fat-soluble vitamins A and D. Excessive amounts can cause toxic accumulation of A and D. (See A, VITAMIN; D, VITAMIN; OMEGA-3 FATTY ACIDS.)

codonopsis
(bonnet bellflower, dang shen)
A flowering, twining herb with heart-shaped, aromatic leaves, *Codonopsis pilosula,* of the Campanulaceae family, originally found in Northeast Asia. The plant's name is the Greek word for bell-like, which describes the bell-shaped flowers. The roots are used in Chinese medicine to prevent gonorrhea and relieve heart palpitations, diabetes, hypertension, breast cancer, diminished sexual desire, amnesia, asthma, insomnia and menstrual difficulties. Some believe codonopsis root may offer a substitute for the widely known stimulant ginseng.

coenzyme
A nonprotein compound that binds with a protein (apoenzyme) to form an active enzyme. Some B-complex vitamins such as pantothenic acid are converted in the body to co-enzymes.
(See also COENZYME A.)

coenzyme A
A compound derived from the B-complex vitamin pantothenic acid required to convert carbohydrates, fats and some proteins to energy.
(See also COENZYME; PANTOTHENIC ACID.)

coenzyme B_{12}
(adenosylcobalamin)
One of two active forms of vitamin B_{12} synthesized after the ingestion of the vitamin. (See B_{12}, VITAMIN; COENZYME.)

coenzyme Q-10 (coQ)
The substance ubiquinone. (See UBIQUINONE.)

coenzyme R
The former name for biotin. (See BIOTIN.)

coix
(Job's tears, yi yi ren)
A flowering, southeast Asian grass named *Coix lacryma-jobi,* or tears of Job, by the Swedish botanist Linnaeus, who created the system of naming and classifying plants. Of the family Gramineae, coix kernels (in Greek, *koix* means palm)

are used in Chinese, Japanese, Indian and Filipino medicine to treat fever, rheumatism, gonorrhea and other ailments.

colombo
(kalumb, calumbo)
A southeast African climbing perennial, *Cocculus palmatus,* whose rootstock is used in herbal medicine to treat diarrhea, nausea and vomiting, fever, dyspepsia and colon disorders.

coltsfoot
(kuan dong hua, British tobacco, foal's foot, flower velure, butterbur)
A flowering, perennial plant, *Tussilago farfara,* of the United States, Europe and the East Indies, whose leaves and flowers are used in herbal medicine for numerous respiratory problems, including pleurisy, bronchial asthma and hoarseness and for diarrhea.

comfrey
(knitbone, bruisewort, healing herb, gum plant, salsify, blackwort, wallwort)
An American and European flowering perennial plant, *Symphytum officinale,* of the family Boraginaceae, whose rootstock is made into a decoction and used as a gargle for sore throat and bleeding gums. When drunk, this decoction is considered by herbalists to remedy various symptoms of indigestion. Comfrey contains calcium, phosphorus, potassium, and vitamins A and C, and when powdered, its rootstock may be applied to minor cuts and burns to promote healing.

Comfrey tea, however, which has been popular for hundreds of years as a therapeutic agent, is now the subject of much controversy because of its pyrrolidine content, a substance that may cause liver dysfunction and cancer. While pyrrolidine and other alkaloids found in comfrey have not been proven to be carcinogenic, herbalists recommend cautious use of comfrey. Comfrey's chief reputation as a healing herb for external use on wounds and broken bones is largely attributable to the plant's allantoin content. Allantoin, a white crystalline substance found in amniotic fluid, is thought to stimulate cell growth.

contraceptives, oral, and vitamin deficiency
Drugs that inhibit ovulation and effectively prevent pregnancy that also depress serum folic acid levels. Therefore they may increase the risk of birth defects related to folate deficiency if pregnancy occurs in women who have recently used these products, also known as birth control pills.

cooking methods' effect on nutrients
The method of preparing foods in order to preserve their vital nutrients. While many people believe that eating vegetables raw is the best way to obtain the nutrients they offer, experts now believe that minimal cooking, which involves the use of heat, may yield optimal results in terms of the food's digestibility and making the nutrients available to the body.

For example, raw carrots are low in fat, but carrots cooked lightly in a microwave oven make the beta-carotene more available. Dr. John W. Erdman, Jr., director of the University of Illinois division of nutritional sciences at Champaign-Urbana, explained in an August 1994 *New York Times* article that, because chunks of raw carrot may not be broken down by digestive enzymes, a person may not be able to absorb more than 1 percent of the carrot's beta-carotene. A cooked carrot preserves the beta-carotene and also offers more available protein and fiber, even though some water-soluble, heat labile vitamin C is sacrificed. Juicing, which does not involve heating but does serve to pulverize food, is another effective way to create bioavailability of nutrients.

In addition, the cooking of vegetables creates a greater availability of starches. A potato eaten raw offers about 30 percent of its starch, but a cooked potato offers 95 percent. Raw cauliflower and broccoli are among other vegetables with high amounts of starch.

If vegetables are boiled, about 50 percent of their vitamins C and B and minerals will be destroyed. Vegetables should be cooked in as little water as possible only long enough to soften them slightly (this result is often called al dente, that is, maintaining some of the crunchiness), whether steaming or microwaving. Of boiling, steaming and microwaving, the last is considered the method that preserves the most nutrients of foods, especially vegetables.

According to Dr. Paul Lachance, chairman of the Food Science Department of Rutgers University, New Brunswick, New Jersey, Chinese wok cooking (also called "stir-frying") and pressure-cooking methods are also recommended. Stir-frying requires no water, and the small amount of oil that is used helps foods retain their nutrients. Beta-carotene, for example, is absorbed best when the vegetable containing it is cooked in oil. A pressure-cooker heats foods quickly, allowing them little or no contact with water. Foods boiled while enclosed in a plastic bag also maintain their nutrients because the nutrients cannot leach into the water.

copper

A metallic element essential in human nutrition. The average adult has stores of about 100 to 150 mg of copper in the liver, brain, heart, kidney and hair. Copper plays an essential role in the utilization of iron in the synthesis of hemoglobin. Copper is also involved in the metabolism of vitamin C, the sense of taste and collagen elastin, bone and myelin (the covering for nerves) development. Copper is involved in a number of enzymatic reactions for the production of energy, oxidation of fatty acids and formation of the skin pigment melanin.

Ceruloplasmin is a substance in the blood containing six atoms of copper that appears to serve as a transport vehicle for the mineral to tissues where it is needed.

Deficiency

Although human deficiencies are rare, malnourished South American children were shown to have anemia, low white blood cell counts, poor bone formation and growth impairment from diets lacking in copper. In adults, deficiencies have been found in patients on total parenteral nutrition (TPN), the intravenous provision of the total caloric needs of a patient who cannot take food orally. A rare inherited disorder, Menkes' steely hair disease, involves impairment of copper utilization. Spue, a malabsorption disease, and the kidney disorder nephrotic syndrome cause inadequate protein and therefore the body may fail to produce sufficient ceruloplasmin necessary for the metabolism of copper. The evidence for an increase in cholesterol, glucose and heart disease in persons whose copper intake is very low has been inconsistent. However, there may be an increased incidence in heart disease for those individuals whose zinc-to-copper dietary intake was elevated. Copper supplementation has experimentally raised HDL ("good" cholesterol) and lowered total cholesterol in copper deficient animals and humans.

Dietary Sources

Liver and other organ meats, shellfish, nuts, legumes, whole-grain cereals and raisins provide the highest dietary levels of copper. Copper intake may be increased by the influence of acidity in the water supply from contact with copper pipes. The federal Food and Drug Administration (FDA) in the Total Diet Study between 1982 and 1986 showed a daily copper intake of 1.2 mg for adult males and 0.9 mg for females. Infant ingestion was 0.45 mg and 0.57 mg daily for infants and toddlers, respectively.

Recommended Daily Requirement

The National Research Council's Food and Nutrition Subcommittee recommends 1.5 to 3 mg per day as a safe and adequate level for copper ingestion for adults, although there has been insufficient data to establish a Recommended Daily Requirement (RDA). There may be an increased need for copper during pregnancy since birth defects have been shown in experimental animals deficient in this mineral. Copper is stored in the liver by the human fetus. For infants 0.6 mg per day is recommended and 0.7 mg for babies six to 12 months. Premature infants and infants exclusively breastfed may need supplementation of copper. The American Academy of Pediatrics recently recommended that infant formulas provide 60 mcg of copper per 100 kilocalories, therefore providing an average 0.4 mg of copper daily. For seven-to-10-year-old children, 1.0 to 2.0 mg per day are recommended and 1 to 1.3 mg per day for preadolescent and adolescent girls.

Supplements

Copper is generally included in multivitamin-mineral supplements. Copper gluconate is preferred over copper sulfate because it is easier to digest.

Toxicity

Wilson's disease is an inherited disorder that causes hepatitis (inflammation of the liver), kidney and neurological dysfunction and degeneration of the lens of the eye from copper excess. Vitamin C may interfere with the absorption of copper, while being of some benefit in Wilson's disease.

Acute poisoning, which may be fatal, is characterized by nausea, vomiting, abdominal pain, diarrhea, headache, dizziness and a metallic taste.

Typical American diets contain less than 5 mg of copper per day. Levels up to 10 mg per day are probably safe for adults. Toxicity is extremely rare in the United States. Elevated copper levels are sometimes found in individuals with the following conditions: viral infections, rheumatoid arthritis, rheumatic fever, systemic lupus erythematosus (SLE), leukemia, some cancers and post-heart attack. It is not known what role copper plays in the presence of disease. It is not clear if copper helps fight these conditions or if it is part of the disease process. Interestingly, drugs containing copper are often helpful in fighting some of these diseases. It has been theorized that copper-containing drugs help repair tissues damaged by many diseases.

coptis

(goldthread, huang lian)

A Chinese herb, *Coptis chinensis,* of the Ranunculaceae family, whose underground stem is used in Chinese medicine to promote lactation and to treat nausea and vomiting, fever, conjunctivitis and bleeding.

coriander

(dhanyaka [Sanskrit])

An annual plant, *Coriandrum sativum,* of the carrot family, with aromatic fruits, grown in Europe, North and South America and the Mediterranean region, whose seeds are used as a spice in (Asian) Indian cuisine and, in herbal and Ayurvedic medicine, as an antispasmodic, carminative and stomachic. Coriander, once considered an aphrodisiac, may also be prepared as a topical treatment for rheumatism.

corn

(maize, yu shu shu)

The plant originating in America and recognized as valuable by Native Americans, *Zea mays,* a cereal grass, whose grain is used to make cornmeal and whose kernels are eaten as a vegetable and used in animal feed. Now cultivated in China and many other parts of the world, corn is also thought to have medicinal properties. Tea made from cornsilk (*yu mi xu,* in Chinese) was used as a diuretic by Native Americans to ease bladder and kidney infections. Invalids were routinely fed corn porridge because it is easy to digest.

cornflower

(cyani, bluebonnet, bachelor's button)

An annual European herb, *Centaurea cyanus,*

whose blue flowers are used by herbalists as a remedy for stomachache or indigestion.

cornus
(shan zhu yu, Japanese cornel, Japanese cornelian cherry)
A Chinese, Korean and Japanese tree or shrub, *Cornus officinalis,* of the Cornaceae family, that bears flowers and fruit. The plant contains a guinol glycoside, perhaps responsible for the use of cornus in Chinese medicine as a remedy for excessive urine discharge. The fruit is also used to treat intestinal worms, vertigo, backache, night sweats, excessive menses and fever.

cottonroot
A biennial or triennial herb, *Gossypium herbaceum,* of the Malvaceae family, native to Asia and cultivated in the United States, among other regions, whose inner root bark is considered in homeopathic medicine to be a treatment for lack of menses, sterility, painful menstruation, ovarian pain, vomiting related to pregnancy and labial abscess.

couch grass
(dog grass, twitch grass, agropyrum)
The plant *Triticum* or *Agropyrum repens,* of the Gramineae family, found in North America and Europe, whose rootstock and rhizome are used in Native American medicine for the treatment of bladder irritation and infection, catarrh, gout, jaundice, and enlarged prostate. Couch grass contains vitamin C, carotene, glucose and other nutrients.

cowslip
(palsywort, herb peter, paigles)
A North American and Arctic flowering perennial, *Primula officinalis,* of the Primulaceae family, known to the Greeks as "Paralysis." Cowslip flowers and leaves are used in Native American medicine as an antispasmodic and sedative, particularly cowslip tea for vertigo, seizures, anxiety, bladder and back pain and palsy. Homeopathic medicine prescribes cowslip tincture for fevers, migraine, neuralgia, eczema and dizziness. In folk medicine, cowslip is also considered an expectorant, diuretic and diaphoretic. The root and rhizome are given as an extract or powder combined with other herbs as a laxative and digestive tonic.

cramp bark
(guelder rose, high cranberry, snowball tree, squaw bush)
A North American flowering, fruit-bearing shrub, *Viburnum opulus*, of the Caprofoliaceae family, with acidic berries high in vitamins C and K. Viburnine, the substance considered medicinal in the plant, is in the dried bark of the stem. Cramp bark and the related *Viburnum prunifolium* (black haw) are prescribed in Native American and herbal medicine for uterine and menstrual problems, including premenstrual syndrome (PMS) and cramps and other gynecological complaints. Cramp bark is also used as an antispasmodic and to treat rheumatism and heart palpitations.

cranesbill
(wild geranium, dovesfoot, storksbill)
An American flowering plant, *Geranium maculatum,* of the Geraniaceae family, whose dried root is used in Native American and herbal medicine as an astringent, especially useful in the treatment of diarrhea, dysentery and infantile cholera, as a styptic, to check hemorrhage, leukorrhea, diabetes, nosebleed, Bright's disease and excessive discharges of mucus.

crataegus
(hawthorn, Chinese hill haw)
Deciduous trees or shrubs of the north temperate

regions, *Crataegus cuneata* and *pinnatifida,* whose ripe fruits in Chinese medicine are used in the treatment of diarrhea, dysentery and stomachache.

crawley
(chickentoe, coral root)
A flowering North American plant, *Corallorhiza odontorhiza,* whose powdered root in warm water is a remedy for fevers, especially because of its diaphoretic and sedative properties, according to herbalists and Native American medicine.

crocus
(saffron)
A flowering plant, *Crocus sativus,* of the Iridaceae family, originally from Asia Minor and named from the Greek word *krokos,* meaning saffron, a popular coloring and food-flavoring agent. In Chinese medicine, the stigmas of the flowers are dried and prepared as a remedy for lack of or irregular menses, asthma, seizures and whooping cough. Crocus is also thought to be a blood and circulation tonic. In Ayurvedic medicine, the herb called *nagakshar* in Sanskrit is known as cobra's saffron.

croton
A Chinese, Burmese, Laotian, Vietnamese and Malaysian evergreen, *Croton tiglium,* of the Euphorbiaceae family, cultivated for its seeds, used in Chinese medicine as a powerful purgative. Croton oil obtained from the seeds is poisonous.

crowfoot
(buttercup)
A perennial flowering herb, *Ranunculus bulbosus,* of the Ranunculaceae family, that grows in colder regions of North America and Europe. Crowfoot parts cause mouth ulcerations when chewed. Once used by beggars to incite pity, crowfoot is prepared

as a tincture in homeopathic medicine for the treatment of alcoholism, chilblains, delirium tremens, epilepsy, jaundice and liver pain, rheumatism, hay fever and other ailments.

cubeb
(Java pepper, tailed pepper)
A flowering, fruit-bearing perennial, *Piper cubeba,* that grows in regions near New Guinea and Sumatra, whose unripe berries resembling black pepper are used in herbal medicine to treat intestinal gas, respiratory congestion and indigestion. Cubeb oil is prescribed for gonorrhea and urinary tract problems.

curculigo
(xian mao)
A tropical flowering herb, *Curculigo orchioides,* of the Hypoxidaceae family, whose underground stem is used in Chinese medicine as a remedy for impotence, lumbago and joint pain, and as a tonic and aphrodisiac.

curcuma
(turmeric, jiang huang, haridra [Sanskrit])
An Indian and tropical, aromatic herb, *Curcuma domestica,* of the Zingiberaceae family. A flavoring and coloring agent, turmeric means yellow in Sanskrit, and had many uses in Hindu traditions. The underground stem is used by Chinese practitioners to promote the manufacture of hemoglobin, dissolve clots and stop bleeding. It is also prescribed for dysentery, stomach disorders and abdominal and chest pain. Native to India, wild turmeric, or *Curcuma aromatica,* treats excessive gas, seizures, liver ailments and other problems.

cuscuta
(tu si zi, devil's guts, dodder, lady's laces, bride's laces)

The plant *Cuscuta japonica,* of the Convolvulaceae family, of both China and Japan, whose seeds are prescribed by Chinese practitioners to treat prostatic inflammation, impotence, premature ejaculation, vertigo, lumbago and nervous disorders.

cyanocobalamin
See B$_{12}$, VITAMIN.

cyathula
(hookweed)
A flowering plant, of the Amarantaceae family, used in Chinese medicine as a laxative and antiarthritic.

cycas
(sago palm, Japanese fern palm)
A type of palm tree, *Cycas revoluta,* of the Cycadaceae family, grown in Japan and southern China, whose seeds are considered by Chinese herbalists to be a tonic, expectorant and antirheumatic.

cymbopogon
(lemon grass, rohisha [Sanskrit])
A grass native to India and Sri Lanka and cultivated in the tropics, *Cymbopogon citratus,* of the Gramineae family, used as a food flavoring and an oil for soap and perfume. Chinese and Ayurvedic herbalists prescribe the plant for coughs, colds and bloody sputum, and as a diaphoretic.

cynanchum
Various species of a northern Chinese and Japanese herb of the Asclepiadaceae family, with a fragrant root and flowers. Cynanchum is prescribed in Chinese medicine to treat urethral problems, fever, cough, pneumonia, difficult breathing and other ailments.

cyperus
(nut grass, sedge root, xiang fu)
A flowering, weedlike plant, *Cyperus rotundus,* of the Cyperaceae family, whose tubers are used in Chinese medicine to ease various menstrual problems, chest pain, dysentery, headache and indigestion.

cypress
(gopher wood)
Originally a Mediterranean tree or shrub, *Cupressus,* of the Coniferous Cupressaceae family, whose cones or nuts are used in Native American medicine and by herbalists to arrest bleeding. Homeopaths prescribe a tincture of cypress berries and leaves for tumors, warts and other ailments.

D

D, vitamin

(vitamin D_1 or calciferol, cholecalciferol [vitamin D_3], ergocalciferol [vitamin D_2])

An essential vitamin manufactured in the skin during exposure to the sun. Dietary supplements may be necessary for those lacking sunlight exposure. Vitamin D is a generic term for a family of compounds known as vitamins D_1, D_2 and D_3. Chemically these substances are called sterols, and their metabolic products have the ability to prevent rickets in children or osteomalacia in adults. Vitamin D is fat-soluble and requires dietary fat that absorbs the vitamin from food sources or supplements in the digestive tract.

Vitamin D_2 is derived from plants and can substitute for vitamin D_3 in the human body. Calcium balance is regulated by the interaction of three hormones, vitamin D, parathormone (PTH) and calcitonin. PTH is secreted by the parathyroid gland and calcitonin, which antagonizes or blocks the effects of PTH, by special cells in the thyroid gland.

Functions of Vitamin D

Considered a hormone, vitamin D is responsible chiefly for regulating the absorption and use of calcium and phosphorous and facilitating the formation of normal bones, cartilage and teeth. Other important functions of vitamin D include maintaining normal nerve conduction and muscle contractions, especially those of the heart muscle. Vitamin D regulates the supply of calcium in the blood and plays a role in the utilization of magnesium.

Some researchers theorize that vitamin D might aid in the prevention or treatment of cancer and assist in regulating the immune system. Vitamin D was formerly advocated as a treatment for lupus vulgaris (tuberculosis of the skin) that is now considered unacceptable. Vitamin D has been reported to lessen the severity of psoriasis.

Vitamin D Deficiency

Rickets is caused by inadequate exposure to sunlight or dietary lack of vitamin D and occurs in childhood. It is characterized by malformed and weak bones because of poor calcium and phosphrous deposition. Defective mineralization of both bones and cartilaginous material in the epiphyseal growth plate becomes apparent as the child grows. Weight-bearing bones buckle, the head becomes malformed, wrists and ankles become enlarged and the sternum bows to resemble a pigeon breast. The severity of the changes varies with the degree of vitamin D deficiency. Early recognition may escape even trained health professionals but should be considered in an infant who is restless, sleeps poorly, sweats profusely, repeatedly turns its head from side to side and has delayed dentition (formation of teeth). The infant will have reduced mineralization of the skull, or craniotabes, and bossing of the skull and delayed closure of the fontanelle. Sitting and crawling skills may be delayed beyond the normal stage of development in which they are usually demonstrated. Costochondral beading, known as rachitic rosary, occurs. Rickets is readily recognized when the toddler develops the typical bowed legs, knock knees and kyphoscoliosis (lateral curvature of the spine with an anteroposterior hump) shortly after starting to walk.

Deficiencies of vitamins C, D and other nutrients often coexist, and symptoms of vitamin D deficiency may mask or modify important symptoms and X-ray findings of scurvy (see ASCORBIC ACID).

With widespread availability of vitamin D-fortified milk, rickets is rarely seen except in northern climates with limited sunlight. The production of vitamin D is blocked or inhibited by multiple factors such as dark skin pigment. The darker the skin, the less readily the vitamin is formed. Malnourished black infants are more prone to rickets than Caucasian or other light-skinned infants. Substances or situations that block the sun's ultraviolet rays include smoke, fog, smog, clothing and windows.

Children with celiac disease or other disorders of fat absorption, and those taking anticonvulsants for seizure disorders, are at risk of vitamin D deficiency and rickets. Although vitamin D supplementation corrects the bone structure, it may be too late to correct deformed bones.

The hallmarks of osteomalacia—softening and deformities of the bones of the arms, legs, spine, thorax and pelvis—result from a deficiency of calcium or vitamin D. Osteomalacia occurs after the epiphyseal growth plates fuse, thus the term "adult rickets." Although bone fractures are uncommon, chronic pain and muscle weakness add to the symptoms of the disorder.

Osteomalacia is commonly confused with osteoporosis, in which bone fractures are common. In the later stage of osteoporosis, muscle weakness is rare, and pain is only present when brittle bones become fractured. Osteomalacia most commonly occurs in women who have had multiple pregnancies and are also vitamin D or calcium deficient.

Aging reduces the ability of the body to manufacture vitamin D. Hearing loss may be related to malformation of the bones in the middle ear or changes that occur to these bones in the elderly. Elderly invalids are also more likely to have inadequate sunlight exposure or have poor dietary intake of required nutrients.

Studies in the United States suggest that 30 to 40 percent of hip-fracture victims have vitamin D deficiencies. Those at risk for vitamin D deficiency are infants, pregnant women and individuals with little or no sunlight exposure, especially the disabled.

Calcitrol, a vitamin D derivative, vitamin D_3, is used in the treatment of osteoporosis in Japan, where estrogen therapy is not well accepted. Calcitrol is also used in Australia and New Zealand. There is a considerable risk of vitamin D toxicity with the use of calcitrol.

In 1992, "The Mediterranean Osteoporosis Study" (in the *British Medical Journal*) failed to show that vitamin D, fluorides or anabolic steroids reduced the incidence of hip fractures in postmenopausal women at increased risk. However, estrogen, calcium or calcitonin were protective, reducing risk by 55, 25 and 31 percent, respectively, in a group of more than 5,500 women.

A contradictory account in 1992 of 138 women studied at Cambridge University similarly reported in the *British Medical Journal* confirmed that increasing vitamin D intake to 400 International Units daily or exposing the skin to sunlight for 30 minutes daily would increase bone density by 5 to 10 percent and reduce the occurrence of bone fractures by an estimated 20 percent.

Vitamin D may be especially important during winter in northern latitudes such as Sweden, where calcium alone increases bone density in the summer, but density is lost during the winter unless 400 units of vitamin D are added to the diet.

Sun-blocking agents with a skin-protection rating of 8 or greater prevent the formation of vitamin D in the skin. It is unlikely that children or most adults would use sunscreens often enough to develop vitamin D deficiency, but some elderly persons concerned about skin cancer may become deficient.

Causes of vitamin D deficiency

Dietary deficiencies of vitamin D are rare in the United States and other developed countries. Intestinal disorders that interfere with dietary absorption usually only are associated with vitamin D deficiency if the afflicted individuals lack sufficient exposure to the sun or have rare disorders of the metabolism. Vitamin D deficiency causes hypocalcemia and hypophosphatemia, or diminished blood levels of calcium and phosphorus. The deficiency in turn causes stimulation of the parathyroid gland. The hormone secreted by the gland pulls calcium

Table 8
COMPARISON OF OSTEOMALACIA AND OSTEOPOROSIS

	Signs and Symptoms	Prevention	Treatment*
Osteoporosis	pain from fractures muscle weakness is rare fractures are common skeletal deformities only related to fractures widespread loss of bone density normal blood levels of calcium, phosphorus and alkaline phosphatase normal or high levels of calcium in the urine	adequate calcium intake (1,000 mg in premenopausal women and 1,500 mg after menopause) + estrogen therapy + regular weight-bearing exercise	calcitonin, calcium, estrogens, fluoride (controversial) vitamin D (used in Japan) is controversial and can be toxic

*[Author's note. The treatments currently available for osteoporosis are either expensive, not very effective, toxic or all of these.]

	Signs and Symptoms	Prevention	Treatment*
Osteomalacia	chronic bone pain muscle weakness (may result in a gait disturbance) fractures are rare skeletal deformities are common bone density loss is usually limited to the spine low calcium and phosphorus blood levels high alkaline phosphatase blood levels low calcium levels in the urine	adequate sunlight and/or vitamin D in the diet or supplements	vitamin D supplements

out of bones to restore the calcium in the blood to adequate levels. This process causes rickets in infants and children and osteomalacia in adults.

Drugs such as the anticonvulsant drug phenytoin (Dilantin) may impair the effectiveness of vitamin D.

Dosage

Dosages of vitamin D are usually expressed as International Units (I.U.) of cholecalciferol, with 400 I.U. being equivalent to 10 mcg of the vitamin. Five to 7.5 mcg (200 to 300 I.U.) should be given only to those infants who are fed unfortified formulas. However, the rare infant with a malabsorption disorder or who is the offspring of a mother with a vitamin D deficiency may require up to 750 mcg or 30,000 I.U. daily for a short period.

Ten mcg (400 I.U.) are recommended during pregnancy and lactation if there is inadequate dietary vitamin D or sunlight. The same amount is generally advisable in the elderly.

When Vitamin D supplements are given to treat deficiency, the dose should be reduced to the Recommended Daily Allowance (RDA) as soon as symptoms are improved and before bone healing is complete, because the effects of vitamin D persist for prolonged periods and may result in elevated calcium levels and kidney damage. If larger than 10 mcg per day of vitamin D are taken for extended periods, blood-calcium levels and 24-hour urine specimens should be monitored frequently. Vitamin D supplements are available in 400 and 1,000 I.U. strengths over-the-counter and 25,000 and 50,000 I.U. by prescription.

A fair-skinned person can probably manufacture 10,000 I.U. of vitamin D in one day. In temperate climates, 10 minutes of sunbathing daily throughout the summer months will provide adequate stores of the vitamin for the colder months. Infants and children who must remain on a milk-free diet can obtain an adequate supply of calcium, vitamin D and other essential nutrients from vegetables, including broccoli, kale, turnip greens or tofu.

Drug Interactions

The cholesterol-lowering drug cholysteramine and mineral oil both interfere with the intestinal absorption of vitamin D. Phenytoin and phenobarbital, drugs used in the treatment of seizures, speed up the metabolism of vitamin D.

Most problems with the use of vitamin D interacting with other drugs occur in the presence of hypercalcemia (elevated blood-calcium levels) and heart or kidney disease. Heart irregularities may occur with the use of digoxin and other digitalis derivatives or verapamil. In the presence of elevated calcium levels associated with the vitamin's use, arrhythmias (heart irregularities) may occur. Thiazide diuretics in the presence of vitamin D may cause hypercalcemia in the presence of hypoparathyroid disease. Persons with kidney failure should avoid taking magnesium-containing antacids with vitamin D.

Toxicity

Vitamin D is highly toxic, especially in infants and children who have developed of hypercalcemia. Sensitive infants may develop high calcium levels with as little as 10 mcg or 400 I.U. daily. Prolonged exposure to excessive doses that may be slightly above 25 mcg (1,000 I.U.) per day for infants may result in mental retardation, lagging physical growth, elfin facies (resembling the facial features of an elf), kidney failure and death. Older children and adults may develop weakness, loss of appetite, vomiting, diarrhea, excessive thirst and urination as well as mental changes associated with elevated blood-calcium levels from doses of vitamin D exceeding 1.25 mg or 50,000 I.U. daily. Prolonged use of megadoses may also result in kidney failure and death. In the absence of severe kidney damage, hypervitaminosis D is usually reversible with cessation of vitamin D.

d-alpha-tocopherol
(natural vitamin E)
See E, VITAMIN.

daily minimal requirements
See RECOMMENDED DIETARY ALLOWANCES.

damiana
The plant *Turnera diffusa,* of the family Turneraceae, native to Texas, southern California, Mexico, South America and the West Indies, whose leaves are made into a tea and used in the treatment of depression, coughing and congestion and as a mild aphrodisiac in the case of decreased sexual desire.

dandelion
(pu gong ying, lion's tooth, blow ball, cankerwort)
The biennial or perennial plant *Taraxacum officinale,* of the family Compositae, originally from Greece. Dandelion may be eaten as a vegetable, made into wine and tea and, in herbal medicine, used for the treatment of bladder, kidney, gallbladder, pancreas and spleen obstructions, stomachaches, hepatitis, high blood pressure, anemia, fluid retention, weight loss and breast cancer.

Dandelion leaves contain vitamins A, B, C and G, sodium, protein, iron, calcium, phosphorus and inulin. Tea, coffee or a vodka beverage made from dandelion root was once dubbed the "life elixir" by advocates of home remedies and was considered a blood purifier; liver, gallbladder, spleen and female organ tonic; and treatment for rheumatism, urinary tract problems and skin diseases. Homeopathic medicine also prescribes dandelion tincture for diabetes, jaundice, neuralgia, night sweats, typhoid fever and mapped tongue.

daruharidra
See BARBERRY.

datura
(downy thorn apple, horn-of-plenty)
A flowering plant, *Datura metel,* of the Solanaceae family, originally thought to be from eastern India or southwestern China, whose leaves, seeds and fruit contain poisonous tropane alkaloids, and whose leaves and seeds are the source of scopolamine, a sedative and motion-sickness drug.

Datura has a strange history of uses, including as a trance-inducer by ancient priests of Apollo in Greece, as a preoperative sedative of the Incas, as a way for robbers in Indian, Malaysian and other cultures to debilitate their victims and as as an intoxicant of African boys during rite-of-passage ceremonies. However, to Chinese Buddhists, datura is considered sacred because they believed rain from heaven fell on the datura plant when Buddha spoke.

In Chinese medicine, the flowers are used for the treatment of nervous disorders, muscle pain, asthma and colds.

decoction
The method of extracting the essences or medicinal properties from hard or coarse herb stems, barks and roots. The herb part or parts may be simmered in water until one-third of the water has evaporated. The herbs are then strained and the liquid retained for use.

dendrobium
(shi hu)
The plants *Dendrobium nobile, monile* and *hancockii,* of the Orchidaceae family, named from the Greek words *dendron* (tree) and *bios* (life). Chinese practitioners use mainly the stem, but also the whole plant, in the treatment of arthritis, fever, impotence, pain and cough.

dentes
The latin word for teeth. Nutritionally, normal dentition (the number and arrangement of teeth) and healthy teeth and gums depend on calcium, which gives the teeth their rigidity, and other nutrients, including vitamin C, for healthy collagen matrix and optimal strength and integrity of teeth and mouth. A lack of protein may result in small, irregularly shaped teeth, a delay in the appearance of teeth and susceptibility to cavities. A lack of vitamin A may contribute to poorly formed teeth and possibly the delayed eruption of teeth, as well as problems involving the keratin matrix of enamel. Magnesium is important for the development of tooth enamel. Phosphorus deficiency may result in poor mineralization, and iron, zinc and fluoride deficiencies may cause susceptibility to cavities.

Dental health requires that individuals:

a)–restrict the ingestion of sweets, especially at bedtime,

b)–drink fluorinated water and provide infants with fluoride supplements if fluorinated water is not available,

c)–restrict the ingestion of sticky foods (such as caramel, nougat, fruits that stick to the teeth longer than required by the normal eating time, etc.), d)–brush the teeth and floss regularly, after every meal and snacks if possible, or rinse the mouth with water,

e)–eat foods containing calcium and phosphorus,

f)–eat high-fiber foods that inhibit dental cavities and stimulate the flow of saliva, such as raw vegetables, and,

g)–when appropriate, substitute low-fat cheese for sweet dessert, because cheese is high in calcium and promotes the formation of acid and saliva that inhibit cavity development. Chocolate, tea, coffee and beer, all of which contain the acid tannin, help prevent cavities. (Children without dietary restrictions may eat regular cheeses.)

denutrition

An alternate term for malnutrition, or a deficiency of nutrients that causes debilitation, weakness, disease processes and other problems. Malnutrition exists in individuals as well as populations throughout the world.

depression

See STRESS.

dermatitis

Skin inflammation characterized by itchiness, redness and various types of eruptions or lesions. Nutrition-related dermatitis may involve desquamating changes of the skin, or abnormally pigmented areas, usually on the legs, thighs, buttocks and extremities, that resemble flaking paint or "crazy pavement." Desquamation on the trunk is associated with kwashiorkor, a severe, life-threatening protein deficiency common to children in many Third World countries.

Dermatitis has many causes, including allergic, hereditary, infectious and psychological. Depending upon the type of dermatitis, vitamins E, A and D salves or creams, mineral ointments and other topical applications, along with alterations in diet and nutrient supplementation, especially in the case of a vitamin or mineral deficiency, may be recommended as treatment.

desmodium

The climbing plants, *Desmodium triquetrum, pulchellum, triflorum* and *styracifolium,* of the Leguminosae family, named from the Greek word *desmos* (chain). In Chinese medicine, desmodium preparations are prescribed for numerous ailments, including intestinal worms, infantile convulsion, indigestion, internal blod clots, dysentery and colic.

dessicated liver

Dried, powdered beef liver available in tablet form in health food stores as an iron and multinutrient supplement.

dhanyaka

See CORIANDER.

diabetes mellitus

A chronic disorder of the body's ability to metabolize carbohydrates. Beta cells in the pancreas fail to secrete an adequate amount of insulin, a hormone essential for maintaining a normal blood-sugar level and the utilization of glucose. Symptoms include hyperglycemia (elevated blood sugar), sugar in the urine, excessive urination, extreme thirst, increase of food intake and genital itching.

It has been speculated that micronutrients, especially zinc and chromium, play a role in the development of carbohydrate intolerance leading to diabetes mellitus, both Type I, insulin-dependent, and type II, non-insulin dependent. Supplementation with micronutrient minerals is considered experimental, and there may be some as-yet-undetermined risk.

Standardized diets, exercise regimes and insulin therapy for people with diabetes are geared toward balancing carbohydrates, proteins and fats and improving glucose utilization. In addition, many nutritionists, homeopaths, naturopaths, herbalists and others offer alternative treatments, especially with herbs that affect blood-sugar levels. Untreated diabetes may lead to coma, acetone (sweet) breath odor, nausea, headache, vomiting, difficulty in breathing, a sense of drunkenness, delirium, weakness or deep coma and subsequent death.

dicalcium phosphate

The substance containing two atoms of calcium used in dietary calcium supplements.

diets, fad

Weight-reduction regimes that become a sensation or popular through the media that may or may not be nutritionally sound. They include liquid formulas, calorie restrictions, fasting techniques and diets emphasizing one type of food or another in the diet over a certain period of time. No one diet is a panacea for people who wish to lose weight, and a healthy nutritional status depends upon biopsychosocial aspects of the individual. Some diets cause a state of ketosis in dieters, which may reduce the desire for food and increase the rate of weight loss. Ketosis is an accumulation of ketones—acetone, betahydroxybutric acid and acetoacetic acid—as a result of inadequate metabolism of fatty acids and carbohydrate deficiency. High-fat diets, starvation, poorly monitored diabetes mellitus, pregnancy and postoperative ether anesthesia are often linked with ketosis.

Other problems frequently exist alongside fad diets. Milkshake-type preparations become boring, weight lost quickly may be as quickly replaced, psychological and other individual factors may not be taken into account and nutrient deficiencies may emerge.

digestion

The body's process of breaking down ingested foods into forms that are most readily absorbed by the gastrointestinal tract and the nutrients distributed throughout body tissues. While salt, glucose and other simple sugars, water and crystalloids can be absorbed intact, fats, starches and protein require considerable breakdown into smaller molecules. Digestion begins with the enzyme ptyalin, in the saliva, that splits starch. The partially digested starch then proceeds to the stomach and the intestines for further breakdowns by other enzymes such as pepsin, lipase, trypsin, invertase, and other enzymatic substances in the pancreatic juices and the epithelial cells of the small intestine. Fats are mostly digested in the small intestine. Proteins go through several digestive stages before they are converted into amino acids. Whatever remaining materials the body has not converted into valuable nutrients become waste material and are eliminated at the end of the digestive tract, through the rectum.

dl-alpha-tocopherol

(synthetic vitamin E)
See E, VITAMIN.

dill weed

The herb *Anethum graveolens,* of the family Umbelliferae, used primarily as a flavoring spice. Dill weed is also an herbal medicine for treating colic, stomachaches, indigestion, abdominal cramps, colds, influenza and coughs. It is also said to increase breast milk.

dioscorea

(yam, shan yao)
The vines *Dioscorea opposita, nipponica, bulbifera, tokoro, japonica* and *hispida,* of the Dioscoreaceae family, found in Korea, Japan and China, whose tubers are edible and also used in Chinese

medicine. The Chinese yam, which contains the anti-inflammatory agent diosgenin, provides preparations for the treatment of numerous ailments, including diarrhea, dysentery, arthritis, rheumatism, rheumatoid arthritis, sore throat, poisonous snakebite, cough and premature ejaculation.

diospyros
(Japanese persimmon)
A Japanese and Chinese deciduous tree, *Diospyros kaki,* of the Ebenaceae family, with edible fruit often made into jam and cosmetic products. In Chinese medicine, diospyros fruit, fruit juice and fruit stalk are used to treat high blood pressure, cough, hiccough and diarrhea.

dipsacus
(Venus' basin, teasel, xu duan)
European, western Asian and North African herbs, *Dipsacus asper* and *japonicus,* of the Dipsacaceae family, named from the Greek word *dipsakos* (thirst). Dipsacus roots are used in Chinese medicine to treat pain, lumbago and excessive menses.

dogbane
(catchfly, bitterroot, honeybloom, milk ipecac, western wallflower)
An American flowering perennial, *Apocynum androsaemifolium,* whose rootstock is used in herbal medicine as an emetic (to induce vomiting), expectorant, stimulant and cathartic. While the leaves appear to be poisonous to animals, the plant with its milky juice is thought to be effective against gallstones, stomachache, constipation and dropsy.

dog poison
(fool's parsley, small hemlock, fool's cicely)
A North American and European annual plant, *Aesthusa cynapium,* whose herb is used in homeopathic medicine to treat nervous stomach and spasms. The leaves and roots, which resemble parsley, are poisonous.

dogwood
(Virginia dogwood, flowering cornel, green ozier, Florida cornel, cornelian tree, budwood, borwood)
Shrubs, trees and herbs of the Cornaceae family, found in Canada and the United States. The *Cornus florida* flowers, according to Native American herbal medicine, have a soothing property similar to camomile (see CAMOMILE) and the bark is used to make a healing ointment. Homeopathic medicine uses tincture of dogwood bark for dyspepsia, fever and pneumonia.

dolichos
(Egyptian bean, hyacinth bean, lablab bean, seim bean)
A tropical bean plant thought to be of Asian origin, *Dolichos lablab,* of the Leguminosae family, whose bean is eaten as a vegetable in India and whose flowers and seeds are used in Chinese medicine to treat poisoning from fish and vegetables, sunstroke, colic, infectious dysentery, cholera and rheumatism.

dolomite
The mineral CaMg $(CO_3)_2$, a calcium magnesium carbonate originating in limestone and crystals. Although in wide use as a calcium supplement, it is not only poorly absorbed, but it often contaminated with lead, which may be toxic.
   (See also CALCIUM.)

dong quai
(tang kwei)
The plant *Angelica sinensis,* of the Umbelliferae family, well known in Chinese traditional medicine as a "female" treatment. The root of the plant is

prescribed for menstrual cramps and other menstrual discomfort, menopausal symptoms, hypertension, insomnia, anemia, constipation and other problems.

(See also ANGELICA.)

don sen
(tang shen)
The *Codonopsis pilosula* plant, of the Campanulaceae family, whose root, similar in action to ginseng, is prescribed in Chinese traditional medicine for strengthening the *chi,* or vital energy throughout the body. Don sen is also used for indigestion caused by excessive gastric acid and as treatment of infections, inflammation and diabetes.
(See GINSENG.)

double-blind study
Also known as an open-label study, a technique for the purpose of scientific experimentation and study in which neither the researchers nor the subjects know which treatment (nutrient, drug, placebo, etc.) the subjects are receiving or participating in. A double-blind study seeks to eliminate any bias on the part of researchers and subjects that may skew the results. When the experiment is over, the treatments and subjects are revealed and the data analyzed.

dragon root
(jack-in-the-pulpit, wake robin)
A North and South American flowering plant, *Arum triphyllum,* of the Araceae family, whose dry root is used in Native American medicine as a stimulant and expectorant, especially in the treatment of asthma, whooping cough, colic, chest pain and other ailments. Homeopathic medicine uses tincture of the plant's fresh tuber or corn for headache, diphtheria, swollen glands, hoarseness, pain in the jaw and numerous other problems.

drynaria
(oak-leaf fern)
The tree *Drynaria fortunei,* of the Polypodiaceae family, whose stem is used in Chinese medicine to treat bleeding, gangrene, kidney weakness and other ailments.

dryobalanops
(Bornean camphor-tree, kapur)
The Malaysian, Javan and Bornean tropical tree, *Dryobalanops aromatica,* of the Dipterocarpaceae family, that yields camphor. In Chinese medicine, camphor preparations treat chicken pox and sore throat and tonify the body.

dyer's broom
(furze, greenweed, waxen woad, dyer's whin)
A northeastern American and European perennial shrub, *Genista tinctoria,* that bears fruit. The shrub's flowering twigs are used in herbal medicine to make tea, considered effective against gallstones, gravel and hypotension. Dyer's broom tea is also a vasoconstrictor with properties similar to those of nicotine.

E

E, vitamin

(d-alpha-tocopherol, or natural vitamin E; dl-alpha-tocopherol, or synthetic vitamin E)
Alpha-tocopherol, the most active of the eight forms of vitamin E found naturally. This fat-soluble vitamin was named from the Greek *tokos,* meaning offspring, and *pherein,* meaning to bear. Vitamin E is absorbed into the lymphatic circulation from the gastrointestinal tract and has been shown to have antioxidant, or protective, actions in the cells. The vitamin is stored in all tissues, and vitamin E deficiency is rare. Approximately three-fourths of the vitamin are excreted in the bile, while the balance becomes a metabolite or altered form in the urine.

Naturally obtained d-alpha-tocopherol is more potent than synthetic dl-alpha-tocopherol, a racemic (optically inactive) mixture. Vitamin E may be the only vitamin in which the natural form is superior to the synthetic.

There have been many unproven claims supporting the supplementation of this vitamin by "megavitamin" promotors for many years. Until recently, medical investigators could find no proven human requirement. Vitamin E is known to be essential for laboratory-animal, but not human, fertility. The results of two Harvard University studies published in 1992 show promising results for the reduction of heart-attack risk in men and women through moderate doses of vitamin E (see CARDIO-VASCULAR DISEASE PREVENTION AND ANTIOXIDANT VITAMINS).

In 1994, diabetes investigators in Boston and Japan have reported preventing some of the most serious complications of diabetes in rats and these same researchers expect to be able to apply the benefits to humans in the near future.

History

In 1922, Evans and Bishop reported failed pregnancies in rats fed diets thought to contain all required nutrients. In 1924, Sure discovered a missing nutrient required for rat reproduction: He named it vitamin E. By 1931, Pappenheimer and Goettsch demonstrated that chicks deficient in vitamin E had abnormal brain development, while rabbits and guinea pigs developed muscular dystrophy. The same year, Olcott and Mattill found a high concentration of vitamin E in the lipids of lettuce. These investigators also demonstrated the antioxidant properties of vitamin E. In 1936, Evans derived the vitamin from wheat-germ oil. By 1938, Fernholz established its chemical structure, and Evans and Calhoun named it tocopherol.

Deficiency

Vitamin E rarely may cause hemolysis (destruction of red blood cells) resulting in anemia in humans with malabsorption problems. It may also cause degeneration of axons of the spinal cord and peripheral nerves. Vitamin E has many other proven deficiencies in animals.

Dosage

The adult estimated daily requirement is 10 to 30 mg per day. The daily requirement is increased by the dietary intake of polyunsaturated fat. Dosages from 100 to 250 I.U. daily, used in the Harvard studies cited above, seemed adequate to reduce heart-attack risk.

Recommended Dietary Allowances

The Food and Nutrition Board Subcommittee on the Tenth Edition of the Recommended Dietary Allowances arbitrarily established a value based on customary American dietary intake of 10 mg for adult men and 8 mg for women, who are generally smaller. The daily requirement is diminished or increased by the amount of dietary intake of polyunsaturated fatty acids (PUFA) varying from 5 to 20 mg per day.

Vitamin E requirements may be increased in persons taking large doses of iron. The daily requirement for vitamin E may be diminished in the presence of diets high in selenium or other antioxidants.

Toxicity

Most individuals can tolerate prolonged ingestion of large amounts of vitamin E, and many authors of vitamin books state there are no proven cases of vitamin E toxicity in doses up to 1,200 units per day. However, doses of 800 to 1,500 International Units or more may depress prothrombin levels, interfere with the action of vitamin K and the clotting of blood. This is especially risky in patients taking oral anticoagulants such as warfarin sodium (Coumadin) to prevent blood clots. Premature infants given vitamin E may develop various adverse effects, including jaundice and thrombocytoopenia (low platelet counts), which may cause bleeding.

In April 1994, the *New England Journal of Medicine* reported an increased risk of hemorrhagic strokes in a study of 29,000 Finnish men taking vitamin E in a cancer-prevention study.

Table 9
RECOMMENDED DIETARY ALLOWANCES FOR VITAMIN E

Age	Milligrams of d-alpha-tocopherol
Birth to 6 months	3
6 to 12 months	4
1 to 3 years	5
4 to 6 years	6
7 to 10 years	7
11 to 14 years	8
Males over 14	10
Females over 14	8
Pregnancy	10
Lactation	11

Table 10
POTENCIES OF VITAMIN E SUPPLEMENTS

1 mg of product	International Units (IU)
d-alpha-tocopherol	1.49*
d-alpha-tocopheryl acetate	1.36**
d-alpha-tocopheryl acid succinate	1.21**
dl-alpha-tocopheryl	1.10*
dl-alpha-tocopheryl acetate	1.00**
dl-alpha-tocopheryl acid succinate	0.89**

*Unstable because of oxidation in the presence of light
**Light stable

There was not an increase in total deaths in the group taking alpha-tocopherol. The authors of this study attributed their finding to the vitamin's effects on platelet function. In the same study, there was a diminished incidence of prostate cancer.

In addition, high doses of vitamin E may cause nausea, flatulence or diarrhea and an allergic contact dermatitis. There are rare reports of heart palpitations that led to fainting. Individuals known to be hypertensive (having high blood pressure) may have a slight rise in their pressure at the onset of vitamin E therapy and should begin with a dose of no more than 100 I.U. and be monitored as they increase the dose.

Dr. H. J. Roberts, of the Palm Beach Institute for Medical Research, an authority on vitamin E, differs in his opinion of the safety of this vitamin. Although premature infants may exhibit low platelet counts, adults may have thrombocytosis (increased platelets). Dr. Roberts attributes cases of thrombophlebitis (blood clots in the deep veins of the legs) that may lead to life-threatening pulmonary emboli (blood clots in the lungs) and gynecomastia (enlarged breasts) to as little as 300 International Units (I.U.) of vitamin E. The Vitamin Nutrition Information Service estimates that in 1990, up to 7.3 million adults took vitamin E supplements, and the majority of those individuals took 400 units daily. Ten percent of the population

Table 11
ADVERSE OR TOXIC EFFECTS OF
VITAMIN E

Blood clots—deep vein thrombophlebitis, pulmonary
   embolism
Decreased blood clotting for individuals taking oral
   anticoagulants
Increased risk of hemorrhagic stroke
High blood pressure
Impaired wound-healing
Allergic contact rash
Gastric distress—nausea, flatulence and diarrhea

took 800 units, and about 3 percent took 1,200
units, although the adult requirement has been
calculated at only 8 to 10 mg.

Chronic excess doses of vitamin E may also
increase the levels of androgenic and estrogenic
hormones and cholesterol, impair wound-healing,
cause hypoglycemi (low blood sugar), lower levels
of thyroid and increase vitamin D requirements.

Vitamin E has been implicated in the deaths of
38 infants given the vitamin intravenously for
reasons not fully understood by the authors.

echinacea
(purple cornflower, black sampson)
A flowering perennial plant, *Echinacea angustifolia,* of the Compositae family, found on western
American prairies whose root is used by Sioux
Indians to treat rabies, snakebites and systemic
poisoning. Echinacea is sometimes considered a
natural antitoxin. Homeopathic medicine prescribes a tincture made of the entire plant for
appendicitis, pus in the blood, gangrene and various types of poisoning, and Russian folk medicine
uses echinacea as both an internal and external
antiseptic.

eclipta
(han lian cao, bhringaraj [Sanskrit])
A flowering weed, *Eclipta prostrata,* of the Compositae family, of India, Japan, China, Taiwan,
Indochina, the Philippines and elsewhere, used by
Chinese and Ayurvedic practitioners as a remedy
for vertigo, bloody vomitus and urine and lumbago.

elder
(elderberry, sambucus)
A North American shrub, *Sambucus canadensis,
nigra, racemosa* and *ebulus,* of the Caprifoliaceae
family, whose root and rootstock, bark, leaf buds,
leaves, flowers, young shoots and berries are considered medicinal by herbalists. In the form of tea,
wine, infusion, decoction and tincture, elder is
used as a remedy for a wide range of ailments,
including urinary and kidney problems, edema,
rheumatism, constipation, neuralgia, sciatica, diarrhea, cholera and headaches attributable to colds.
In the *canadensis* species of elder, internal use of
fresh plant parts can cause poisoning. In the *nigra,*
berries must be cooked before eating or making
juice. The berry seeds of the *racemosa* are poisonous, and the berries of the *ebulus* are poisonous.

elecampane
(deviat sil [Russian], pushkaramula [Sanskrit], elf
dock, scabwort, aunee, horseheal)
A perennial herb, *Inula helenium,* of the Compositae family, that resembles horseradish and grows
in northern Asia, Europe and eastern North
America. The use of elecampane root in Ayurvedic
and Native American medicine includes treatment
for respiratory, breast and liver diseases, dyspepsia
and malignant fever. Homeopathic tinctures are
prescribed for erysipelas, sciatica, cough, back
ache, toothache and cramps.

electrolytes
See CHLORIDE; POTASSIUM; SODIUM.

elettaria
See CARDAMOM.

elsholtzia

An aromatic Chinese herb, *Elsholtzia splendens,* of the Labiatae family, named for the German botanist and physician John Sigismund Elsholtz (1623–1688). The seeds are used in Chinese medicine as a remedy for typhoid, stomachache and colds.

emilia

(Cupid's shaving brush)
A tropical herb, *Emilia sonchifolia,* of the Compositae family, eaten in salad in Indochina, whose leaves are used by Chinese practitioners to reduce fever and as a remedy for dysentery.

enriched foods

See THIAMINE.

enzymes

Complex proteins in living cells that are catalysts for temperature-sensitive biochemical reactions. Several hundred enzymes are recognized to date, although it is believed that nearly 1,000 exist in mammals. An example of an enzyme is ptyalin. Ptyalin, a component in saliva, splits starch and begins the process of digestion. Other digestive enzymes are amylases, pepsins, lipase, trypsin, chymotrypsin, carboxypeptidase, enteropeptidase, maltase, lactase, sucrase and nucleosidases.

epazote

(Mexican wormseed)
The plant *Chenopodium ambrosioicles,* of the Chenopodiaceae family, that grows in Central America (and is also cultivated in China), whose aerial portions and seeds are used in herbal medicine to treat flatulence and worms.

ephedra

See MA HUANG.

epilepsy

See ANTICONVULSANT DRUGS AND VITAMIN INTERACTIONS.

epimedium

(lusty goatherb)
A North American and Chinese herb, *Epimedium pimedium grandiflorum* and *sagittatum,* of the Berberidaceae family, that contains vitamin E, oleic and linolenic acids and other biochemicals. Epimedium is used in Chinese and western herbal medicine to stimulate the production of androgen and is therefore considered effective against male problems such as impotence and prostate and testicular ailments. Other medicinal uses of epimedium include treatment for hypertension, bronchial asthma and weakness in kidney function.

ergocalciferol

See D, VITAMIN.

ergot

(mother of rye, cockspur rye, hornseed, smut rye)
A fungus, *Claviceps purpurea,* that is a source of LSD and ergotamine tartrate, which is listed in the United States Pharmacopoeia (USP) and used to treat migraine and cluster headaches and after childbirth because it induces vasoconstriction and uterine contraction. Trade names for this drug are Ergostat, Ergomar and Gynergen.

In western herbal medicine, the dried sclerotia of ergot is also used to treat headaches and prevent hemorrhage after childbirth and menstrual problems. Ergot poisoning may be caused by overdose of the drug or by ingesting rye bread contaminated by the *Claviceps purpurea* fungus. Symptoms of ergot poisoning include vomiting and abdominal cramps, excessive thirst, diarrhea, dilated pupils, remarkable weakness, twitching extremities, absence of urination, sometimes seizures and, as a secondary condition, gangrene may develop in the extremities. Treatment may include gastric lavage, a saline cathartic, anticonvulsants and inhaled amyl nitrate, though ergot poisoning may be fatal.

eryngo
(rattlesnake master)
The flowering plant *Eryngium aquaticum,* of the Umbelliferae family, that grows in the New Jersey Pine Barrens and to southern and western locations, with a tuberous, parsniplike root, considered in Native American and homeopathic medicine the useful part of the plant. Tincture of eryngo root provides a treatment for influenza, gleet, gonorrhea, constipation or diarrhea, cough, conjunctivitis, urinary incontinence and sexual weakness, among other ailments. It is also used for sluggishness of the liver and jaundice.

essential fatty acids
(linoleic, linolenic, arachidonic acids)
See FATTY ACIDS.

eucalyptus
(blue gum, fever tree)
The aromatic evergreen tree, and sometimes shrub, native to Australia and cultivated in numerous other regions, *Eucalyptus globulus,* of the myrtle family. The oil from the *globulus species'* mature leaves is a popular ingredient in over-the-counter preparations such as cough drops for respiratory distress. Tea made from the leaves should not be ingested, but rather inhaled to open and soothe mucus-laden nasal and bronchial passages. There are about 600 species of the myrtle (Myrtaceae) family. Certain species attract bees that yield eucalyptus honey. The eucalyptus has a peppermint-lemon fragrance.

Native American medicine prescribes eucalyptus oil, leaves and bark preparations for bronchitis, asthma, diphtheria, malaria and neuralgia. Homeopathic medicine uses the essential oil and fresh leaves for bladder infections, dysentery, strychnine poisoning, syphilis, worms, kidney diseases, aneurism, gout and many other ailments.

eucommia
(du zhong)
A Chinese deciduous tree, *Eucommia ulmoides,* of the Eucommiaceae family, whose bark is used in Chinese medicine to treat hypertension, back ache, impotence and the threat of miscarriage.

evening primrose
(sundrops)
One of many flowering, perennial herbs, *Oenothera biennis,* of the *Onagraceae* family, that grows in the United States, whose leaves and bark provide Native American and homeopathic preparations to treat nervousness, gastrointestinal disorders, nervous or spasmodic cough, diarrhea, hydrocephaloid and gynecological complaints.

exercise and supplements
Special needs for physically active individuals based on sound nutritional principles. The nutrients required are the same for men and women, athletic or non-athletic. The degree of one's physical activity determines the required quantity of some nutrients, especially sodium, potassium, thiamin, riboflavin and niacin. An ideal diet designed to meet the increased needs of an athlete should provide the requirements without the need for supplements. However, because few people eat all the foods necessary to provide the ideal balance of nutrients, vitamin and mineral supplements can satisfy dietary gaps. Adequate hydration (water) is also essential because of extra losses that occur during vigorous exercise.

Sodium and potassium help maintain normal body water balance. Though these minerals are lost in sweat, the losses are usually quite small and are easily replaced by normal diet. Salt tablets should not be used.

In some situations, well-balanced diets are abandoned. For example, wrestlers may be on low-calorie diets for weight-class maintenance but continue to expend high amounts of energy. Many athletes mistakenly believe that vitamins are a direct source of energy. They are not. Vitamin supplements in excess of the recommended dietary allowances (RDAs) will not enhance performance, increase strength or endurance, prevent injury or illness, provide energy, or build muscles.

There are instances where taking supplements may make sense. Athletes who are at highest risk for iron deficiency and who may need supplementation include females who lose iron through menstrual bleeding, those males and females who eat no red meat, marathon runners who may damage red blood cells by pounding their feet on the ground during training, endurance athletes who may lose significant amounts of iron through heavy sweating and teenagers who are growing rapidly. Iron should always be used under a physician's observation because of the possible increased risk of toxicity (see IRON). There are reports of athletes taking up to 10,000 milligrams of vitamin C daily. Not only has no benefit to taking such massive doses of vitamin C or any other vitamin been proven, there also may be considerable risks from taking megadoses. Clearly, research on both physical and psychological effects of vitamin C is needed.

Some women who exercise strenuously stop menstruating. This condition, called "athletic amenorrhea," is caused by diminished estrogen production. Since estrogen deficiency is a major risk factor for developing osteoporosis, these women may be at increased risk for the early onset of osteoporosis. Therefore, calcium supplements become beneficial to those women.

Athletes are more prone to zinc deficiency because of losses through sweat and urine. Most individuals generally do not get the RDA of this important mineral; however, meat, eggs, and seafood are excellent sources of zinc and may help offset a deficiency. In some causes supplements may be necessary.

Chromium is important for the utilization of glucose and supplements seem to be safe. However, whole wheat, peanuts, prunes, apples, mushrooms and wine are good sources of this mineral.

(Adapted with permission from a lecture by Laura Tedesco, R.D., C.D.E., nutritionist at the Joslin Center for Diabetes at Saint Barnabas, Toms River, New Jersey.)

eyebright

The herb *Euphrasia officinalis,* of the Scrophulariaceae family, whose aerial portions are used in western herbal medicine to treat inflammations, sinus congestion and conjunctivitis. Eyebright may be taken internally or used externally, primarily as an eyewash.

eye diseases

Dysfunction and other detrimental conditions of the eye. Night blindness, inadequate night vision, has long been recognized to be related to vitamin A deficiency. Vitamin E deficiency in premature babies is a suspected cause of retinal damage that may lead to blindness. Cataracts and macular degeneration are causes of diminished vision and blindness that may be prevented or delayed by improved nutrition, including adequate amounts of the antioxidant vitamins.

Two studies on vitamins and cancer were conducted by the National Eye Institute and the Chinese Academy of Medical Sciences in Beijing, China, and reported in 1993. In the first study, 2,141 45-to 74-year-olds were given two brand-name multivitamins plus 25,000 International Units (I.U.) of beta-carotene or a placebo for five years. The older individuals, aged 65 to 74, had a 43-percent reduction in vision-limiting nuclear cataracts, a type of cataract that clouds the center of the lens of the eye. In the second study group, 3,249 Chinese were given 2.3 mg of riboflavin (vitamin B$_2$) and 40 mg of niacin daily for five years. These are approximately twice the United States Recommended Daily Allowances (RDA). Those individuals had about a 50 percent reduction in the nuclear cataracts (see also RIBOFLAVIN). Interestingly, persons taking other antioxidants, 25,000 I.U. of beta-carotene, 30 I.U. of vitamin E and 50 mcg of selenium, indicated no reduction in their chances of developing the cataracts, but they did have a reduced risk of stomach cancer. It must be recognized, however, that the Chinese population studied were undernourished, which may have influenced their chances of having eye problems.

(See also A, VITAMIN; E, VITAMIN; NIGHT BLINDNESS.)

F

false unicorn
(helonias)

The plant *Chamaelirium luteum,* of the Liliaceae family, whose root is considered by herbalists to be a uterine tonic, diuretic and antiworm remedy. Not to be confused with *Helonias bullata,* an endangered species according to the federal government, false unicorn is also prescribed for "morning sickness" during pregnancy, stomachaches, anorexia, lumbosacral pain, intestinal parasites, lack of menses and menstrual pain.

fast foods

Meals consisting mainly of hamburgers, fried chicken, french fried potatoes and soft drinks produced extremely quickly and provided "over the counter." The highly successful industry has created much concern over the nutritive quality of the food choices, most fried and garnished with cheese, bacon, mayonnaise and other substances of questionable nutritive value. Nutritionists suggest that the intake of fast foods, also including pizza, submarine sandwiches and hot dogs, should be limited and the intake of healthier choices of foods emphasized.

fat

Vital dietary macronutrients including grease, oil, lipids (fat or fatlike substances) that are not water-soluble. Chemically esters of glycerol with fatty acids, triglycerides or neutral fat. Fats, which yield 9 kilocalories of energy per gram, should compose 20 to 30 percent of a normal diet. Most fats ingested in the diet are in the form of triglycerides. Triglycerides contain both saturated and unsaturated fatty acids. Saturated fats, such as palmitic and stearic, are usually solid at room temperature. Monosaturated fats are liquid at room temperature and harden or thicken when refrigerated. Polyunsaturated fats, including oleic and linoleic, are liquid at room temperature.

Deficiency

Insufficient dietary fat can lead to deficiencies in vitamins A, D, E and K, the fat-soluble vitamins. These vitamins require fat for absorption from the gastrointestinal tract and utilization by cells. Deficiencies can cause problems with bone development, night blindness and skin disorders (see A, VITAMIN; D, VITAMIN; E, VITAMIN; K, VITAMIN).

Excess or Toxicity

Although fats are a vital component of the diet, excessive intake of dietary fat has been linked to breast and colon cancer. Excessive dietary fats may bind to calcium and interfere with calcium absorption.

fatigue

Tiredness attributable to long periods of work or other activity, stress or the effect of a psychotropic drug. Profound tiredness and weakness may also be the result of malnutrition, the general deficiency of proteins, carbohydrates, minerals and vitamins; a disease process such as anemia, cardiac damage and oxygen and endocrine insufficiency; and psychogenic, environmental or physical challenges. Nutritionists may be consulted as part of the health-care team for individuals suffering any form of fatigue, including chronic fatigue syndrome, in order to determine if dietary factors are involved and whether the diet should be altered and supplements administered.

(See also CHRONIC FATIGUE SYNDROME.)

fat-soluble vitamins

Vitamins A, D, E and K stored in fat, or lipid, tissue as well as some organs, especially the liver. These vitamins are insoluble in water and require dietary fats and bile acids to be absorbed through the intestinal tract membranes. Excess intake of these vitamins may cause toxicity because of their ability to be stored. (See A, VITAMIN; D, VITAMIN; E, VITAMIN; K, VITAMIN.)

fatty acids

Straight chain monocarboxylic acids, many of which occur naturally in fats. Essential fatty acids for the synthesis of prostaglandins (potent biochemicals important for a variety of physiologic processes) and membrane structure, include polyunsaturated arachidonic, linoleic and linolenic acids. These essential nutrients must be supplied by the diet, although arachidonic acid can be made in the body from linoleic acid. Requirements of essential fatty acids are 1 to 2 percent of dietary calories in adults and 3 percent for infants. Pyridoxine, vitamin B_6, is required for the metabolism of essential fatty acids.

Deficiency

Essential fatty-acid deficiency characterized by failure of growth and skin rashes is found in formula-fed infants on a skim-milk formula low in linoleic acid.

FDA

See FOREWORD.

fennel

(hui xiang, finocchio, shatapushpa [Sanskrit])
A perennial European herb, *Foeniculum vulgare,* of the carrot family, similar to celery but with an anise-like taste and aromatic seeds. Italians eat fennel cooked or raw, especially in salad, in the tradition of the Ancient Romans, who believed fennel was dietetic. The Ancient Greeks thought eating fennel gave them courage and longevity. Northern Indian cuisine uses fennel seeds mixed with tiny hard candies and shreds of coconut as an after-dinner "digestive." In herbal medicine, fennel is known to promote digestion, relieve intestinal gas, freshen the breath and promote lactation in nursing mothers. The seeds may be eaten or made into a tea, which is also considered a calmative. In addition, fennel is used as an expectorant and antispasmodic.

fenugreek

(methi [Sanskrit])
A flowering annual plant, *Trigonella foenum-graecum,* of the Leguminosae family, whose name in Latin means Greek hay. Native to Asia, fenugreek seed was used as medicine by the Ancient Egyptians and Hippocrates. Modern herbal medicine prescribes fenugreek preparations for tuberculosis, bronchitis, fever, gout, neuralgia, sciatica, fistula, swollen gland and other sufferers. Some believe fenugreek to be an aphrodisiac.

fern, female

(brake fern, stone brake, rock polypod)
An American perennial, *Polypodium vulgare,* whose rootstock is used in herbal medicine to expel worms (particularly tenia worms) and treat respiratory problems, jaundice, fever, diminished appetite and hoarseness. The medicinal use of the rootstock of male fern, or *Dryopteris filixmas,* was documented by the Ancient Greeks and Romans as an anthelmintic, though a prolonged male fern content in the body may cause poisoning, blindness and death.

Osmunda regalis, known by many names including buckhorn brake, water fern or king's fern, is a European and African perennial used to treat internal obstruction, coughs and jaundice. The cinnamon fern, or *Osmunda cinnamomea,* native to North America, is similar in usage to, but somewhat less effective than, buckhorn brake, and when boiled in milk, it yields a mucilage that can counteract diarrhea.

fertility and vitamins
Research in the 1920s identified vitamin E as essential to reproduction in animals. Despite intense scrutiny since, this finding has remained unproved in humans.

ferula
See ASAFOETIDA.

feverfew
(featherfew, pyrethrum, febrifuge)
A European and American flowering plant, *Pyrethrum parthenium,* of the Compositae family, used in Native American and homeopathic medicine as a remedy for tension, poor circulation, dizziness, ill effects of opium, colic, flatulence, indigestion, colds, worms, menstrual problems, rheumatism, convulsions, delirium and St. Vitus' dance (chorea).

fiber, dietary
Parts of food not readily absorbed that resist chemical digestion enzymes in the gastrointestinal tract and promote healthful bowel elimination. Dietary fibers are principally complex carbohydrates including cellulose, hemicellulose and lignin, polysaccharides, gums, mucilages and pectin. These substances are obtained from wheat, oats or algae. Lignin is a noncarbohydrate constituent in plant cell walls. Intestinal microorganisms can convert small quantities of dietary fibers to fatty acids that can be absorbed.

Some food labels may still list fiber content as "crude fiber," but this term in nutritionally obsolete. There is no accurate relationship between dietary and crude fiber.

Benefits
Dietary fibers are hygroscopic, or absorb water, adding moisture and bulk to the stool, thereby improving bowel function.

Sources
The average American consumes an average of 15 to 25 grams of fiber daily. The National Research Council recommends that adequate fiber be obtained from consumption of natural foods rather than by taking proprietary supplements. Fiber-rich foods include oat bran, whole-wheat and whole-grain breads and cereals, fruits containing pectin, especially apples, and legumes. There is evidence that diets rich in plant fiber reduce the incidence of heart disease, gallstones, diverticulosis, colon cancer and diabetes. Questions remain whether fiber alone or other related dietary changes are responsible for these protective effects. It is theorized that adequate fiber promotes rapid passage of suspected carcinogens through the digestive tract, reducing the opportunity for toxins to come in contact with mucosal surfaces in the bowel. Softer stools with increased mass may also dilute the concentration of carcinogens.

Excess
More than 50 grams of fiber daily may cause intestinal distress. Although rare in the United States, excessive fiber intake may bind with calcium and trace minerals reducing absorption of iron and zinc.

fibrocystic breast disease
See BREAST DISEASE AND VITAMINS.

ficus
Old World trees, shrubs and plants of the Moraceae family, with edible fruits. The stems, leaves, roots and fig of the *Ficus pumila,* or creeping fig, grown in East Asia, are used by Chinese practitioners for the treatment of hernia, rheumatism, fever, sore throat, dysentery and inflammation of the bladder.

The *Ficus retusa,* also known as Indian laurel and Malayan banyan, an evergreen tree that grows between India and New Guinea, is used for toothache, swollen feet, rheumatism and pain.

fig
See FICUS.

fillers
Lactose, starch, sugar and other substances added to foods, drugs and supplements to increase bulk, strength, viscosity, opacity and weight.

firmiana
(phoenix tree, Chinese parasol tree)
An East Asian deciduous tree, *Firmiana simplex,* of the Sterculiaceae family, whose seeds, fruits and roots are used in Chinese medicine to treat swellings, mouth abscesses in children and skin disorders.

fish oil
See OMEGA-3 POLYUNSATURATED FATTY ACIDS.

flavonoids
A group of antioxidants including quercetin, kaempferol, myricetin, apigenin and luteolin, found in vegetables, fruits, tea and wine. Dutch researchers found a reduction in coronary artery risk among a group of 805 high-risk men aged 65 to 84 as reported in the British Medical Journal, *Lancet.* There was no significant reduction in cardiac problems in a control group of 693 with no previous cardiac history. It is postulated that flavonoids reduce or prevent oxidation of low-density cholesterol (LDL), inhibiting the build-up of atherosclerotic plaque.

(See also BIOFLAVONOIDS.)

flax
(linseed, lint bells, winterlien)
A North American and European flowering annual, *Linum usitatissimum,* of the Linaceae family, cultivated for its bast fiber and seed. In herbal medicine, a decoction of ripe seeds (immature seed pods may cause poisoning) is used as a remedy for cough, digestive and urinary disorders and other problems. Linseed oil, commonly known as an oil-paint thinner, is used to help eliminate gallstones. When eaten, the seeds work as a laxative by swelling in the intestines, thus promoting elimination of feces.

In Ayurvedic medicine, flax tea may be taken as a laxative, expectorant and decongestant, and flax seeds are thought to be energizing and of therapeutic value in relieving asthma and chronic cough.

fluid balance
See ELECTROLYTES.

fluoride
A binary compound of the nonmetallic, gaseous element fluorine. Fluoride ions combine with bones and teeth to strengthen them. Fluoridation of community water supplies to a level of 1 part per million have achieved a 50 to 75 percent reduction in dental caries (cavities). In nonfluoridated areas, infants and children are usually given daily vitamin supplements containing fluoride or fluoride alone.

Fluoride used experimentally to treat osteoporosis has been disappointing. Although fluoride stimulates bone growth, the resulting bone formation may be poorly mineralized and may be structurally unsound. However, when fluoride is combined with calcium supplements and vitamin D, there may be decreased fractures. The addition of estrogen therapy to the above regimen may be even more effective.

Table 12
ESTIMATED SAFE AND ADEQUATE DIETARY INTAKE OF FLUORIDE*

Birth to 6 months	0.1–.5 mg
6 to 12 months	0.2–1.0 mg
1 to 3 years	0.5–1.5 mg
4 to 6 years	1.0–2.5 mg
7 to 11 years	1.5–2.5 mg
Adults	1.5–4.0 mg

*Because there is insufficient information on which to base Recommended Dietary Allowances (RDA) for fluoride, a range is given.

Toxicity

Fluorosis, or fluoride toxicity, results from excess doses of supplements, or accidental ingestion of fluoride containing insecticides and rodenticides or chronic inhalation of industrial gases or dusts. Fluorine and fluorides are cellular poisons that inhibit the breakdown of glucose. They react with calcium to form insoluble compounds and cause hypocalcemia (decreased calcium). Characteristic findings indicate osteosclerosis and osteomalacia resulting in skeletal changes, such as dense bones, neurologic complications due to bony overgrowth and calcification of ligaments. Anemia, weight loss and weakness may also occur. Mottling of teeth may result if excessive fluoride is ingested during the formation of enamel.

Acute poisoning causes severe abdominal pain, nausea, vomiting and diarrhea. Calcium loss causes tetany, convulsions and eventually death from cardiac or respiratory arrest.

fluorine
See FLUORIDE.

folacin
See FOLIC ACID.

folate
See FOLIC ACID.

folic acid
(folacin)

A substance first extracted from spinach leaves in 1941, named from the Latin word *folium* for leaf, and found to be a treatment for some types of anemia. This water-soluble compound is absorbed from the upper part of the small intestine and converted to its chemically active form by interactions with vitamin B_{12}, vitamin C and niacin.

The U.S. Public Health Service advises all women of child-bearing potential to consume at least 400 mcg of folic acid daily to reduce their risk of having a fetus affected by neural tube defects. It is estimated that at least a 50 percent reduction in neural-tube defects, including spina bifida and anencephaly, can be achieved by this recommendation.

The American diet often fails to provide the required amount of folic acid from leafy vegetables, nuts and oranges or orange juice (see Table 13).

Sources of Folic Acid

The average American diet contains only 0.2 mg of folate. Therefore the Food and Drug Administration (FDA) has proposed fortification of various foods such as enriched breads, rolls and buns; enriched flour and self-rising flour; enriched cornmeal; enriched rice; and enriched macaroni products. Each product will be required to be fortified

Table 13
FOLIC ACID CONTENT OF FOODS

Total Cereal		
1 cup		
466 mcg		
Grape-Nuts cereal	1 cup	402 mcg
Lentils	½ cup	179 mcg
Dry beans	½ cup	120–160 mcg
Spinach (cooked)	½ cup	131 mcg
Asparagus (cooked)	½ cup	121 mcg
Wheaties cereal	1 cup	102 mcg
Turnips (cooked)	½ cup	85 mcg
Iceberg lettuce	1 cup	76 mcg

with folic acid equivalent to 140 mcg/100 grams of the product.

Cooking vegetables usually reduces the folate content to such an extent that in many cases the cooking water contains more of the vitamin than the cooked vegetable. In one study, samples of raw spinach averaged approximately 142.9 mcg of total folate per 100 grams of the vegetable. But after cooking, the spinach retained only 31.2 mcg of the vitamin, while the cooking water contained 92.4 mcg. However, asparagus and brussels sprouts retained approximately 84 percent and 73 percent, respectively, of precooking folate content.

Folic Acid Deficiency

The body stores from three to six months' worth of folate. Deficiencies usually result from malnutrition or malabsorption of the vitamin in the diet. However, there are situations in which drugs or some medical disorders (see Table 15) interfere with the utilization of available vitamin. Pregnancy, some malignancies, increase folate requirements. Some liver diseases cause folate deficiency by increasing excretion of folic acid in urine and feces. Since vitamin B_{12} is required for cells to utilize folic acid, a vitamin B_{12} deficiency also causes symptoms of folate deficiency.

Approximately half of all pregnancies are unplanned. As mentioned above, neural-tube birth defects are caused by a folate deficiency. It is wise for all women of child-bearing age to have adequate folic acid in their diets. But doses of folic acid greater than 1 mg per day may mask the symptoms of pernicious anemia (vitamin B_{12} deficiency-related anemia), allowing permanent neurological damage to progress unrecognized. The dose recommended to prevent folate deficiency must be balanced against dangerous higher levels.

Dosage of Supplements

The Public Health Service (PHS) and the American Academy of Pediatrics recommend a daily dose of 0.4 mg. The pediatric group also recommends against taking multivitamins that contain vitamin A to achieve the required folate.

Folic Acid Toxicity

Megadoses from 5 to 15 mg may cause kidney toxicity with increased diuresis and hypertrophy, or enlargement, of the kidneys indicated by an increase in blood urea nitrogen and creatinine levels. These abnormalities are evidence of kidney failure. Folate excesses can also cause central nervous system inflammation resulting in muscle spasms, aggressive behavior, malaise, depression, irritability and altered sleep patterns with increased dreams or insomnia.

Table 14
THE EFFECTS OF COOKING ON FOLIC ACID CONTENT OF FOODS

Vegetable	raw vegetable	after cooking	lost
Asparagus	174.7	146.3	16%
Broccoli	169.2	64.7	62%
Brussels sprouts	88.5	64.7	27%
Cabbage	29.6	15.9	46%
Cauliflower	56.3	42.2	25%
Spinach	142.9	31.2	78%

Average folic acid content of 4 samples Micrograms per 100 grams of vegetable weight

Table 15
CAUSES OF FOLIC ACID DEFICIENCY

(The anemias caused by folic acid deficiency can be improved by folic-acid supplementation.)

Dietary overcooking of foods (folate is destroyed by heat), inadequate food intake, chronic alcoholism

Malabsorption tropical and nontropical (celiac) sprue, disorders scurvy (vitamin C-poor diets are usually also low in folate))

Drugs that compete for absorption
   phenytoin (Dilantin)
   primidone (Mysoline)
   barbiturates, i.e., phenobarbital
   oral contraceptives
   cycloserine (Seromycin)

Table 15 (cont)
CAUSES OF FOLIC ACID DEFICIENCY

Drugs that cause inadequate utilization, or a block in metabolism of the vitamin

    folic acid antagonists:

        methotrexate and related drugs (used as chemotherapeutic agents in the treatment of some cancers, certain types of arthritis and psoriasis)

        pyrimethamine (for treatment of malaria and toxoplasmosis)

        triamterene (component of the diuretic Dyazide and Maxide)

        pentamidine (protocidal drug for the treatment of pneumocystis carinii pneumonia most frequently seen in AIDS patients)

        trimethoprim (antibacterial drug used alone or with the sulfa drug sulfamextoxazole in Bactrim or Septra)

    anticonvulsants

    enzyme deficiencies:

        congenital

        acquired (liver diseases)

    vitamin B_{12} deficiency

    alcohol

    ascorbic acid (vitamin C) deficiency

    amino acid excesses in the diet (glycine, methionine)

Increased requirements

    pregnancy (especially multiple pregnancies)

    malignancies (malignant tissues, especially lymphoproliferative or myeloproliferative disorders)

    infancy

    increased hematopoiesis (blood production) that occurs with hemolytic anemias, chronic blood loss, scurvy, increased metabolism (hyperthyroidism)

Increased excretion

    vitamin B_{12} deficiency that prevents the ability to incorporate folate in cells

    liver disease

food additives

Chemicals or substances added to foods and medications as coloring or flavoring agents, preservatives, sweeteners or to improve consistency.

Adverse reactions are rare from the approximately 2,800 substances approved by the Food and Drug Administration (FDA). An important and potentially life-threatening reaction can occur in persons susceptible to the preservatives known as sulfiting agents. Sulfite additives can cause asthma and anaphylaxis (a form of life-threatening shock), with symptoms including a flushed feeling, drop in blood pressure and tingling sensations.

Dyes approved in the Food, Drug and Cosmetic Act (FD&C) of 1938 are derivatives of coal tar. Tartrazine, or FD&C yellow dye number 5, is frequently implicated as a cause of hyperactivity in children and asthma. However, less than 10 percent of individuals suspected of having adverse reactions to these additives reacted when challenged in a controlled study. Aspirin-sensitive asthmatic patients should be aware of the rare possibility of cross-reactivity between tartrazine and aspirin.

Parabens, a group of preservatives in creams and ointments, are strong skin sensitizers and can worsen the condition for which they are prescribed. Parabens can cause urticaria (hives) or angioedema (swelling of body tissues) when medications containing them as preservatives are injected. Oral ingestion of these substances does not seem to cause adverse reactions. Sodium benzoate, a chemically related substance, may cross-react with the parabens and can also cause asthma.

Butylated hydroxanisol (BHA) and butylated hydroxytoluene (BHT) are used in low doses as antioxidants in grain products including breakfast cereals and have not been shown to cause any allergic problems. However, since antioxidants are thought by some to prevent cancer and herpes infections and to retard aging, they are often used in megadoses in various health food preparations that may be toxic.

Nitrate and nitrite preservatives commonly used in lunch meats and hot dogs may cause migraine headaches and may be carcinogenic. Monosodium glutamate, the cause of "Chinese restaurant syn-

drome," may rarely cause asthma, hives or angio-
dema.

The azo dye amaranth (FD&C Red No. 5) was
banned by the United States in 1975 because it
was suspected of being a carcinogen. Aspartame
(Nutrasweet) is often blamed for adverse effects,
but except for a few cases of urticaria (hives),
there is no scientific proof of ill effects. Tartrazine
is also frequently implicated in causing urticaria
and angioedema. Well-controlled studies such as
those at the Scripps Clinic and Research Foundation in San Diego, California, have rarely confirmed the suspicions. These dyes do play a role
as sensitizers in allergic dermatitis. They are often
suspected of inducing adverse effects both in the
skin and when ingested. Skin reactions are relatively common; when used in foods and medications, the dyes are rarely proven to be the source
of the adverse effect.

food allergy

Adverse reactions to food or food additives caused
by exposure to an allergen to which an individual
is susceptible. However, many persons refer to
any adverse food reaction as an allergy. There are
basically two groups of food reactions, allergy-
based or "hypersensitivity" reactions and nonallergic, or food "intolerances." When foods thought
to cause allergic reaction are avoided, overall nutrition may suffer if adequate substitutions are not
made in the diet. A person suffering from many
food allergies is clearly at risk of nutrient deficiency, a condition that may compound distress
by causing a myriad of ill effects.

Incidence

Hippocrates (460–370 B.C.) described stomach distress and hives from cow's milk. Galen (A.D. 131–
210) recognized allergic symptoms in a child from
goat's milk. Since early in the 20th century, medical reports carry descriptions of many similar reactions. Prevalence of true allergic reactions to food
is unknown, but studies estimate the incidence of
food allergy in about 1 percent in the general

Table 16
FDA-APPROVED ADDITIVES THAT CAN
CAUSE ADVERSE REACTIONS

Butyl paraben*
Ethyl paraben*
Metabisulfite
Methyl paraben*
Monosodium glutamate (MSG)
Nitrates
Nitrites
Potassium sulfite
Propyl paraben*
Sodium benzoate
Sulfur dioxide
Sulfur sulfite
Yellow dye #5 (tartrazine)

*Parabens are derivatives of parahydroxybenzoic acid.

public. Adverse food reactions of all types, including nonallergic causes, may reach as high as 10
percent among infants if all adverse reactions are
included.

Peak sensitivity to foods occurs at about age
one in 3 to 4 percent of infants. Experts believe
that 70 to 80 percent of babies outgrow their food
allergies. In double-blind food challenges, it was
demonstrated that only one-third of the patients
thought to have allergies to a food actually had an
adverse effect to a suspected food.

In a study of five hundred consecutive newborn
infants followed over a three-year period, 142 (28
percent) were suspected of having an allergy to at
least one food. However, only 27 (5 percent)
reacted when challenged to that food or foods.

True allergy involves an allergen-antibody reaction. A food allergic reaction sets off a complex
series of events when the food allergen comes in
contact with the immune system as it is passing
through or being absorbed by the gastrointestinal
tract. Once absorbed into the bloodstream, the
allergens attach themselves to receptors on mast
cells and basophils in other target organs, the skin,
respiratory tract and circulatory system, triggering
the release of potent chemicals called mediators.

In turn, the mediators bring on the allergic symptoms—sneezing, itching, hives, wheezing and shortness of breath or, in the most severe expression of allergy, acute shock or anaphylaxis.

Anaphylaxis, which may be fatal, seldom occurs and can usually be treated successfully if epinephrine is given immediately. Despite that fatalities are rare, some experts believe that more children and adolescents die from food allergy than bee-stings.

Foods That Most Commonly Cause Anaphylaxis

Only a few foods cause the vast majority of food allergic reactions. Similar properties among these food allergens are their glycoprotein composition, their water-solubility and heat and acid stability. Purified food allergens have been isolated from codfish, soybeans and peanuts. In most foods, only a small fraction of the available protein is allergenic.

Cooking may alter proteins and therefore lessen the allergenic potential of some foods, such as milk.

However, heating milk containing lactose (milk sugar) or milk altered by cooking actually increases the allergenic potential.

In children, most reactions are caused by eggs, cow's milk, and peanuts. In adults, the chief sources of allergic reactions are fish, shellfish, tree nuts and peanuts. Interestingly, various animal products do not always cross-react. Persons may be allergic to milk, but usually are not allergic to beef or inhaled cattle dander. Also, individuals with egg allergy are rarely allergic to chicken meat or inhaled feather allergens.

Many women in the United States consume large amounts of peanuts, especially in peanut butter, as a source of protein while breast-feeding. Peanut allergen in the breast milk may then sensitize the infant prone to peanut or other allergy.

Nuts, peanuts, eggs or milk were responsible for 13 fatal or near-fatal reactions in one group of allergic children. All children in the group had asthma, and most had prior reactions to the same foods.

Outcome and Treatment of Food Allergy

Epinephrine (Adrenalin) is available in spring-loaded, self-injecting syringes (Ana-Kit and Epi-Pen are two commercial brands available by prescription). Children weighing less than 30 kilograms (66 pounds) should receive a reduced dose.

Most children who died in the group mentioned above were in school or other public places at the time of the allergic reaction. Those who were immediately given an injection of epinephrine survived. Onset of a severe reaction usually occurs within minutes, but may be delayed for 30 minutes or more. In the group of 13 patients mentioned above, none of the individuals who died had received an epinephrine injection before severe respiratory distress developed. An initial reaction may be mild for an hour or more and then suddenly worsen.

In the group of fatalities, half suffered a rapid progression of respiratory difficulty before death. The other half had a two-part response: early oral itching and abdominal distress, with minimal symptoms for one to two hours before the onset of rapid deterioration and death. Therefore, it is imperative that anyone who has symptoms of a food allergy be given epinephrine as soon as possible and transported to an emergency medical facility on an urgent basis and observed for at least several hours.

Prevention of Food Allergic Reactions

Adults and children of reading age who have known food allergies should read labels carefully and become familiar with all the alternate names used for some foods. They must ask about ingredients of any foods ordered in a restaurant. Foods are often added unexpectedly; for example, peanut butter may be added to chili for flavoring. The Canadian Restaurant and Foodservice Association has a program in which designated employees of participating members are knowledgeable about all ingredients on their menu.

For persons who have had a prior food reaction and were diagnosed with positive tests for a particular food by a qualified allergist, avoidance of that food is paramount. However, if one showed a positive allergy test but no past reactions to a particular food, that food does not have to be avoided.

Immunotherapy (Allergy Shots) for Food Allergy

Studies are being done to develop a safe method to desensitize food allergic persons. HOWEVER, AT THE PRESENT TIME, ALLERGY SHOTS FOR FOOD ALLERGIES SHOULD NEVER BE ATTEMPTED EXCEPT UNDER RESEARCH CONDITIONS. THE RISK OF FATAL ANAPHYLAXIS IS GREAT.

Testing for Food Allergy

Many individuals who have positive tests to foods can eat those same foods without having a reaction. A history of a prior food reaction usually precedes a fatal attack.

Nonallergic Food Reactions

Various other mechanisms are responsible for an individual's adverse reaction to a food: toxicity to or poisoning by contaminated foods; drug-induced effects such as those following ingestion of caffeine; metabolic or enzyme deficiencies, such as the diarrhea induced by the inability to digest lactose (milk sugar) in a person with the lactase enzyme deficiency.

Typical descriptions of adverse reactions to a food include food hypersensitivity, food anaphylaxis, food intolerance, food toxicity (poisoning), food idiosyncrasy, anaphylactoid food reaction, pharmacologic food reaction and metabolic food reaction.

Rashes, diarrhea, colic and runny nose are often attributed to allergies, but are rarely proven to have origins in allergy.

food groups

See Appendix 1 Food Pyramid.

forskohlii

An Ayurvedic preparation including the herb *Coleus forskohlii,* which contains a diterpene forskohlin. (A terpene is a member of the $C_{10}H_{16}$ family of hydrocarbons.) According to literature on Ayurvedic herbal products from India, this diterpene promotes nearly all pharmacological activities of the herb.

forsythia

(lian qiao, weeping golden bell)
A northern Chinese shrub, *Forsythia suspensa,* of the Oleaceae family, named for British horticulturist William Forsyth (1737–1800). In Chinese medicine, the fruits, leaves, leaf stalks and roots are used for preparations to treat fever, measles, skin disorders, inflammatory conditions, headache, sore throat, lymphatic tuberculosis, pinworm, jaundice and colds, among others.

foxglove

(digitalis, ladies' glove, dead men's bells, purple foxglove, fairy fingers)
Originally a European biennial, sometimes perennial, plant, *Digitalis purpurea,* of the snapdragon family, prized for its bell-shaped or finger-shaped (*digitus* in Latin) flowers and as a source of the drug digitalis, recognized in the United States Pharmacoepia (USP). Digitalis, made from the plant's dried and powdered leaves, contains cardiotonic glycocides, namely digitoxin and digoxin, that increase the heart muscles' ability to contract and thereby increase the heart's output. Digitalis is used in the treatment of congestive heart failure, atrial fibrillation and flutter and paroxysmal atrial tachycardia, and also as a diuretic.

Foxglove's medicinal properties were first documented by Welsh physicians in 1250 and in William Withering's book published in 1785.

Digitalis poisoning may develop from an accumulation of digitalis in the system. Symptoms include irregular pulse, nausea and vomiting, diarrhea, headache, partial heart block and a slowing of the heart rate. Patients on digitalis therapy should be taught to take their pulse, include high-potassium foods in their diet and be aware of the symptoms of digitalis poisoning. The treatment of poisoning may include the administration of digoxin immune Fab (fragment antigen binding), a biological substance under the trade name Digibind.

Digoxin is also obtained from *Digitalis lanata,* and is marketed as the cardiac stimulant Lanoxin.

Herbalists recommend medical direction for the use of digitalis, and add that touching the plant itself has been known to cause skin rashes, nausea and headache.

free radicals
See ANTIOXIDANTS.

fritillaria
(chuan bei mu)
A western North American, European, Asian and North African bulbous herb, *Fritillaria cirrhose, verticillata* or *thunbergii,* of the Liliaceae family, whose bulbs are used in Chinese medicine to treat cough, bronchial and pulmonary conditions, colds, stomachache, breast inflammation and painful menses. *Fritillus* in Latin means checkerboard, which describes the markings on some of the plant's flowers.

fumitory
(smoke of the earth)
A flowering annual found all over the world, *Fumaria officinalis,* of the Fumariaceae family, known also as *fumus terrae,* smoke of the earth. In herbal medicine, the flowering herb is dried and prepared as a remedy for liver and gallbladder conditions and scabies and other skin problems. Used also as a laxative and diuretic, fumitory in excessive doses may cause stomach pain and diarrhea.

G

G, vitamin

An obsolete name for riboflavin or vitamin B_2.

galangal

(catarrh root)

A Southeast Asian, Chinese, Indonesian and Iranian perennial, *Alpinia galanga,* whose rootstock has been considered medicinal since the Middle Ages, when it was thought to be an aphrodisiac. Galangal prescriptions given by practitioners of herbal medicine are similar to those of ginger. (See GINGER.)

garden nightshade

A flowering plant, *Solanum nigrum,* of the Solonaceae family (see also BELLADONNA) and native to regions of the United States, whose leaves are used in Native American and herbal medicine as a sedative and narcotic. Homeopathic tinctures of garden nightshade are prescribed for chorea, headache, heartburn, meningitis, night terrors, stammering, hydrocephalus, mania, peritonitis, tetanus and other ailments. The berries, poisonous until boiled, contain solanine, a toxic alkaloid, which is used to treat fever, diarrhea, heart disease and to dilate the pupils. The juice of the plant is used for kidney, liver, spleen, bladder and skin problems. Ointments and poultices are also made of garden nightshade for herpes, burns, joint pain, swellings and other irritations.

gardenia

(zhi zi, cape jasmine)

A popular flowering plant, *Gardenia jasminoides,* of the Rubiaceae family, originally from China and named after American physician Alexander Garden (1730–1791) who corresponded with the famous botanist Linnaeus. The fruit, seeds, flowers and roots are used in Chinese medicine as treatment for jaundice, gonorrhea, rheumatism, bleeding, abscesses and other problems.

garlic

See ALLIUM.

gastrodia

(tian ma)

An East Asian orchid, *Gastrodia elata,* of the Orchidaceae family, whose underground stem is used in Chinese medicine to treat headache, vertigo, rheumatism, paralysis and lumbago.

gelatin

A glutinous material derived by boiling collagen obtained from the skin, white connective tissue and bones of animals. Gelatin is used by the pharmaceutical industry in the manufacture of capsules for drugs and supplements.

generic products

Non-brand name drugs or supplements that contain similar active ingredients or nutrients as name-brand products and generally are less expensive. Capsules, tablets, fillers, binders or special time-release mechanisms may alter the amount of active drug absorbed and/or the time or rate at which the absorption occurs, thereby affecting the products' effectiveness. Major manufacturers claim that their brand-name products are superior to generics, but many of the same companies also make a line of generic drugs and supplements.

Theoretically, there should be no difference. But potent drugs such as heart and thyroid medications may differ significantly in their potency, and most physicians prescribe brand-names for these drugs. Vitamin and mineral supplements that meet United States Pharmacopoeia (USP) standards for dissolution are probably as effective as similar name brands. The USP is a legally recognized publication of standards and is updated regularly.

genetic code

The biochemical basis of heredity in which codons of DNA and RNA determine the specific amino acids sequence in proteins. Cancer may begin as an alteration in the genetic code that controls the characteristics of each cell. Antioxidants, including vitamin E, are thought by some researchers to protect a person's genetic code against these modifications. Some even feel that vitamin E can convert minor abnormalities back to normal.

(See also ANTIOXIDANTS.)

gentiana
(gentian)

A flowering herb of temperate and arctic regions and certain tropical areas, *Gentiana macrophylla, scabra* and *triflora,* of the Gentianaceae family. Gentian is named for Gentius, king of Illyricum (the area formerly known as Yugoslavia) who allegedly discovered the medicinal plant 2,000 years ago. In Europe, gentian-root powder put in wine was considered a treatment for a number of ailments, including stomach and joint pain. In Chinese medicine, gentian is used as a remedy for rheumatoid arthritis, eye inflammations, convulsions, tuberculosis and other problems because it contains gentianine, an anti-inflammatory alkaloid. Gentian violet, from the dried rhizome and roots of *Gentiana lutea,* is the coal-tar dye $C_{25}H_{30}ClN_3$ used as a histology, cytology and bacteriology stain. It is also a topical anti-infective by the chemical name hexamethylpararosaniline chloride.

germanium
(germanium dioxide or GE-132)

A mineral with dangerous adverse effects and unproven claims to boost the immune system in fighting cancer and AIDS. In 1988, the Food and Drug Administration banned importation of the substance following reports of weight loss, fatigue, anemia, kidney failure and death.

ghee

An Ayurvedic preparation of heated, unsalted butter, used plain or varied by adding licorice, calamus root or gotu kola. Ghee is considered a flavor-enhancer of foods; a tonic for increased intelligence, understanding and memory; and a digestive, laxative and detoxifier of the system. Also a remedy for peptic ulcers, colitis and wounds, ghee is said not to affect cholesterol level.

ginger
(sheng jiang, sheng jiang pi, African ginger, black ginger, race ginger)

Originally a tropical Asian perennial, *Zingiber officinale,* of the family Zingiberaceae, now cultivated in many parts of the world. A popular cooking spice, ginger root, as it is commonly called, is also highly regarded as medicinal, especially as a "warming" agent that promotes digestion of fatty foods and counteracts flatulence.

In Chinese medicine, ginger tea is prescribed for colds and mucus congestion, nausea, hangover, menstrual cramps and other problems; ginger tea serves also as a bladder, kidney and uterine tonic. Ginger is also eaten as a vegetable in several Oriental cuisines.

In Ayurvedic medicine, ginger (*sunthi,* in Sanskrit) is touted as the best kitchen remedy for cough, colds, sinusitis and congestion. A paste made of ginger powder is used for relief of headache, and adding ginger to foods serves to promote digestion, elimination and body heat in cold weather.

Ginger oil, baths and compresses are used in Japan as topical applications for a wide range of ailments, including earache, flu, pain, sinusitis, kidney problems and gout, among others.

According to the *New England Journal of Medicine* in 1983, ginger capsules were discovered to be effective against vertigo and motion sickness.

gingko biloba
(maidenhair tree)
Originally an eastern China, fruit-bearing deciduous tree, *Ginkgo biloba,* of the family Ginkgoaceae, whose fruit's kernels are eaten as a delicacy and also are said to expel intestinal worms and aid digestion. Young fruits and fruit pulp are used in Chinese medicine to treat tuberculosis and other pulmonary complaints, gonorrhea, kidney and bladder problems and vaginal discharge.

ginseng
(ren shen, five finger root, sang, ninsin, panax, pannag, red berry, root of life, man root, immortality root, vidari-kanda [Sanskrit for Indian ginseng])
An Asian and North American perennial plant, both wild and cultivated, *Panax quinquefolius,* or *Panax ginseng (shinseng),* of the family Araliaceae, valued as an herbal medicine. Ginseng root is used in many cultures as a stimulant, general tonic and sometimes an aphrodisiac. According to allopathic (western) medicine, evidence supporting ginseng is controversial. With its adaptogenic (antistress) properties called ginsenosides, ginseng root may be eaten raw or processed for storage as dried root (usually in the form of tea, pills or tablets) or liquid put into capsules.

Some of the acclaimed therapeutic uses of ginseng include the treatment of impotence, infertility, uterine disorders and other sexual complaints (Chinese, Tibetan, Native American), senility, hypoglycemia, arteriosclerosis, exhaustion, mental illness, stomach disorders, headache, fever and cough. Contemporary Russian scientist I. I. Brekhman's research found that ginseng may also be used as a stress-reliever, because it has positive effects on the adrenal cortex of the brain, which produces hormones that fight stress. Therefore Brekhman believes ginseng may help the body resist illness.

At the Third International Ginseng Conference in Korea in 1981, ginseng was touted by Japanese scientist Dr. M. Kimura, who used it to treat patients with diabetes, and Dr. Morio Yonezawa, who reported that ginseng extract administered by injection seemed to prevent radiation-induced bone-marrow damage in patients exposed to radiation. Dr. Yoon Seok Chang, of the Seoul National University Hospital in Korea, concurred, revealing two comparative studies done on 50 patients with cervical cancer also treated with radiation. Chang reported that red panax ginseng taken orally by these patients restored their bone-marrow functions. Some scientists in the United States maintain that ginseng is a placebo, while others, like the Chinese doctors and herbalists, call it "the king of medicines."

In Ezekiel 27:17, ginseng (often written as "pannag") was traded at the marketplace of Israel. Ginseng—from the Orient, eastern Canada, the United States, or the ginseng plantations in Russia—is available all over the world. Homeopathic practitioners prescribe trituration and tincture of the root for appendicitis, lumbago, rheumatism, sciatica, general weakness and other ailments. Other Native American uses include treatment of asthma, whooping cough, nervous disorders, poor appetite, gout, cardiac weakness, indigestion, colds and neuralgia.

In Ayurvedic medicine, vidari-kanda (known as Indian ginseng) is from the plant *Ipomoea digitata,* of the Convolvulaceae family, and is used as a nutritive tonic, aphrodisiac and diuretic.

Legend (and perhaps reality) has it that Panax ginseng plants emit light at night, possibly attributable to the plant's alleged ability to give off organic radioactive rays like those of Gartwitch rays of onions, said to promote the life processes in cells. Furthermore, ginseng plants are believed to move of their own accord during the night, possibly because their roots shift. Dr. James Duke, a researcher of the U.S. Department of Agriculture's Economic Botany Laboratory, experimented with 100 ginseng plants and discovered that about half the plants did in fact move during the night. When he replanted the ones that had been somehow disturbed, they moved again. Dr. Duke did not come to any precise conclusions about this phenomenon.

Some writers have noticed that ginseng does not seem to have an effect on individuals who are usually energetic and active. Llynn' Newman, certified nutritionist/herbalist and holistic counselor of Long Island, New York, wrote that ginseng, which supports all bodily functions, is contraindicated for those with high blood pressure and women with cysts, and it is not to be taken in conjunction with caffeine, citrus or vitamins.

gleditsia
(honey locust)
A Chinese deciduous tree, *Gleditsia sinensis,* of the Leguminosae family and named after the German botanist Johann Gottlieb Gleditsch (1714–1786). The roots, bark, fruits, seeds, leaves and thorns are considered medicinal by Chinese practitioners, and are made into preparations for excess mucus, intestinal worms, fever, swellings, indigestion, wounds and other ailments.

glehnia
(bei sha shen)
A Korean, Taiwanese, Chinese and Japanese plant, *Glehnia littoralis,* of the Umbelliferae family, whose roots are used by Chinese practitioners as a tonic for the liver and kidneys and to treat pulmonary complaints and chest pain.

glycemic index
Physiological measure of the human body's ability to derive glucose (sugar) from foods containing carbohydrate. The index is the ratio of serum glucose in the blood derived from food to that derived from a solution of pure glucose, measured over a two-hour period after ingestion.

Table 17
GLYCEMIC INDEXES OF FOODS

100%	80–90%	70–79%	60–69%
Glucose	Carrots	Bread	Bananas
	Corn flakes	(whole meal)	Beetroot
	Honey	Broad beans	Bread (white)
	Maltose	(fresh)	Mars bar
	Parsnips	Millet	Muesli
	Potatoes	Potato (new)	Raisins
	(instant	Rice (white)	Rice (brown)
	mashed)	Swede	Ryvita
		Weetabix	Shredded wheat
			Water biscuits

50–59%	40–49%	30–39%	20–29%
All-bran	Beans	Apples	Fructose
Buckwheat	(canned	(Golden	Kidney
Digestive	navy)	Delicious)	beans
biscuits	Orange	Blackeye	Lentils
Oatmeal	juice	peas	
biscuits	Oranges	Butter beans	**10–19%**
Peas (frozen)	Peas	Chick peas	Peanuts
Potato chips	(dried)	Haricot beans	Soya beans
Rich tea	Porridge	Ice cream	(fresh and
biscuits	oats	Milk (skim)	canned)
Spaghetti	Potato	Milk (whole)	
Sucrose	(sweet)	Tomato soup	
Sweet corn	Spaghetti	Yogurt	
Yam	(whole		
	meal)		

glycyrrhiza

(gan cao, kum cho, sweetwood, Chinese licorice)
A Mediterranean, Asian and southern European herb, *Glycyrrhiza glabra,* of the Leguminosae family, whose roots are used in Chinese medicine to treat peptic ulcers, poor appetite, heart palpitations, weakness, dizziness, productive cough and hemorrhoids. A licorice and soybean decoction was considered an antidote for various poisons in 18th-century China. According to recent research, the roots are effective against cocaine hydrochloride and chloral hydrate, snake venom, tetanus and globefish toxins.

Cough medicines often contain licorice flavoring. In Africa, glycyrrhiza stems and roots are made into an infusion and used as a remedy for pulmonary tuberculosis, eye diseases and appendicitis. Dried, powdered glycyrrhiza root is used in Vietnam as a purgative, diaphoretic and diuretic. A glycoside called glycyrrhizine, with a licorice flavor, is found in the plant and believed to be 50 times sweeter than sugar.

Licorice may be contraindicated for persons with hypertension because it may cause salt retention, excess potassium loss and elevated blood pressure.

goat's rue

A southern European, western Asian and North American flowering perennial, *Galega officinalis,* poisonous to sheep who graze on it but considered therapeutic by herbalists. The medicinal herb is used, albeit rarely, in the treatment of diabetes, fever, worms and poisoning.

goiter

Enlarged thyroid gland often caused by an iodine deficiency, usually occurs where the iodine content of a normal diet is low. Goiter was endemic to the Great Lakes region (prior to the introduction of iodized salt) and still occurs elsewhere in the world, especially in such mountain regions as the Alps, Pyrenees, Carpathians, Andes and Himalayas, where as many as 10 percent of the population have the disorder.

(See also IODINE.)

goldenrod

(blue mountain tea)
A North American flowering perennial herb, *Solidago canadensis* or *juncea* (two of about 100 species), of the family Compositae, whose leaves and tops are used in Native American and other herbal medicine practices for the treatment of bladder stones, hay fever and colds related to tuberculosis. Homeopathic practitioners prescribe tincture of aromatic goldenrod flowers or infusion of dried leaves and flowers for painful urination, protein in the urine, enlarged prostate, gout, deafness, croup, rheumatism, scrofula, sciatica and scanty urine. Russian herbalists used goldenrod for lack of menses, diarrhea and cystitis.

goldenseal

(orange root, tumeric root, yellow puccoon,
ground raspberry, jaundice root, eye balm, Indian plant)
A North American fruit-bearing perennial, *Hydrastis canadensis,* of the family Ranunculaceae, whose root is valued in Native American and other herbalist medicines as a treatment for colds, stomach ulcers, tonsillitis, grippe, diphtheria, scarlet fever, smallpox, intestinal catarrh, gonorrhea, gleet, bladder ulcers and other illnesses. Homeopathic practitioners prescribe goldenseal root tincture for alcoholism, asthma, cancer, constipation, lupus, sciatica, syphilis, sore throat, uterine problems, liver disorders, including jaundice, and other ailments.

In Ayurvedic medicine, goldenseal is used for obesity, malaria, pyorrhea, hepatitis, diabetes, ulcers, infectious fever, swollen glands and various other afflictions. Like synthetic antibiotics, goldenseal's antibiotic action may be detrimental to good intestinal flora.

Goldenseal preparations are also used as a topical antibiotic and for insect bites, eczema and ringworm.

goldthread
(vegetable gold, canker root, mouth root)
An evergreen perennial, *Coptis groenlandica,* of the Ranunculaceae family, found in the northern United States, Canada, Siberia, India and Iceland, whose root is considered medicinal by Native American and other herbalists. Goldthread (often combined with goldenseal) is used as a tonic and relief from the desire for alcohol. Goldthread is also used to promote appetite and digestion and prevent pinworms.

gotu kola
(brahmi [Sanskrit])
A bitter, cooling Ayurvedic herb, *Hydrocotyle asiatica,* of the Umbelliferae family, used as a nervine, rejuvenative, alterative and diuretic. Gotu kola is said to relieve stress, quiet the mind, alleviate sinus congestion, develop memory and intelligence, and promote sleep. The Sanskrit name is derived from the word *Brahma,* meaning cosmic consciousness.

GRAS list
Food additives *"Generally Recognized As Safe"* authorized by Congress in 1958. The additives selected for this list were chosen because of their absence of known adverse or toxic effects rather than scientific proof of their safety. Motivated by the discovery that cyclamate artificial sweetners caused cancer in laboratory animals, the Nixon administration charged the Food and Drug Administration (FDA) with the responsibility of reevaluating the GRAS list. In 1969 a panel of experts—the Select Committee on GRAS Substances of the Federation of American Societies for Experimental Biology—was assigned this task. By 1980, 305 of 415 substances studied were considered safe enough be given Class 1 status. Although additional research was recommended for 68 Class 2 substances, including vitamins A and D, they were approved for use at current levels. Caffeine, BHA, and BHT were listed as Class 3 ingredients that required additional studies within a given time frame; however, they were allowed to be used pending the outcome of those studies. Salt and four starches were placed in Class 4 with limitations on quantities or certain restrictions. Eighteen substances were recommended for removal from the GRAS list because of insufficient evidence for safety. More than 1,700 food additives are currently on the GRAS list.

gravelroot
(Joe-Pye weed, queen-of-the-meadow, purple boneset)
A North American perennial, *Eupatorium purpureum,* of the Compositae family, named for Joe Pye, a Native American healer who successfully treated typhus fever with gravelroot, and for an Ancient Roman king, Mithridates Eupator, who also used gravelroot as medicine. While large doses of gravelroot induce vomiting, the plant is used therapeutically to relieve calculus, or stones and gravel, in the urinary tract, rheumatism, gout, low back pain, fever and frequent nighttime urination.

growth factors
Poorly understood compounds in food that are known to play a role in the development of some animal species, but requirements in human nutrition are unconfirmed. Growth factors include asparagine, bifidus factor, biopterin, chelating agents, cholesterol, coenzyme Q (ubiquinones), hematin, lecithin, lipoic or thioctic acid, nerve-growth factors, *p*-aminobenzoic acid, various pep-

tides and proteins, pimelic acid and pteridines. It is theorized that humans synthesize these substances in sufficient amounts to satisfy normal growth.

guaiac
(guayacan, lignum vitae, pockwood, guaiacum)
A resin from the trees of the *Guaiacum genus,* such as *G. sanctum* or *G. officinale,* used in allopathic medicine for testing for occult blood in feces. In herbal medicine, guaiac resin (from *G. officinale*) is used as an antiseptic, diaphoretic, diuretic and stimulant, especially in the treatment of syphilis, gout, catarrh and skin diseases.

guggul
(Indian bedellium)
An Ayurvedic preparation made from the gum resin of the tree, *Commiphora mukul,* of the family Burseaceae, containing guggulsterones, isolated substances in the gum gugul resin, considered therapeutic as a rejuvenative, alterative, antispasmodic and expectorant. Guggul is marketed under the trade name Gugulmax.

H

hair analysis

Specimens of human hair examined chemically for the presence of vitamins, minerals and toxins in an attempt to diagnosis various diseases, deficiencies or toxicities. Hair analysis is an unproven technique plagued by inconsistencies in results of hair samples from the same individual in one or more laboratories. However, there may be some validity to public health studies of hair for environmental heavy-metal exposure in various populations. Individually, great caution should be exercised in assigning any value to the results of hair analysis in determining nutritional status.

hair loss

Rarely related to vitamin or mineral deficiency. Vitamin A deficiency may cause hair loss and dandruff to occur, although vitamin A toxicity may have the same result. The anemia that results from a lack of vitamins B_6, B_{12}, folic acid or iron may cause inadequate oxygenation of blood supplying the scalp and affect the appearance of hair or its growth. Biotin deficiency, which is extremely rare, causes hair loss. Scurvy, or severe vitamin C deficiency, causes the hair to split and break below the surface of the skin, resulting in an abnormal circular hair pattern. Copper deficiency, or molybdenum toxicity that interferes with the utilization of copper, causes hair loss. Since copper is also a hair pigment, deficiency may also result in loss of hair coloring. Zinc helps maintain the oil-secreting glands attached to hair follicles, and deficiency is another correctible cause of baldness and dry scalp.

haritaki

(Chebulic myrobalan)

An Ayurvedic herb, *Terminalia chebula*, of the Combretaceae family, used as a rejuvenative, astringent, nervine and laxative.

hawthorn

(May bush, whitethorn, quickset, thorn-apple tree)

A British and European flowering, fruit-bearing shrub or tree, *Crataegus oxyacantha*, of the Rosaceae family, whose flowers and fruits are used by herbalists to regulate cardiac activity, myocarditis, nervous cardiac problems, insomnia and arteriosclerosis. In Ayurvedic medicine, hawthorn is considered a heating agent, stimulant, antispasmodic and diuretic. Chinese practitioners also use the hawthorn plant known botanically as *Crataegus pinnatifida,* or *shan zha.*

headaches

Acute or chronic aches or pain in the head attributable to illness, stress, strain, injury and other problems, but that also may be caused by vitamin A toxicity. Niacin can also cause headaches in therapeutic doses necessary for cholesterol reduction but probably not in doses within the Recommended Daily Allowance (RDA). Vitamin E in doses exceeding 800 I.U. may cause headaches. (See A, VITAMIN.)

hearing loss

Diminished sense of hearing or profound loss, or absence of the sense of hearing. While aging, injury, disease processes, drug reactions and other factors may be responsible, hearing loss may result from vitamin D deficiency, which causes loss of calcium in bones. Therefore, vitamin D is essential to maintain the integrity of the small bones of the middle and inner ear. The cochlea in the inner ear is especially susceptible and may become porous and unable to transmit messages to the hearing center in the brain. Vitamin D supplementation may improve hearing in only those individuals whose loss is secondary to D deficiency. For unknown reasons, an iodine deficiency may result in a rare but correctable type of hearing loss.

heart disorders

See CARDIOVASCULAR DISEASE PREVENTION AND ANTIOXIDANT VITAMINS.

hedyotis

(oldenlandia)

Tropical herbs of the Rubiaceae family, including *H. corymbosa* (or *Oldenlandia corymbosa*) and *H. diffusa,* used in Chinese medicine as treatments for stomach disorders and intestinal diseases, and some believe it to be a cure for cancer. Indian practitioners use hedyotis as a remedy for fever, malaria and depression.

hemochromatosis

Inherited or acquired disorder in which excessive iron in the form of a complex molecule known as hemosiderin accumulates in body tissues. This potentially fatal condition causes tissue damage and disrupts function in the liver, pancreas, heart and pituitary gland. Cirrhosis of the liver, congestive heart failure, diabetes, sexual failure, loss of body hair and bronze pigmentation of the skin are signs.

Primary hemochromatosis is the inherited autosomal recessive form of the disorder and is more common. There are several acquired forms

including one that can occur from excessive blood transfusions and excessive use of iron supplements. (See IRON.)

hemoglobin

Oxygen containing pigment of erythrocytes, or red blood cells. Formed in the bone marrow as a conjugated protein consisting of an iron-containing pigment called heme and a simple protein, globulin. In the lungs, hemoglobin combines with oxygen to form oxyhemoglobin. In the tissues, oxyhemoglobin liberates oxygen in exchange for carbon dioxide. As red blood cells age, they eventually disintegrate, and liberated hemoglobin is removed from circulation by cells of the reticuloendothelial system, especially the liver and spleen. The iron is stored and reused. The globin is converted to amino acids and also re-utilized. (See ANEMIA, MACROCYTIC; ANEMIA, MICROCYTIC.)

hemosiderin

A storage form of iron. Complex granules containing about 33 percent iron by weight, polysaccharides and proteins accumulate in tissue cells of the spleen, liver, and bone marrow. (See HEMOCHROMATOSIS, IRON.)

hemp seed

The seed of the hemp plant, *Cannabis sativa,* of the mulberry family, that can be used whole or ground into a flour. Hemp seed is high in essential fatty acids and ranks second (soybean is first) in protein content. The psychoactive compound tetrahydrocannabinol (THC) in the leaves and flowers of the hemp plant, also known as marijuana, is not found in any appreciable quantity in the seeds, stalk or fiber.

During the Han Dynasty in China, imperial court documents indicate that since 2737 B.C. or earlier hemp was used to alleviate labor pains and as a treatment for general pain, rheumatism and fevers. As a top-notch source of protein, sterilized hemp seeds may be eaten raw or roasted (they are said to taste somewhat like sunflower seeds) or ground into flour and substituted for about one-fourth the flour called for in any recipe.

In 1794, George Washington said, "Make the most of the hemp seed, and sow it everywhere." Although the seeds, oils, paper, clothing fibers, biomass fuel and other commercial and industrial uses of hemp are relatively free of THC, hemp cultivation remains illegal: One cannot grow hemp without also growing its leaves and flowers containing THC, labeled a "controlled dangerous substance." Cannabis extracts and derivatives had been included in clinical and over-the-counter pain remedies until 1976, when the government pronounced marijuana illegal and decided to restrict its use to people suffering from certain diseases. Medicinal uses of the marijuana leaves, particularly for the treatment of the ocular pressure caused by glaucoma; nausea and vomiting caused by chemotherapy in cancer patients; and to relieve the muscle spasms of multiple sclerosis, were banned in 1992 under the Bush administration's war on drugs.

Hemp agrimony (*Eupatorium cannabinum,* also called water maudlin and sweet-smelling trefoil) is a European perennial used by herbalists. The leaves are made into an infusion for treating liver ailments and rheumatism, and a decoction of the rootstock acts as an expectorant. Hemp agrimony is also thought to be effective against constipation and, as a topical remedy, wounds, swellings and other external problems.

Hemp nettle is not of the *Cannabis genus,* but an annual weed known as *Galeopsis tetrahit,* or bastard hemp, of North America, especially Alaska and Canada, used by herbalists for excess bronchial phlegm, anemia, spleen disorders and tuberculosis.

henbane
See HYOSCYAMUS.

hesperidin
Bioflavonoid found in lemons and oranges. (See BIOFLAVONOIDS.)

hibiscus
A genus, *Hibiscus,* including about 200 species, the medicinal of which are *H. abelmoschus* (or musk-mallow), *bancroftanius, esculentus, mutabilis, palustris, rosa-sinensis, sabdariffa, sagittifolius, surattensis, syriacus* and *tiliaceus.* Musk-mallow, also known as Syrian mallow, rose mallow and musk seed plant, is an annual or biennial plant of Egypt, the East and West Indies and India whose seeds are used as a nervine, stomachic, breath-freshener, aphrodisiac and antispasmodic. In Chinese medicine, Chinese hibiscus (*H. rosa-sinensis*) leaves and flowers are remedies for mumps and fever, and *H. syriacus,* or rose-of-sharon, bark, roots and flowers are for dysentery, nausea and internal bleeding. Chinese practitioners also prescribe *H. mutabilis,* or cotton rose, leaves and flowers for pain, excess phlegm, copious menses, dysuria, snakebite and inflammatory problems.

In Ayurvedic medicine, *H. rosa-sinensis,* of the Malvaceae (mallow) family, is used as an alternative, refrigerant, hemostatic and emmenagogue (to induce menses).

holistic medicine
The practice of considering all aspects of an individual—physical, emotional, cultural, spiritual, sociological and economic—in the prevention and treatment of health problems. Many branches of holism incorporate the mind-body connection, that is, the theory that patterns of thinking and behavior affect a person's physical state, traditionally known as "mind over matter." Holistic concepts have been a part of medical and health disciplines and many other human activities since ancient times. The Ancient Greek physician Hippocrates said: "I would rather know what type of person has a disease than what type of disease a person

has." Holistic techniques have finally begun to influence modern physicians, nurses, therapists, social workers and others, and to encourage the development of new ideas. Among the holistic leaders of today are Dr. Bernie Siegel, Dr. Deepak Chopra, Dr. Wayne Dyer, Louise Hay, Dr. Visant Lad, Thomas Moore, Dr. Dean Ornish, Melody Beattie and many others, all of whom have also become popular authors.

holly
Plants of the genus *Ilex* of the Aquifoliaceae family, including *I. pubescens* (*mao dong qing,* in Chinese medicine), *aquifolium* (English holly), *opaca* (American holly), *vomitoria* (Indian black drink), *verticillata* (winterberry or feverbush) and *paraguariensis* (yerba). Various species' parts are used by herbalists to treat a range of ailments, such as gout, stones, arthritis, worms, dyspepsia and other problems.

(See also YERBA SANTA.)

hollyhock
(althea rose, malva flowers, rose mallow)
A perennial flowering Chinese herb, *Althaea rosea,* of the mallow family, found in India and southern Europe and cultivated elsewhere, whose flowers are used as a tea by herbalists to alleviate throat and mouth inflammation.

holy thistle
See BLESSED THISTLE.

homeopathy
A type of medical practice founded by Dr. Samuel Christian Friedrich Hahnemann (1755–1843), based on the theory that "like cures like," that is, a large dose of a drug or other substance that can produce symptoms when given to a healthy person will in a tiny dose cure a sick person with the same symptoms. Modern homeopaths often prescribe tinctures of various herbs and combinations of herbs.

hops
A perennial plant, *Humulus lupulus,* of the Moraceae family, cultivated in the United States and other parts of the world for the manufacture of beer and ale. The hops contain lupulin, a yellow, bitter, kidney-shaped grain often preferred over the hops itself. Native Amerian practitioners prescribe lupulin tincture for delirium tremens, anxiety, worms and pain associated with gonorrhea.

In folk medicine, a root decoction of hops treats both jaundice and dandruff, and homeopathic treatments with hops include dyspepsia and gonorrhea.

Hops' conelike fruit produced by the plant's female flowers is used medicinally as a nervine. Hops tea, for example, is said to calm the nerves as well as treat diarrhea and insomnia, relieve flatulence, intestinal cramps, coughs, excess uric acid and water retention.

hordeum
See BARLEY.

horehound
(marrubium)
A mostly European and North American perennial, *Marrubium vulgare,* of the Labiatae family, named from the Hebrew word *marrob,* or bitter juice. Native American, Ayurvedic and other herbal medicine practitioners use horehound as a cough remedy, expectorant, diuretic, diaphoretic, tonic and stimulant. It has also been prescribed for calming cardiac activity and to restore homeostasis (the body's natural balance) in glandular secretions.

horse chestnut
(buckeye, Spanish chestnut)
An eastern European, Asian and North American deciduous tree, *Aesculus hippocastanum,* of the

family Hippocastanaceae, whose leaves, bark and fruit are used medicinally by herbalists. Varicose veins, hemorrhoids, neuralgia, diarrhea, bronchitis and other ailments have been treated with horse chestnut.

horseradish

A European and Asian perennial, *Armoracia lapathifolia,* or *Cochlearia armoracia,* of the Cruciferae family, cultivated in the United States and most parts of the world. The hot-tasting grated root may be mixed with vinegar and sugar or honey and used as an herbal remedy for pulmonary complaints such as asthma and coughs, gout, rheumatism and bladder infections. Horseradish, commonly eaten as a condiment, may also be made into a tincture, which homeopaths prescribe for other problems including urinary gravel and disorders, scurvy, cataract, colic, headache, toothache, protein in the urine, corneal spots and other eye afflictions and ulcers. Russian *hren* (horseradish) is a rich source of vitamin C and, in Russian folk medicine, used to treat a sluggish liver and dropsy.

horsetail

(shave grass, pewterwort, bottlebrush)
A perennial plant, *Equisetum arvense,* of the family Equisetaceae, whose outer layer contains silica, an astringent substance. Homeopaths and other herbalists including Native Americans use horsetail preparations to treat eye and skin problems, dropsy, gravel, foul perspiration, kidney ailments, urinary pain or difficulty and bleeding.

In Ayurvedic medicine, horsetail is used as a diuretic, diaphoretic and alterative.

horseweed

(fleabane, butterweed, colt's tail, pride weed, Canada fleabane, bloodstaunch)
A North and South American and European flowering annual, *Erigeron canadensis* or *Conyza canadensis,* of the Compositae family, used in herbal medicine as an astringent, diuretic and styptic. Ailments treated with horseweed include diarrhea, dysentery, hemorrhoids, menstrual irregularities, bladder problems, rheumatism and internal bleeding.

houseleek

(thunder plant, Jupiter's beard, hens and chickens)
A European flowering perennial, *Sempervivum tectorum,* of the orpine (Crassulaceae) family, whose leaves are made into infusions or decoctions for internal or external use and prescribed by herbalists to treat shingles, skin problems, hemorrhoids, worms and other ailments.

human milk

See MILK, HUMAN.

humulus

See HOPS.

hydnocarpus

(chaulmoogra tree)
A tree, *Hydnocarpus anthelmintica,* of the Flacourtiaceae family, found in Burma, India and Thailand, whose seeds and seed oil are used by Chinese practitioners for the treatment of leprosy, syphilis, intestinal worms, scabies, gout and rheumatism.

hydrangea

Deciduous or evergreen shrubs of the Saxifragaceae family, including *Hydrangea aspera, strigosa, heteromalla* and *macrophylla,* that are considered medicinal by Chinese practitioners. Named from the Greek words *hydros* and *aggos,* meaning water and jar, hydrangea is used in the treatment of bladder stones, wounds, malaria and certain heart diseases.

hydroxycobalamin
See B$_{12}$, VITAMIN.

hyoscymus
(henbane, stinking nightshade)
A poisonous flowering, foul-smelling plant, *Hyoscyamus niger,* of the Solanaceae family, used as a hallucinogenic during the Middle Ages in Europe, smoked by priestesses at the Oracle of Delphi, and the contemporary source of the narcotic and antispasmodic drug hyoscyamine. While henbane is primarily a narcotic painkiller, Chinese practitioners and other herbalists use it to treat scrotal and breast swellings, gout, painful joints, headache, asthma, toothache, epilepsy and coughs.

Henbane poisoning, similar to atropine poisoning, is characterized by dry mouth; burning pain in the throat; blurred vision; thirst; hot, flushed, dry skin; rapid heart rate; palpitations; restlessness; convulsions; confusion; mania; and delirium, though death is rare. Induced vomiting, stomach lavage and intravenous administration of phyostigmine salicylate may reverse the poison's effects.

hypervitaminosis
Toxicity from any vitamin, but especially the fat-soluble vitamins A and D. (See A, VITAMIN; D, VITAMIN; MEGAVITAMINS.)

hyssop
Mainly a southern European, flowering perennial, *Hyssopus officinalis,* of the Labiatae family, named from the Hebrew word *ezeb,* referred to in Psalm 51:7 as a plant used to purify the body. In Native American medicine, the tops and leaves provide ingredients for a stimulant, aromatic, carminative, tonic and expectorant, especially helpful in treating asthma and pulmonary ailments, high blood pressure, poor circulation, jaundice, gravel, scrofula and epilepsy. In Ayurvedic medicine, hyssop is considered an anthelmintic, diaphoretic and diuretic as well.

I

Iceland moss

(eryngo-leaved liverwort, Iceland lichen)

A lichen—a combination of a fungus and an alga living symbiotically on a surface—found in arctic and mountainous regions, including Iceland, Asia, northern North America, Great Britain and Europe. Iceland moss, *Cetraria islandica,* of the Parmeliaceae or algae family, is considered nutritive because it contains polysaccharides and iodine, but herbalists may prescribe it also as an anti-emetic and demulcent. As a decoction, it is thought to be helpful for pulmonary insufficiency and other upper respiratory problems such as cough, hoarseness and bronchitis, and sometimes for tuberculosis. Iceland moss tea stimulates the flow of breast milk and regulates stomach acid. In order to be used as a food, the plant must be boiled a very long time. Prolonged usage and/or excessive amounts of Iceland moss may induce gastrointestinal and hepatic disturbances. In Ayurvedic medicine, Iceland moss is characterized as cooling, salty, sweet and astringent and used as a tonic, demulcent and alterative.

illicium

(star anise, true anise, Chinese anise, Japanese anise)

A southern Chinese and northeastern Vietnamese plant, *Illicium verum* and *anisatum,* that bears star-shaped fruit used as an aromatic flavoring for liqueurs (such as anisette) and as a spice. The fruit oil of *I. verum* serves as an antidote for poisoning and a treatment for rheumatism in Chinese medicine. The *I. anisatum* plant, not used internally, is prescribed as a topical medicine for skin disorders.

immune system and vitamins

The effects nutrients have on the body's innate ability to ward off disease, such as the fact that vitamin A and beta-carotene improve immune function in measles, respiratory infections and AIDS, possibly reducing deaths. Healthy skin plays an important function in the immune system by acting as a protective barrier against invading microorganisms and vitamin A plays an important role in maintaining the skin.

Immune function deteriorates with age. Many feel that the antioxidant vitamins C and E help preserve immune functions and prevent cancer by blocking the actions of free radicals. Free radicals appear to stimulate the production of prostaglandins, which are involved in inflammatory changes in the tissues and infection.

Vitamin C has long been promoted for its possible protection against the common cold. While this alleged benefit has not been proven, the vitamin does play a role in the production of certain antibodies and interferon. A group of Belgians over age 70 given zinc supplements had a greater immune response to tetanus vaccine and seemed to mount a better response to fighting infection. Pyridoxine, vitamin B_6 deficiency, may have a negative effect on the immune system.

(See also, A, VITAMIN; ANTIOXIDANTS; ASCORBIC ACID; E, VITAMIN; FREE RADICALS.)

imperata

(lalang)

A weed-grass with sharp blades, *Imperata cylindrica,* of the Gramineae family, named for Italian physician and naturalist Ferrante Imperato. In Chinese medicine, the stems, roots and flowers are prescribed as treatments for ailments including kidney, lung and liver diseases, influenza, nosebleed, fever and productive cough. Extracts of lalang are said to have anticancer and antiviral properties, and herbal remedies of lalang are used in Japan, Indochina, the Philippines and Malaysia.

imperial masterwort
A wild, European perennial, *Imperatoria ostruthium,* whose rootstock is used in herbal medicine for gout, cough, poor appetite, cramps, congestion, rheumatism, bronchitis and fever.

Indian turnip
(bog onion, wakerobin, dragonroot)
A perennial, *Arisaema triphyllum,* native to the states east of Louisiana, Kansas and Minnesota, whose partially dried rootstock is used by herbalists after the examples set by Pawnee and Hopi (Native American) tribes. The Pawnee made a powder of the root and applied it to the head as a remedy for headache, and the Hopis mixed it in water for temporary or permanent sterility—a surprising method of birth control. In the 19th century, Native Americans thought the Indian turnip effective against rheumatism, whooping cough and asthma.

indigo, wild
(horsefly bush, rattle bush, yellow indigo)
A southern and eastern United States fruit-bearing, flowering perennial, *Baptisia tinctoria,* of the family Leguminosae, whose root bark and leaves are considered medicinal by Native American herbalists. Indigo tea was given to smallpox sufferers, and according to research done at the Flower Hospital in New York, indigo is an effective remedy for dysentery, colitis, follicular tonsillitis, quinsy, eruptive diseases and ulcerations.

Homeopathic medicine prescribes indigo in the treatment of influenza, mumps, cancer, plague,

typhus, worms, variola, threatened miscarriage and hysteria, among other ailments. Indian and Pakistani practitioners use *guli* or *nil-nilika* (common and Indian indigo) to treat cardiac, liver, spleen, kidney and bladder diseases and nervous disorders including epilepsy.

(See also INDIGOFERA.)

indigofera
A tropical shrub, *Indigofera tinctoria,* of the Leguminosae family, known for its blue dye, used in Chinese medicine for dysentery and liver diseases. In Ayurvedic medicine, indigofera is considered an antibiotic, laxative and alterative.

infections
See IMMUNE SYSTEM AND VITAMINS.

infusion
A liquid or tea made by steeping the leaves of various herbs in boiling water.

inositol
(*myo*-inositol)
Substance chemically related to glucose and essential for the growth of human cells. There are nine isomers of inositol but only *myo*-inositol is of importance to plant and animal metabolism. However, although there is no recommended daily allowance, scientists have discovered that inositol is necessary for the metabolism of calcium in cells. Therefore, it may be considered an essential nutrient in the future. The substance was first discovered in the urine of diabetics more than 100 years ago. However, it was not until 1941 that Gavin and McHenry discovered important metabolic actions in rats. Research by Eagle and colleagues demonstrated a human need by studying tissue cultures. Since bacteria in the human gastrointestinal tract and the manufacture of inositol in

cells seems be adequate, it does not satisfy the definition of a vitamin.

Uses

There are no definite indications for the use of inositol. However, there is preliminary evidence that inositol may benefit some persons with diabetic neuropathy, kidney failure and galactosemia, an inherited metabolic disorder. However, there also may be toxic effects in the latter two disorders (see below).

Inositol is present in human breast milk and may be an important nutrient for infancy. Inositol supplementation appears to be beneficial in low birth-weight infants with respiratory distress syndrome.

Toxicity

Although inositol is generally considered nontoxic, in the presence of kidney failure there may be a dangerous buildup of inositol in the blood. Despite the possibility of beneficial effects of inositol as discussed above, in some cases there may be toxic effects on nerve tissues which may contribute to the development of uremic polyneuropathy. This disorder is characterized by numbness and weakness of the extremities.

insomnia

Inability to sleep. (See TRYPTOPHAN.)

International Unit (I.U.)

Unit of biological material established by the International Conference for the Unification of Formulas. It is used to measure vitamins, enzymes, hormones and other substances.

intrinsic factor

See B$_{12}$, VITAMIN.

inula

Old World and Asian subtropical and temperate herbs including *Inula britannica* and *helenium,* of the Compositae family, used in Chinese and Ayurvedic medicine. The *I. britannica* plant and its roots are considered remedies for hay fever, asthma and bronchitis, and *I. helenium* roots, known as elecampane (*pushkaramula,* in Sanskrit) are used to treat cholera, dysentery, intestinal worms, malarial fever, snakebite and insect stings.

(See ELECAMPANE.)

iodine

A nonmetallic element of the halogen group essential in nutrition for the synthesis of thyroid hormones that control human metabolism. The halogen elements also include bromine, chlorine, fuorine and astatine, all of which form salts with sodium and other metals. Iodine is an essential mineral for all animal species. Iodine is usually in the form of inorganic iodide salts that are readily absorbed and transported to the thyroid gland for utilization and also concentrated in salivary and gastric glands. Excretion of unused iodides are metabolized by the kidneys and lost in the urine. Organically bound iodine-amino acid complexes are less efficiently absorbed, and some are lost in the feces.

Deficiency

Goiter is the most noticeable example of iodine deficiency that causes hypothyroidism, or underactive thyroid gland. The most serious instance is cretinism, a congenital form of mental retardation. Chinese researchers found that dietary iodine given during the first and second trimesters of pregnancy reduced birth defects associated with cretinism by 400 percent. Only 2 percent of the Chinese infants given the supplement early in pregnancy had neurologic problems at birth compared to 9 percent in those supplemented only in the last trimester.

Dietary Sources

Seafoods and water are chief sources of iodine in coastal areas. In mountainous or inland areas, sometimes called the "goiter belt," iodized salt that contains 76 mcg of iodine per gram of salt is the chief source. Milk and other dairy products absorb iodine from iodine-containing disinfectants used on cows, milking machines and storage tanks. Also, iodine is added to animal feeds.

Recommended Allowances

Levels of iodine necessary to prevent goiter are estimated by measuring urinary output. A minimum intake of 50 to 75 mcg of iodine daily is needed to maintain an adequate urinary excretion of the mineral. The U.S. Recommended Daily Allowance (RDA) has been set at 150 mcg for adults to assure an adequate margin of safety.

An extra 25 mcg of iodine is recommended during pregnancy and 50 mcg for nursing mothers.

Toxicity

Iodine intake up to 2 mg per day has not seemed to cause ill effects in Americans. However, bread fortified with 2 to 4 mcg per gram of dry bread fed to a group of Tasmanian Islanders (where there is an endemic high level of goiters) caused a doubling of the usual incidence of thyrotoxicosis.

ipecacuanha

The plant *Cephaelis ipecacuanha,* of the Rubiaceae family, grown in Brazil, and used in allopathic (United States Pharmacoepia), herbal and Ayurvedic medicine as a popular emetic and source of emetine (to induce vomiting). Syrup of ipecac is used primarily to induce the vomiting of noncaustic poisons (including contaminated food and certain drug overdoses). It is also considered an expectorant in the case of intestinal amoebas and as a remedy to relieve asthma and severe congestion.

ipomoea

(vidari-kanda [Sanskrit])

A tropical American plant of the Concolvulaceae family, including *Ipomoea batatas* (sweet potato), *aquatica* (kangkong) and *hederacea.* While some species of ipomoea have hallucinogenic properties, others, such as *I. batatas,* are cultivated and the tuberous roots eaten as a vegetable. The nutritious sweet potato (whose leaves are also considered a vegetable) provides feed for livestock and a stomach, spleen and kidney tonic prescribed by Chinese practitioners. Kangkong, both vegetable and medicine, is thought to be a tonic, laxative and food-poisoning antidote. The seeds of *I. hederacea* induce menses and abortion and counteract constipation, intestinal worms and scanty urine. The plant itself is used as a purgative.

In Ayurvedic medicine, vidari-kanda (*Ipomoea digitata*) provides a nutritive tonic, diuretic and aphrodisiac.

Irish moss

(carrageenan)

A colloid (a substance whose particles are distributed throughout another substance), named after Carragheen (near Waterford), Ireland. The colloid is extracted from red algae and used commercially as a food stabilizer or thickener. In Ayurvedic and other herbal medicine, Irish moss—*Chondrus crispus,* of the Gigartinaceae family—is nutritive because of its iodine, amino acids, polysaccharides and other biochemical constituents, and considered an effective demulcent, emollient, tonic, antitussive and laxative. Herbalists prescribe Irish moss for patients suffering from lung irritations and diseases, dry throat and cough, ulcers and dysentery. Ayurvedic practitioners believe Irish moss to be a sweet, heating agent with nutritive, demulcent and emollient capabilities.

iron

A metallic element commonly found in soil, combined with other minerals and as salts and in mineral waters. Widely used in medicine, it is essential in humans for hemoglobin, cytochrome and other enzymes essential for life. Its chief roles are in the transport of oxygen to the tissues and in oxidation reactions in the cells.

As much as 30 percent of iron is stored in the spleen, liver and bone marrow as ferritin and hemosiderin. Iron is absorbed from the intestinal mucosa or lining and regulated by a complex balance between total iron stores, the amount and type of iron in food and by other dietary factors. Although the ability to absorb more iron increases in the presence of iron deficiency, eventually there may be insufficient dietary supply to keep up with iron loss to prevent anemia.

Historical Background

Iron has been known since ancient times and used in tools and weapons. In the Egyptian Ebers papyrus, an ointment containing rust was mentioned as a treatment for baldness. Male impotency was treated with an iron and wine solution in early Greece. In the 17th century, chlorosis, a condition later recognized as being related to iron deficiency, was treated empirically with iron. Chlorosis, a disorder in which a greenish-yellow skin discoloration was frequently seen in adolescent females in the past, is rare today.

A case of iron overload was first described in 1871. Although the first nutritional study on iron deficiency was reported in 1895, it was not until 1932 that the value of iron therapy was proven.

Recommended Daily Allowances (RDA)

The RDA for iron is based on achieving iron stores of 300 mg to meet the nutritional requirements for healthy people. That level of stored iron is sufficient for several months of an iron-deficient diet. To maintain adequate stores, the RDA for healthy menstruating adolescent and adult women is 15 mg daily. The RDA for postmenopausal women and adult men is 10 mg daily.

The daily dietary allowance of 1.0 to 1.5 mg of iron per kilogram of body weight should be sufficient for most infants. During pregnancy, an estimated total requirement of 1,040 mg of iron is needed to allow for an expanding need for mother, placenta and fetus. Although there is no need for routine supplementation during the first trimester, additional iron is necessary during the later stages of pregnancy. An average increment of 15 mg daily throughout pregnancy should satisfy the requirements of most women.

A diet needs to contain 30 to 90 grams of meat, poultry or fish, all of which provide heme iron, a complex molecule that is highly absorbed. Ascorbic acid (vitamin C) found in plant foods improves the absorption of non-heme iron and is beneficial for people not consuming adequate animal protein. However, there is probably no benefit to adding vitamin C to the easily absorbed ferrous-sulfate form of iron found in most supplements.

Deficiency

As iron deficiency progresses, iron stores are at first diminished without functional impairment. Eventually there is a reduction in quantity of erythrocytes, or red blood cells, and hemoglobin, and the red cells become smaller than normal. The World Health Organization has established that anemia occurs when hemoglobin concentration falls 13 grams/decaliter in adult men and 12 grams in nonpregnant women. During pregnancy 11, 10.5 and 11 grams of hemoglobin respectively, for the

Table 18
MOST COMMON OCCURRENCES OF IRON DEFICIENCY IN THE UNITED STATES

Stage of life	Cause
early childhood (6 months–4 years)	Low iron content of milk is inadequate to meet needs of rapid growth
adolescence	Rapid growth requiring increasing number of red blood cells
childbearing age	Menstrual blood loss
pregnancy	Expanding blood volume of mother, fetus and placenta, blood loss at delivery
Women peri- or post-menopausal women	Abnormal vaginal bleeding (cancer must be ruled out)
Adult men and post-menopausal women	Abnormal blood loss from gastrointestinal tract (cancer must be ruled out)

first through third trimester, are the lower levels of normal.

Iron deficiency may result in reduced physical tolerance even before a fall in hemoglobin is seen. Changes in several constituents of the immune system may also occur, although resistance to infection is questionable. Children may experience apathy, attention deficit, irritability and difficulty learning.

Iron is also essential, with protein, vitamin E and zinc in the metabolism of vitamin A. A high calcium intake may interfere with the absorption of iron and other minerals.

Dietary Iron and Supplements

Iron supplements are preparations or natural sources of the mineral iron that are added to the diet, especially in the incidence of anemia or other indication of iron deficiency. The only times that iron supplementation are recommended for healthy people is during infancy and pregnancy. However, because of poor dietary habits, many menstruating women should probably take iron supplements also. The average American diet fails to provide adequate iron during pregnancy, and these women should receive daily supplements of 15 mg. Although menses is usually absent during lactation, nursing mothers should continue taking iron supplements for about three months postpartum because of the blood loss during delivery.

In the United States wheat flour is enriched with 20 mg of iron per pound. In Sweden and some other countries, an even greater amount of iron is added. Since ferrous sulfate imparts an undesirable taste to bread, reduced metallic iron is used. However, this form of iron is not well absorbed, and commercially available bread is now about equal to beef in iron content and only 1 to 12 percent is absorbed by normal persons. Iron-deficient individuals do absorb a somewhat greater amount.

The second National Health and Nutrition Examination Survey (NHANES II), reported in 1987, showed that not only did supplement-takers consume greater quantities of vitamin C, fruits and vegetables than non-supplement users, but users of vitamin supplements with iron did not have significantly higher levels of iron in their bodies than non-users.

Once the cause of iron deficiency has been found and corrected, the anemia is usually easily corrected by the oral supplementation of iron salts, usually ferrous sulfate. Ferrous sulfate is easily absorbed, and about 20 percent of the iron in each tablet is absorbed. This salt is the standard by which other iron salts are measured. Large quantities of vitamin C increase absorption of iron. Constipation and gastric upset are the most frequent adverse effects of iron supplements. Iron-deficient persons who require full therapeutic doses should start with one tablet daily and gradually increase to the full adult dose of three tablets daily. Most persons can tolerate the 40 to 50 mg of elemental iron required. There may be a vast difference in cost for various iron preparations, but there is little if any therapeutic benefit to the more expensive forms.

If ferrous sulfate causes sufficent gastric irritation to be intolerable, ferrous succinate, lactate, fumerate, glycine sulfate, glutamate and gluconate are absorbed almost as well as the sulfate form, but none are clearly superior. Ferric iron salts, however, are less well absorbed.

Although ascorbic acid increases absorption of iron, preparations that combine iron with vitamin C, molybdenum, copper, cobalt, folic acid and vitamin B_{12} are more expensive and may have some other disadvantages. Enteric coated and timed-release iron preparations should be avoided, because they release the iron in the area of the small intestine with a lower rate of absorption, or they may pass through the intestine too quickly to be absorbed at all.

Liquid iron preparations are available for children and the dosage requirement is generally half the adult dose for weights from 30 to 80 pounds of body weight and full adult dose over 80 pounds. Liquid iron sulfate should be sipped through a straw to prevent staining of the teeth. It is essential to take iron supplements for a minimum of six to

12 months to provide for the replenishment of the body iron stores that are diminished in the presence of anemia. In the existence of chronic blood loss, continuous iron supplementation may be necessary.

Iron dextran (Imferon) injections are rarely required and should be reserved for those persons who are unable to tolerate or absorb oral tablets. Those conditions that may require the intramuscular or intravenous routes for giving iron include: malabsorption disorders such as ulcerative colitis, Crohn's disease, colostomy or ileostomy patients or those rare persons whose iron stores are so severely depleted that large amounts of iron must be administered urgently. Rarely, large doses of injected iron dextran have been reported to cause formation of a sarcoma, a form of malignant tumor. Therefore, injectible iron should be reserved for those persons whose need is absolute.

Toxicity

In normal persons, the possibility of iron toxicity from food sources is remote. In the past there were reports of poisoning from home brews made in iron vessels. However, there are approximately 2,000 cases of iron poisoning in the United States each year from supplements. Most of these occur accidently in children. Three grams of ferrous sulfate, or about nine tablets, can cause death in a two-year-old child.

Primary hemochromatosis is an inherited metabolic disorder in which excessive iron accumulates in the tissues, causing cirrhosis of the liver, congestive heart failure and bronze pigmentation of the skin. Less commonly, there are several acquired forms, one of which can occur from excessive blood transfusions (see HEMOCHROMATOSIS).

Iron supplements cause a grayish-black stool that should be distinguished from the black, tarlike stool that occurs from a bleeding ulcer.

ironweed

A flowering perennial, *Veronica fasciculata,* of the Compositae family, found on prairies, riverbanks and roadsides in the eastern, southern and some western parts of the United States, whose bitter root and leaves are used in Native American medicine as treatment for various gynecological problems, chills and bilious fever, scrofula, dyspepsia and syphilis.

isoniazid

Antimicrobial drug used in the treatment of tuberculosis. However, peripheral neuritis is a common adverse affect that can be prevented by taking pyridoxine (vitamin B_6).

ivy American

(woodbine, Virginia creeper, wild wood vine)
A flowering, fruit-bearing vine, *Vitis quinquefolia,* of the Vitaceae (grape) family, considered in Native American and homeopathic medicine to be a tonic, expectorant and astringent. The bark and twigs are prepared as a syrup, which is prescribed for scrofula, dropsy, cholera, hoarseness, hydrocele and lung diseases.

ixora

Evergreen trees or shrubs, both cultivated and wild, of the Rubiaceae family, such as *Ixora chinensis,* named after a Malabar (from the Malabar Coast, a region of southwest India) god and used by Chinese practitioners to treat rheumatism, pain, abscesses and contusions.

J

jalap

An annual vine, *Ipomoea jalapa,* of the Convolvulaceae family, native to Mexico (Xalapa), with a tuberous root that is used in herbal medicine as a carthartic.

(See also IPOMOEA.)

Japanese turf lily

(dwarf lilyturf, creeping lily root)
The plant *Ophiopogon japonicus,* of the Liliaceae family, whose bulbs are considered a nutritive Yin tonic by herbalists. Turf lily is prescribed for dryness in the body (membranes lacking moisture), dry cough, asthma, insomnia, anxiety and paranoia. Yin represents darkness, cold and wetness in Chinese cosmology. Also considered the "feminine passive" principle in nature, yin combines with yang ("masculine active") to produce all life.

jasmine

(yellow jessamine, yasamin [Arabic])
A fragrant, flowering shrub, *Jasminum officinale,* of the Oleaceae family, whose oil extract is used in perfumes and whose flowers are used in herbal medicine as a calmative. In Ayurvedic medicine, jasmine flowers are also thought to promote menses and to act as an alterative, refrigerant and nervine.

jimson weed

(stinkweed, mad-apple, stinkwort, devil's trumpet, Jamestown weed, nightshade, thornapple, apple Peru)
Annual shrubs and trees of the Solanaceae (nightshade) family, especially the flowering, malodorous *Datura stramonium,* found largely in North and South American fields, gardens, waterfronts and waste areas. Early American colonists discovered jimson weed growing on ship rubbish near Jamestown, Virginia, and called it "Jamestown weed." While jimson weed leaves and seeds may be considered an opium substitute for cases of epilepsy, delirium tremens, mania and general pain, herbalists have pronounced the plant dangerous. An overdose may be fatal. Tincture of jimson weed has been prescribed for hiccough, meningitis, hydrophobia, tetanus, typhus, chorea, catalepsy, apoplexy, angina pectoris, sun headache, enuresis, chronic laryngitis, spasmodic cough and asthma. Jimson weed cigarettes have been used by smokers with asthma.

External uses of the plant by Native Americans include placing crushed leaves and seeds on bruises, saddle sores and swellings and rattlesnake and tarantula bites. The plant, found in varying amounts in hay, is poisonous to horses, cattle and geese.

In October 1994, an outbreak of jimson weed use by teenagers in New Jersey, Connecticut and New York was reported in local newspapers. In New Jersey, the possession or ingestion of jimson weed is illegal, punishable by a maximum of $1,000 fine and six months in jail. One 14-year-old boy became severely ill after eating 30 to 60 jimson weed seeds, and other youngsters had to be hospitalized after eating or smoking the weed.

Not considered a narcotic, the poisonous jimson weed contains toxic chemical properties called alkaloids, which attack the body's central nervous system. Possible adverse effects include hallucinations, tachycardia, dry mouth, blurred vision, elevated body temperature, seizures and other problems that may be life-threatening.

The English settlers of Jamestown used to boil the spring sprouts of jimson weed and eat them as a vegetable. This caused hallucinations and strange, silly behavior that escalated in a matter of days to self-destructive behavior, choking and wallowing in their own waste. The victims were then confined.

jin bu huan

An herb used in traditional Chinese medicine for relief of insomnia and pain. Life-threatening heart irregularities have been reported in children ingesting from seven to 60 tablets of jin bu huan. Cases of hepatitis have also been attributed to this herb.

juglans
(English walnut, Persian walnut)
An Asian and European fruit-bearing tree, *Juglans regia,* of the Juglandaceae family, named from the Latin *Jovis glans* (nut of Jupiter) and considered by the Ancient Greeks and Romans to be a symbol of fertility. Chinese practitioners and other herbalists use the walnut's kernels as a tonic and to increase the flow of urine and the kernel oil to treat intestinal worms and skin diseases. Originally, the walnut was thought to resemble the brain and thus was used in various ways to treat brain disorders.

Walnuts, commonly eaten as snack food or used as an ingredient in spreads, desserts, stuffings and many other foods, contain fats, protein and, like other nuts, the B-complex vitamins niacin, thiamine and riboflavin, and the minerals calcium, iron, copper, manganese and phosphorus.

juncus
(bog rush, Japanese-mat rush)
A Japanese, Chinese, Korean and North American plant, *Juncus effusus* or *decipiens,* of the Juncaceae family, used in the making of tatami floor mats and lampwicks. In Chinese medicine, juncus pith is prescribed for the treatment of cough, pharyngitis, memory loss, insomnia and anxiety.

juniper
(hapusha [Sanskrit])
A North American, European and Asian flowering, fruit-bearing evergreen shrub, *Juniperus communis* and *oxycedrus,* of the Cupressaceae family, used in Chinese herbal medicine to treat bleeding and coughs. Other herbalists use juniper berries and twigs in preparations for the treatment of gastrointestinal cramps, gas, inflammations and infections, gout and rheumatism, tuberculosis and other ailments. In Ayurvedic medicine, juniper berries, in various species of the Coniferae family, are used as a diuretic, diaphoretic, carminative and analgesic.

K

K, vitamin

(phytonadione, vitamin K_1; menadione, vitamin K_3)

A group of compounds with a common basic structure that act as a co-factor for the enzyme system essential for normal blood-clotting. Since vitamin K is produced by bacteria in the intestines, it does not strictly fit the definition of a vitamin. Only about half of the daily requirement is satisfied by intestinal flora. Dietary sources are necessary to prevent vitamin K deficiency. Vitamin K is also found in various foods of plant origin (see Table 19).

Actions

Under normal conditions, in the presence of bile, pancreatic juice and dietary fat, vitamin K is absorbed from the jejunum and ileum of the small bowel. Once absorbed, vitamin K is transported in lymphatic fluid to the liver, where it is concentrated and then widely distributed to body tissues.

In the tissues, vitamin K is associated with cell membranes, most importantly with endoplasmic reticulum and mitochondria. Normally 30 to 40 percent of absorbed vitamin K is excreted in the feces and 15 percent in the urine as metabolic products.

In the liver, vitamin K plays an important role in the actions of prothrombin (coagulation factor II), factors VII, IX, X and proteins C, S and Z. Although these proteins are still synthesized in the absence of vitamin K, they are inactive. In the presence of vitamin K, prothrombin is converted to thrombin, an enzyme. Thrombin in turn converts fibrinogen to fibrin to form a blood clot.

Other proteins that depend on vitamin K are found in bone, kidney and other tissues. Combining with calcium, these proteins help in the formation of bone crystal. Possibly they play a role in the synthesis of some phospholipids and may serve other functions.

The drug warfarin (Coumadin) is the most commonly prescribed oral anticoagulant whose action is based on its ability to counter the effects of vitamin K. Related compounds are the basis for some rat poisons that cause rats to bleed to death. Vitamin K does not reverse overdoses of the injectable anticoagulant heparin.

Vitamin Requirements

The primary criterion for determining the adequacy of vitamin K in humans is based on the maintenance of adequate prothrombin concentrations. Studies have demonstrated that individuals deprived of dietary sources of vitamin K develop clotting problems that can be corrected with resumption of an adequate diet or supplementation of vitamin K. Because there is synthesis of vitamin K by bacteria in the gut of vitamin K-deprived individuals, there is a need for dietary sources of the vitamin.

Studies have also shown that a dietary intake of about 1 mcg per kilogram (1 kilogram = 2.2 pounds) of body weight daily maintains normal blood clotting in healthy adults. Therefore the Recommended Dietary Allowance, or RDA, for a 79-kilogram (174-pound) male is 80 mcg per day and 65 mcg for a 63-kilogram (139-pound) woman.

Ill elderly patients with inadequate prothrombin respond to vitamin K supplementation, but a well-nourished, healthy geriatric population does not appear to need supplements. Trauma, physical dehabilitation, kidney failure and prolonged use of broad-spectrum antibiotics may cause vitamin K deficiency. Antibiotics often destroy the normal intestinal bacterial flora (which synthesize vitamin K) along with the pathogenic (disease-causing) germs. Malabsorption syndromes such as celiac disease disrupt the absorption of adequate vitamin K from the gut. A relative deficiency may occur in the presence of excessive doses of other fat-soluble vitamins A, D or E.

There are insufficient data to establish the RDA during pregnancy or lactation. The diets of pregnant and lactating females appear to exceed the RDA established for adult women. Therefore no supplementation is recommended.

A healthy newborn infant has low plasma prothrombin levels, and levels in premature infants may be inadequate to prevent hemorrhage. Newborn infants are now routinely given 0.5 to 1.0 mg of vitamin K by intramuscular injection. Pre-term infants are given 1 mg or more. The dose may be repeated in one week if needed. Breastfed infants, especially those delivered at home, may be especially prone to vitamin K deficiency. An intake of 5 mcg of vitamin K as phylloquinone or menaquinone per day is recommended for the first six months of life and 10 mcg during the second six months. The recommended amount in infant formulas is 4 mcg of vitamin K per 100 kcal.

RDA for older children is the same as adults, 1 mcg per kilogram of body weight.

Dietary Sources

Green leafy vegetables, some legumes and vegetable oils are the best dietary sources of vitamin K. However, vegetable oils lose much of their vitamin K content when exposed to light. Higher amounts of vitamin K are found in the outer leaves of vegetables while lower amounts are found in inner leaves. Climate and soil conditions may influence amounts of vitamin K in foods. Lesser amounts are found in milk and other dairy products, meats, eggs, cereals, fruits and vegetables. Breast milk is relatively poor in vitamin K content.

In the United States, the usual healthy adult diet contains an average of 300 to 500 mcg of vitamin K. Some studies suggest that these amounts are overestimated. Although a survey demonstrated that only one in 12 persons in the United States consumed green leafy vegetables on a specific day in 1977, deficiencies in Americans appear to be rare.

Preparations

There are several structurally different analogues of vitamin K. Phytonadione, or vitamin K_1, has the quickest onset of action and the most prolonged duration, and it is the most potent of all vitamin K products. It is also safer for newborns than menadione, vitamin K_3.

Toxicity and Other Adverse Effects

With the exception of patients requiring anticoagulants (in which case excessive vitamin K may neutralize the drug's effectiveness), there appears to be no deleterious effect from ingestion of large amounts of oral vitamin K.

Intravenous injections of phytonadione can cause flushing of the face, excessive perspiration, chest tightness, cyanosis, vascular collapse and shock, and severe allergic reactions, including fatal anaphylaxis. Administration of menadione to a person with glucose-6-phosphate dehydrogenase (G6PD) deficiency (a genetic disorder of metabolism) or to newborns may cause hemolytic anemia (destruction of red blood cells) and jaundice. These conditions do not occur with the use of phytonadione. Despite studies questioning the safety of vitamin K administered to newborns, scientists at the National Institute of Child Health and Human Development have concluded that there is no apparent association between vitamin K given to prevent bleeding disorders in infants and an increased risk of childhood cancers.

Herbal teas may contain coumarin derivatives, such as tonka beans, melilot, or sweet clover, and sweet woodruff may be dangerous in patients taking anticoagulants such as warfarin (Coumadin).

kaempferia

An Old World, tropical herb, *Kaempferia galanga,* of the Zingiberaceae family, whose underground stems are used by Chinese practitioners to treat constipation, angina pectoris, headache, toothache

Table 19
PROVISIONAL TABLE ON THE VITAMIN K₁ CONTENT OF COMMON FOODS

Food (estimated portions)†	Vitamin K₁ (mcg/100 gm) median (range)
Abalone (3½ oz.)	23
Algae	
Green laver	4
Purple laver	1385
Konbu	66
Hijiki	327
Amaranth, raw leaf	1140
Apple	
fleshy portion (1 medium)	0.4 (0.1–0.7)
Green peel	60
Red peel	20
Apple juice (3½ fl. oz.)	0.1 (0.01–0.2)
Applesauce (½ cup)	0.5
Apricots, canned with skin (4 halves)	5
Artichoke, globe (1 very small)	14
Asatsuki, leaf	190
Ashitaba, leaf	590
Asparagus, raw (7 spears)	40
Avocado, peeled (1 small)	40
Banana, raw (1 medium)	0.5
Basella, raw leaf	160
Beans (½ cup)	
Blackeyed, dry	5
Kidney, dry	19
Lentil, dry	22
Lima, dry	6
Navy, dry	2
Pinto, dry	10
Soybean, dry	47
Soybean, dry, roasted	37
Beans, pod, raw (1 cup)	47 (40–60)*
Beef, ground, regular, raw (3½ oz.)	0.5 (0.3–0.5)
Beet, raw (½ cup)	3 (0–5)
Bell tree dahlia	
Raw leaf	630
Cooked leaf	1110
Blueberries, canned (⅔ cup)	6
Bread, assorted types (4 slices)	3
Broccoli, raw (½ cup)	205 (147–230)

Table 19 (continued)
PROVISIONAL TABLE ON THE VITAMIN K₁ CONTENT OF COMMON FOODS

Food (estimated portions)†	Vitamin K₁ (mcg/100 gm) median (range)
Broccoli, cooked (½ cup)	270
Brussels sprouts, sprout (5 sprouts)	177 (175–300)
Brussels sprouts, top leaf (5 sprouts)	438 (400–475)
Butter (6 Tbsp.)	7 (6–8)
Butterfly bream (3½ oz.)	0.2
Cheese, Cheddar (3½ oz.)	3 (2–3)
Cabbage	
raw (1½ cups shredded)	145 (46–584)*
Red, raw (1½ cups shredded)	44 (30–57)*
Sauerkraut (1 cup)	25
Turnip	2
Cantaloupe, fresh (⅔ cups pieces)	1
Carrots	
Raw (1⅓ medium)	5 (4–11)*
Cooked (⅔ cup slices)	18
Cauliflower	
Raw (1 cup)	5
Cooked (1 cup)	10
Celery, raw (2½ stalks)	12 (5–18)
Cereal	
Bran flakes (2½ cups)	2
Corn flakes (4 cups)	0.04
Puffed rice (7 cups)	0.08
Puffed wheat (7 cups)	2
Shredded wheat (4 oz.)	0.7
Total brand (4 oz.)	0.7
Chayote	
Raw leaf	200
Cooked leaf (½ cup pieces)	270
Chicken meat, raw (3½ oz.)	0.1 (0.01–0.2)
Chili con carne (3½ oz.)	2
Chingentsuai, raw green	120
Chive, raw (33 Tbsp. chopped)	190 (130–250)
Chrysanthemum, garland	350
Clam (4 large or 10 small)	0.2
Coffee (10 cups brewed beverage)	10 (<0.005–20)

Food (estimated portions)†	Vitamin K_1 (mcg/100 gm) median (range)
Cola	
Regular (3½ fl. oz.)	<0.005
Diet (3½ fl. oz.)	<0.005
Coleslaw (¾ cup)	57
Coriander	
Raw leaf (6¼ cups)	310
Cooked leaf	1510
Corn, sweet, raw (½ cup)	0.5
Crackers	
Graham (14 crackers)	0.5
Saltines (33 crackers)	2
Cranberry juice (3½ fl. oz.)	<0.005
Cranberry sauce (⅓ cup)	1
Cucumber	
Raw (1 cup slices)	19 (5–50)*
Raw, peel only	360
Fleshy portion only	2
Eel (3½ oz.)	0.02
Egg	
Yolk (5 large)	2 (0.01–4)
White (3 large)	0.01 (0–0.02)
Eggplant, raw (1¼ cups pieces)	0.5
Endive, raw (2 cups chopped)	231
Flour (1 cup)	
Barley	1
Buckwheat	7
Rice	0.04
Wheat	0.6 (0.1–1)*
Fruit cocktail, canned (½ cup)	0.8
Fruit spread, assorted flavors	0.5
Fungi	
Shitake, raw	0
Shimeji	0
Nameko	0
Ginger ale	
Regular (3½ fl. oz.)	0.01
Diet (3½ fl. oz.)	<0.005
Grape juice (3½ fl. oz.)	0.2
Grapes, fresh (1 cup)	3
Grapefruit, fresh (½ medium)	0.02

Table 19 *(continued)*
PROVISIONAL TABLE ON THE VITAMIN K₁ CONTENT OF COMMON FOODS

Food (estimated portions)†	Vitamin K_1 (mcg/100 gm) median (range)
Grapefruit juice (3½ fl. oz.)	0.2 (0.02–0.3)
Honey (5 Tbs.)	0.02 (0.01–0.02)
Horse, meat (3½ oz.)	2
Itohiki-natto	10
Kaiwaredaikon, raw leaf	80
Kale, raw leaf (¾ cup)	817 (724–1139)*
Kiwi fruit (1 medium)	25
Komatsuna, raw leaf	280
Leek, raw (1 cup chopped)	14 (10–18)
Lemon, fresh (2 medium)	0.2
Lemonade (3½ fl. oz.)	0.03
Lettuce (1¾ cups, shredded)	
Raw, heading & bib	122 (70–850)*
Red, leaf	210
Mackerel (3½ oz.)	5
Malabar gourd, raw leaf	22
Margarine (7 Tbsp.)	51 (4–97)*
Mayonnaise (7 Tbsp.)	81
Meatloaf (3½ oz.)	6
Milk, cow:	
Chocolate, 2% Fat (3½ fl. oz.)	0.4
Dry, whole (1 cup)	2
Skim (3½ fl. oz.)	0.02 (0.01–0.03)
Whole, 3.5% fat (3½ fl. oz.)	0.3
Millet, dry (3½ oz.)	0.9
Mint	
Raw leaf	230
Cooked leaf	860
Mituba, raw leaf & stalk	370
Miso, dry (½ cup)	11
Mushroom, raw (1½ cups)	0.02 (0.02–<1)
Mustard greens, raw (1½ cups)	170
Nightshade	
Raw leaf	620
Cooked leaf	700
Oatmeal, instant, dry (1 cup)	3
Octopus (3½ oz.)	0.07
Oils (7 Tbsp.):	
Almond	7
Canola (Rapeseed)	141

Food (estimated portions)†	Vitamin K_1 (mcg/100 gm) median (range)
Corn	3
Olive	49 (42–55)
Peanut	0.7
Safflower	11 (9–12)
Salad	148
Sesame	10 (5–15)
Soybean	193
Sunflower	9
Walnut	15
Onions, (⅔ cup, chopped)	
White, raw	2 (0.2–5)*
Green scallion, raw	207 (170–243)
Welsh (white)	5
Welsh (green)	243
Orange, fleshy portion (1 medium)	0.1 (0.01–0.1)
Orange juice, fresh (3½ fl. oz.)	0.1 (0.04–0.1)
Osh, raw leaf	310
Oyster (7 medium)	0.1
Pacific Saury (3½ oz.)	0.02
Parsley	
Raw leaf (1½ cups chopped)	540 (350–730)
Cooked leaf	900
Parsnip	1
Pea	
Raw	36 (33–39)*
Pod, raw	25 (20–50)
Green, cooked (⅔ cup)	23
Peaches	
raw (1 medium)	3 (2–3)
Peanut, raw	0.2
Peanut butter (6 Tbsp.)	10
Pear, canned (½ cup)	0.5
Pecan, dry	10
Pepper, raw, green (1 cup, chopped)	17 (2–30)*
Perilla, raw, leaf	650
Pickle, dill (1 medium)	26
Pineapple, fresh (½ cup, pieces)	0.1

Food (estimated portions)†	Vitamin K_1 (mcg/100 gm) median (range)
Pineapple juice, canned (3½ fl. oz.)	0.7
Pistachio nut (170 nuts)	70
Plum, fresh, raw (2 medium)	12
Pork, meat (3½ oz.)	0.07 (0.03–0.1)
Potato, baked flesh and skin (1 med)	4
Potato, baked skin only	0.3
Potato, sweet, canned (1 cup)	4
Potato, raw (1 potato)	0.8 (0.2–4)*
Potato chips (4 oz.)	10
Potato, french fries (20 pieces)	5
Prawn (3½ oz.)	0.03
Pretzel (4 oz.)	1
Prune juice, canned (3½ fl. oz.)	0.6
Pumpkin, canned (½ cup)	16
Purslane, raw	381
Radish, raw (22 radishes)	0.1
Rice, white (½ cup)	1 (0.05–2)*
Rice cake	0.6
Roctish	
Raw leaf	290
Cooked leaf	420
Sake (3½ fl. oz.)	<0.005
Salmon, pink (3½ oz.)	0.4
Samat	
Raw leaf	350
Cooked leaf	960
Sardine (3½ oz.)	0.09
Sesame seed, dry (11 Tbsp.)	8 (2–14)*
Sour cream (8 Tbsp.)	1
Soy milk (3½ oz.)	3 (2–5)*
Spaghetti, dry (3½ oz.)	0.2
Spaghetti sauce, meat-based (4 oz.)	4
Spinach	
Raw, leaf (1½ cups)	400 (240–1220)*
Raw, stalk	6
Squid (3½ oz.)	0.02

Table 19 (continued)
PROVISIONAL TABLE ON THE VITAMIN K₁ CONTENT OF COMMON FOODS

Food (estimated portions) †	Vitamin K₁ (mcg/100 gm) median (range)
Squash, summer	
Fleshy portion	3 (1–4)
Peel only	80
Swiss chard, raw leaf	830
Tea	
Black, Brewed (3½ oz.)	0.05
Black, Leaves (Dry)	262
Decaffeinated, Brewed (3½ oz.)	0.03
Green, Leaves (Dry)	1428
Tofu (½ cup)	2
Tomato	
Ripe (1 tomato)	6 (6–7)*
Juice, canned (3½ fl. oz.)	4 (2–6)*
Sauces (3½ fl. oz.)	7 (1–13)
Top shell	3
Toumyao (Chinese)	380
Tuna, bluefin (3½ oz.)	0.03
Turkey, meat (3½ oz.)	0.02
Turnip	
Raw	0.09 (0.09–<1)
Greens, raw (1½ cups, chopped)	251 (192–310)*
Tziton, raw leaf	250
Watercress, raw (3 cups)	250 (88–390)*
Wine (3½ oz.)	<0.005
Yellowtail, young (3½ oz.)	0.08
Yogurt	
Low fat (3½ oz.)	0.3 (0.2–0.3)
Fruit flavored (3½ oz.)	0.7

Reference: Booth S.L., Sadowski J.A., Weihrauch J.L., Ferland G. Vitamin K₁ (Phylloquinone) content of foods: A provisional table. *J Food Comp Anal* 1993;6:109–20.

† Calculated based on estimated portions to equal 100 gm from Pennington J.A., Church H.N.: *Food Values of Portions Commonly Used,* 14th & 15 Editions, J. P. Lippincott Company, 1985.

*More reliable in comparison to the other data based on the analytical quality control criteria.

(Table from Coumadin Patient Guide with permission from DuPont-Pharm.)

and cholera. Kaempferia also serves as a flavoring agent for rice and as an ingredient in cosmetics.

kalanchoe
(air plant, Mexican love plant, life plant, good luck leaf)
A pantropic (though mainly African) plant, *Kalanchoe pinnata,* of the Crassulaceae family, whose leaves are used in Chinese medicine to treat coughs, headache, skin diseases and other ailments.

kale
A hardy cabbage, *Brassica oleracea acephala,* of the Cruciferae family, eaten as a vegetable or taken in tablet form as a supplement mainly for its calcium, vitamin A, ascorbic acid, thiamine, riboflavin, niacin and folacin content. The particularly high calcium content (common to dark-green leafy vegetables) has been recognized as an anti-colon-cancer agent, an antistress mineral, often called "nature's tranquilizer," and a preventive against osteoporosis in certain women.

katphala
See BAYBERRY.

kava kava
(kawa)
A Polynesian herb, *Piper methysticum,* of the Piperaceae family, whose root is considered a remedy for insomnia and anxiety by herbal medicine practitioners. It is also prescribed as a painkiller and, because it has antiseptic and diuretic properties, for urinary tract infections. Regular use of kava kava, however, may cause toxins to build up in the liver.

Pippali, an Ayurvedic medicine (*Piper longum* of the same family as kava kava) is said to be an expectorant, stimulant and aphrodisiac. The Sanskrit word *pippali* means "long pepper."

kelp

A variety of brown seaweeds of the order Laminariales, found largely in cold and temperate seas, and whose ashes are recognized as a source of iodine, potash and soda. Iodine is an essential component of thyroxine, the active substance produced in the thyroid gland. Kelp in tablet or other supplemental form is helpful in any iodine deficiency, including hypothyroidism and goiter.

Kempner's Rice Diet

A treatment for psoriasis, hypertension and renal disease. Developed by American physician Walter Kempner (1903–   ). This diet, consisting of only rice, fruit juices and sugar with vitamin and iron supplements, is generally considered a nutritionally poor diet with no therapeutic value.

Keshan disease

A type of cardiomyopathy, a form of heart disease primarily occurring in children on a selenium-poor diet. First recognized by Chinese scientists in 1979, in areas with soil poor in selenium, such as parts of China, New Zealand and Finland.

(See also SELENIUM.)

khus-khus

(vetiver)

A tropical and subtropical Asian and East Indies perennial grass, *Vetiveria zizanioides,* whose aromatic root is made into a tea considered to be a general tonic.

kidney disorders and vitamin requirements

The process of renal dialysis removes metabolic products derived from ascorbic acid (vitamin C), folic acid and pyridoxine (vitamin B_6). One hundred to 300 percent of the Recommended Daily Allowance (RDA) of the nutrients should be given to renal-dialysis patients. With the possible exception of vitamin E, there are no other increased needs for vitamin supplementation with dialysis.

kidney liver leaf

(choisy, noble liverwort)

A flowering, evergreen plant, *Hepatica americana* and *nobilis,* of the Ranunculaceae family, used in Native American herbal medicine as a liver tonic and remedy of liver diseases. Homeopathic medicine also prescribes liver leaf for bronchitis, sore throat and dyspepsia.

knotweed

(bian xu, knotgrass, pigweed, birdweed, beggarweed, crawlgrass, ninety-knot)

An annual plant, *Polygonum aviculare,* cultivated throughout the world and whose flowering herb is used by herbalists as a remedy for diarrhea, dysentery, enteritis, bronchitis and other respiratory problems, jaundice, internal bleeding (including bleeding stomach ulcers), cholera infantum and other ailments.

In addition, *Polygonum hydropiper* and *punctatum,* also called smartweed, are used in decoctions for hemorrhoids and scabies, as well as for gargle and rubefacient, a local irritant that produces reddening of the skin for therapeutic purposes.

knoxia

An Asian Indian herb, *Knoxia corymbosa,* of the Rubiaceae family, whose tuberous root is used in Chinese medicine for inflammation, abdominal dropsy and excretory-system problems. The herb is named for R. Knox of Sri Lanka.

kola tree

(cola, kola nut, caffeine nut, guru nut)

A South American, West African and West Indies tree, *Cola acuminata,* of the family Sterculiaceae, whose nuts contain caffeine and flavoring agents used in pharmaceutical preparations and in carbonated beverages. Caffeine, recognized by the United States Pharmacopoeia (USP), is an alkaloid that acts as a stimulant to the central nervous system, the stomach, fatty acids in plasma and basal metabolic rate. Caffeine, also a diuretic, decreases sleep time, may increase blood-sugar level and enhances endurance and reaction time in athletes.

Herbal medicine practitioners prescribe kola nut seeds as a cardiac tonic, pain reliever, especially of neuralgia and migraine, and an antidepressant.

While caffeine is found in coffee, tea, chocolate and cola drinks, and in Anacin, Excedrin and other over-the-counter medicines, it is also available in pill or tablet form under the brand names Vivarin and No-Doz specifically for antifatigue use.

An excess of 250 mg is usually considered an overdose of caffeine that may lead to caffeine intoxication (caffeinism). Symptoms include restlessness, flushing, frequent urination, twitching, increased heart rate and/or irregularities, agitation and other problems. Delirium, convulsions, nausea, vomiting and respiratory and cardiovascular collapse may result. Treatment may include gastric lavage and the administration of phenobarbital or diazepam, and cardiopulmonary resuscitation (CPR).

Korsakoff's syndrome
See ALCOHOLISM; THIAMINE.

kousso
An Ethiopian flowering tree, *Hagenia abyssinica,* whose flowers are used in herbal medicine as an anthelmintic, especially for tapeworms.

Krebs, Ernst
See AMYGDALIN.

kudzu
(kuzu, ge gen)
An herb, *Radix puerariae,* containing varying quantities of the chemical daidzin in its roots, leaves and flowers. Listed in the Chinese pharmacopeia about 1,400 years ago, kudzu is reported to reduce the craving for alcohol in abusers. Studies on Syrian Golden hamsters, one of the rare instances of animals who prefer drinking alcohol to water, demonstrated a markedly decreased desire to drink alcohol in those given the extract or purified daidzin.

The root of the kudzu plant *Pueraria thunbergiana* yields a concentrated starch that is often used as a thickener in foods and for its high mineral content in tea and soup for sufferers of flu, colds and gastrointestinal ailments.

In Chinese medicine, pueraria root, or *ge gen,* is from the *Pueraria lobata* plant and used to treat chills, fever, poor circulation, high blood pressure, excessive thirst and muscle ache.

Ayurvedic practitioners use kudzu, of the *Pueraria tuberosa* plant of the Leguminosae family, as a tonic, diuretic and diaphoretic.

kumari
See ALOE.

L

labeling requirements
See Appendix 8; Foreword.

Labrador tea
(wild rosemary, continental tea, marsh tea)
A North American evergreen shrub, *Ledum latifolium,* of the Ericaceae family, whose leaves are made into a tea and considered by Native American herbalists to be therapeutic in the treatment of respiratory infections. Homeopaths prescribe a tincture of the entire plant or of the leaves and dried twigs for asthma, gout, intoxication, tuberculosis, varicella, tinnitus, ear inflammation, deafness, foot and joint pain and, in a decoction used externally, for problems including eczema, pediculosis, prickly heat and other skin eruptions and wounds. Practitioners of folk medicine also use Labrador tea for headache, stomachache, diarrhea, rickets and urinary tract weakness, among other problems.

lacto-ovo vegetarian
Person whose diet includes vegetables, milk products and eggs, but who avoids meat, sea food and poultry. (See VEGETARIAN DIETS.)

lactovegetarian
Person who eats vegetables and milk products, but avoids eggs, meat, fish and poultry. (See VEGETARIAN DIETS.)

lady's mantle
A North American, European, northern Asian and Greenland flowering perennial, *Alchemilla vul-*garis or *xanthochlora,* of the Rosaceae family, whose aerial portion is prepared as a tea and used by herbalists to treat menstrual problems, rheumatism, gastrointestinal disturbances, poor appetite and external problems including wounds.

Silvery lady's mantle, or *Alchemilla alpina,* is used as lady's mantle and for the treatment of intestinal gas.

lady's slipper
(nerve root, yellow moccasin flower, Noah's ark)
European, Asian, tropical and North American orchids (Orchidaceae family), especially *Cypripedium pubescens,* whose root is valued by Native American, Ayurvedic and other herbalists and homeopaths as a nervine, tonic and antiperiodic. Uses of lady's slipper as a tincture, decoction or infusion include pain relief and the treatment of anxiety, nervous headache, nervous depression and restlessness, hysteria, chorea, nervous stomach, fever, convulsions, delirium tremens, epilepsy, neuralgia, stye and other ailments.

laetrile
See AMYGDALIN.

larch
An American and European tree, *Larix europaea,* of the pine family, whose bark, resin, young shoots and needles are used by herbal practitioners to make a diuretic extract and a decoction that may be added to bath water as a stimulant. The resin, called "Venice turpentine," derives its reputation from European folk medicine in which a certain number of drops mixed with honey are considered

effective against tapeworm, suppressed menses and bloody diarrhea.

larkspur
(knight's spur, lar's heel, lark's claw)
A European and North American flowering annual herb, *Delphinium consolida,* of the Ranunculaceae family, whose roots and seeds have been considered medicinal by Native American, Russian, folk-medicine herbalists and others, although extremely cautious use is advised by these practitioners because delphinium is poisonous. Limited amounts of preparations made from the larkspur herb, flower and other parts may be effective in the treatment of cramps, pleurisy, headache, convulsions, amenorrhea, Parkinson's disease, paralysis and other ailments.

laurel
(bay leaves, bay laurel, sweet bay, Indian bay, Roman or Grecian laurel)
An evergreen bush or tree originally cultivated near the Mediterranean Sea, *Laurus nobilis,* of the Lauraceae family, whose leaves are used in Ayurvedic medicine as a carminative, stimulant and expectorant, and by other herbalists to promote digestion.

lavender
A shrub, *Lavandula vera, officinalis* and *angustifolia,* of the Labiatae family, originally from the Mediterranean area and cultivated in Europe and the United States for its aromatic flowers. In Ayurvedic medicine, lavender is used as a carminative, diuretic and antispasmodic. Other practitioners also consider lavender an antidepressant, nervine, tonic, stimulant and stomachic. Flowers and leaves are used in oil preparations for flatulence, migraine, vertigo and fainting. European herbalists find lavender an effective appetite stimulant and reliever of colic. Lavender is also a main ingredient in the Chinese medicinal oil known as "white flower oil," prescribed for headache, nervousness, upset stomach and other problems. It is also used as an external treatment of insect bites (lavender contains insect- and moth-repelling camphor), cuts and bruises. Lavender tea is considered a vermifuge, i.e., an agent that eliminates intestinal worms.

laxative effects on nutrients
Mineral oil binds to fat-soluble vitamins A, D, E and K and linoleic acid, an essential fatty acid. This binding prevents absorption of the nutrients as they pass through the intestine and they are lost in the stool. Chronic use could result in deficiencies from these vitamins, especially night blindness from lack of vitamin A, bone disorders from inadequate vitamin D and hemorrhage from insufficient vitamin K.

Other laxatives also effect changes in the intestinal mucosa, or lining, causing poor or inadequate absorption of not only the fat-soluble vitamins but also other vitamins and minerals.

lead
A metallic element, known in Latin as *plumbum,* whose compounds are poisonous. It is unknown if traces of this mineral are essential in human nutrition. If required, it is sufficiently plentiful in food, water and air to satisfy human needs.

Forty cases of lead poisoning were reported in California children in 1991 when they were given ethnic folk remedies. Most of these cases were from powders given for digestive problems in Mexican children ranging in age from eight months to five years.

lecithin
A group of fatty substances (named from the Greek word *lekithos,* meaning egg yolk) called phospholipids, or phosphoglycerides, found in egg

yolk, natural oils (such as soybean) and in blood, bile, nerves, brain and various animal tissue. Phospholipids are formed in all cells of the body, though the ones that enter the bloodstream are mainly produced in the liver and intestinal mucosa.

The main function of phospholipids is to maintain the structural integrity of the cells. Lecithin is also a natural bile component important in the metabolism of fat in the liver, and it helps dissolve gallstones. Of the various phospholipids, the lecithins reach the most areas of the body. As a food additive, especially in cheese, margarine and sweets, lecithin performs as an emulsifier and antioxidant.

When hydrolyzed, lecithin produces stearic acid, glycerol, phosphoric acid and choline. Lecithin is a source of the B vitamins cholin and inositol, and it is capable of breaking down fat and possibly cholesterol that clogs arterial walls.

Available in health-food stores as capsules or in granulated form, lecithin was championed by the late American nutritionist Adelle Davis as a dietary supplement that indicated effectiveness for individuals who suffered heart attacks caused by high blood cholesterol. Davis believed granular lecithin, which may be added to breads, pancakes, casseroles, soups, milkshakes, meatloaf and many other recipes, is more valuable than lecithin capsules.

lemon

The yellow, acid fruit of the *Citrus limon* tree, of the Rutaceae family, used as a home remedy both internally and externally. With enough of a vitamin C content to prevent or treat scurvy, lemon juice added to hot water is considered therapeutic for colds and coughs (for persistent cough, honey may be added to the mixture), headache, sore throat and rheumatism. Once commonly called a "physic," lemon juice in water was thought to promote digestion and elimination. Lemon also serves as a substitute for vinegar, spices and aromatic substances for individuals who cannot tolerate the

latter, and lemon is safe for use by people with diabetes. A distinct disadvantage of drinking large amounts of lemon juice or sucking lemon juice directly from the lemon, however, is the potential erosion of tooth enamel.

Lemon juice is also used as an astringent, an enema, on warts and corns and as a hair rinse. Lemon powder helps arrest bleeding.

(See also LIME.)

lemon balm
(melissa, balm)
An Old World perennial, bushy herb, *Melissa officinalis,* of the Labiatae family, known for its lemony, aromatic leaves. In Ayurvedic medicine, lemon balm is thought to be a diaphoretic, carminative and nervine. Many other herbalists use lemon balm for a number of healing purposes, particularly nervous disorders, after the example set by 9th- and 10th-century Arabian physicians who prescribed it for heart palpitations and anxiety. Because it is a mint, lemon balm infusion (tea) is prescribed for stomachache, fever, depression, tension and irregular menses. The external uses of lemon balm include the treatment of herpes simplex, rheumatism, neuralgia and wounds.

lemongrass
(rohisha [Sanskrit])
A tropical grass, *Cymbopogon citratus,* of the Graminaceae family, known for its essential oil whose odor is reminiscent of lemon or verbena. Ayurvedic practitioners use the pungent, bitter herb as a diuretic, diaphoretic and refrigerant.

leonurus
(motherwort, yi mu cao)
An herb found in northeastern Asia, Japan and Taiwan, *Leonurus sibiricus* or *heterophyllus,* of the Labiatae family, named from the Greek words meaning lion's tail because of the plant's form.

Leonurus seeds are used in traditional Chinese medicine to treat problems involving urination and menstruation and to cool the body.

lepidium

(peppergrass)

An herb, *Lepidium apetalum,* of the Cruciferae family, grown in temperate regions and known for its mucilage. Chinese practitioners prescribe lepidium root for colds, cough and excessive sputum production.

leverwood

(hop horn beam, ironwood, deerwood)

A North American tree, *Ostria virginiana,* of the Betulaceae family, whose inner wood and bark are used in Native American and homeopathic medicine for the treatment of fever, stomach ache, neuralgia, headache, liver problems, lumbago and malarial anemia.

licorice

(sweetwood, sweet licorice, gan cao, yasthi madhu [Sanskrit])

An Asian and southern European perennial, *Glycyrrhiza glabra,* among other species of the Leguminosae family, whose root and rootstock are well-known for their flavor when used in cough medicines, syrups, lozenges, liqueurs and candies. While licorice taken in large amounts can cause salt retention, elevated blood pressure and excessive potassium loss through the urine, it is used as a demulcent and mild expectorant, called glycyrrhiza.

Herbalists prepare the dried root of licorice as a remedy mainly for respiratory problems such as bronchitis, cough and congestion, and for stomach and intestinal complaints such as ulcers and constipation.

Licorice grows wild in India and Pakistan. In Ayurvedic practice, licorice is considered a demulcent, tonic, laxative and expectorant with cooling, sweet and bitter properties. Therapeutic use includes the treatment of hyperacidity, painful urination and general debility. Licorice, which may also be added to ghee (see GHEE), is thought to be a rejuvenative food and an agent to calm the mind, increase cerebrospinal and cranial fluid, improve vision, hair, complexion and voice, tone the mucous membranes, relieve muscle spasm and promote a sense of contentment. However, Ayurvedic practitioners do not recommend licorice for those suffering from edema, high blood pressure or osteoporosis.

life root

(golden senecio, squaw weed, ragwort, false valerian, cocash weed, female regulator)

North American perennial flowering herbs of the genus *Senecio,* such as *S. aureus,* of the Compositae family, whose root and herb are considered medicinal by homeopaths, Native American and other herbalists. Although senecio is mainly prescribed for a number of gynecological problems, including painful menses, adverse effects of menopause and weak ligaments of the uterus, it is also used to treat atonic, enlarged prostate, pulmonary complaints, renal colic, sciatica, pain in the spermatic cord, gravel, diarrhea, stones, gonorrhea, dysuria, kidney inflammation, angina pectoris, liver disturbances, ulcers, colitis and many other ailments.

ligusticum

(lovage, chuan xiong)

Asian and European perennials of the *Ligusticum genus,* such as *L. striatum* and *L. wallichii,* whose root or rhizome is used by traditional Chinese practitioners and other herbalists to treat pain, headache, poor circulation, scanty menstrual flow, gout and rheumatism. Lovage has long been known in many countries' legends as an ingredient in love potions.

(See also LOVAGE.)

ligustrum
(nu zhen zi, Nepal privet, glossy privet, white wax tree)

A Chinese, Japanese and Korean evergreen tree, *Ligustrum lucidum,* of the Oleaceae family, whose bark, leaves and fruits are used by Chinese and other herbalists as a diaphoretic, tonic, painkiller and treatment for coughs, swelling, vertigo, fever and headache.

lilium
(lily bulb, bai he)

A Chinese flowering plant, *Lilium brownii* or *colchesteri,* of the Liliaceae family, whose bulb scales are used by traditional Chinese and Ayurvedic practitioners and other herbalists as a demulcent, nutritive tonic, nervine and treatment for urinary problems, deafness, gas and respiratory complaints.

lime
The yellowish-green fruit *Citrus acida* (also *C. aurantifolia*) from tropical citrus trees of the Rutaceae family, that is a source of vitamin C. Ayurvedic and other herbalists use lime as a refrigerant, carminative and expectorant.

Lime is also the alternate name of calcium oxide (USP), a substance recognized in the United States Pharmacopoeia as an ingredient obtained from limestone and used in the making of mortar and cement. Lime water is an alkaline solution of calcium hydroxide in water that is used as an antacid.

linden
(lime blossom, linden flower, American basswood, spoonwood, wycopy, lime tree)

Various species of trees of the *Tilia* genus, such as *T. cordata, americana* and *europaea,* whose flowers, leaves and inner bark are considered of medicinal value by Native American and other herbalists. Linden is commonly prescribed for nervous disorders including epilepsy, colds, cough, hoarseness, mucus congestion, gynecological problems, neuralgia, hives, peritonitis, rheumatism, headache, sterility and absence of menses. A combination of linden charcoal and goat's milk is administered to individuals with tuberculosis.

In addition to medicinal preparations, linden trees provide honey touted as excellent by many herbalists. Linden tar can be applied to eczema, and soft, light linden wood with its fine grain attracts carvers.

lindera
(wu yao)

A Chinese and Taiwanese fragrant shrub, *Lindera strychnifolia,* of the Lauraceae family, named for Swedish physician J. Linder (1676–1723), whose roots are prepared as medicine by traditional Chinese herbalists for the treatment of intestinal worms, indigestion, abdominal inflammation, hernia, asthma, cholera, menstrual pain and urinary-tract weakness.

linoleic acid
An essential fatty acid required for maintaining the integrity of cellular membranes. Human deficiency was not discovered until the early 1970s when hair loss, scaly skin and poor wound-healing was noted in a group of hospitalized patients fed intravenously with fat-free fluids. Chronic users of the laxative mineral oil and persons with chronic diarrhea, especially in cystic fibrosis, may be lacking this nutrient.

linum
See FLAX.

lion's root
(cancer weed, white lettuce, prenanthes serpens)

A North American perennial herb, *Nabalus serpentaria,* of the Compositae (suborder Chicoraceae) family, whose milky juice is used by Native American and other herbalists as an astringent and antiseptic, especially in the case of diarrhea and dysentery. Homeopaths also prescribe tincture of lion's root for constipation and ophthalmia.

lipids
See FAT.

litchi
(lychee, li zhi he)
A southern Chinese fruit of the *Litchi chinensis* tree, of the Sapindaceae (soapberry) family, with a hard reddish covering and white, sweet flesh around a large seed, also called a litchi nut. While litchi nuts are a popular addition to desserts in Chinese cuisine, Chinese practitioners use the fresh fruit as a tonic and treatment of cough and diarrhea, the seeds as painkillers and for treatment of testicular inflammation, ulcers, hernia and lumbago, and the fruit with skin and leaves as a remedy for poisonous animal bites.

lithium
A metallic element, named from the Greek word *lithos,* meaning stone. It is unknown if traces of this mineral are essential in human nutrition. If required, it is sufficiently plentiful in food, water and air to satisfy human needs. Drugs containing lithium salts are used in the treatment of bi-polar (also known as manic) depression.

L-lysine
(α,ϵ-diaminocaproic acid)
An essential amino acid required for the synthesis of proteins needed for optimal growth in infants and to maintain nitrogen balance in adults. Lysine has been reported to suppress herpes simplex infections but studies have failed to confirm this benefit.

lobelia
(ban bian lian, Indian tobacco, pukeweed, gagroot, vomitwort, bladderpod, wild tobacco)
A tropical and temperate herb, *Lobelia chinensis* or *inflata,* of the Campanulaceae (also listed as Lobeliaceae) family, named for Flemish botanist Matthias de Lobel (1538–1616). The lobelia plant contains lobeline, a chemical derived from the dried leaves and tops of the herb that acts like nicotine, although lobelia is less potent. In Ayurvedic medicine, the pungent, heating qualities of *L. inflata* are used as an antispasmodic, emetic, expectorant and diaphoretic. Other herbalists consider lobelia one of the best emetics (hence the name "pukeweed," etc.). Lobelia is also commonly employed in antismoking regimes. Pure lobeline relieves asthmatic symptoms and respiratory difficulties in newborns and individuals under anesthesia. There is some controversy among herbalists regarding lobelia toxicity: Some believe the herb is poisonous and in large doses may cause paralysis, vomiting and collapse, while others have not experienced any problems resulting from lobelia. Other uses of the herb include treatment of tetany and food poisoning, and as a catalyst for other herbs in medicinal formulas.

lonicera
(honeysuckle, jin yin hua)
An East Asian and North American flowering plant, *Lonicera japonica,* of the Caprifoliaceae family, named for German physician and naturalist Adam Lonicer (1528–1586). In traditional Chinese medicine, the whole plant is used to treat fever and scanty flow of urine and prevent diarrhea, while the flowers are used for fever, headache, dysentery and arthritis, and twigs for boils and pain in the bones.

lophatherum
An Asian and Australian grass, *Lophatherum gracile,* of the Gramineae family, used by Chinese

herbalists in the treatment of anxiety, scanty or bloody urine and fever. The root is thought to induce abortion as well as assuage problems during labor.

loquat
(pi pa ye)
The plant *Eriobotrya japonica,* of the Rosaceae family, whose leaves and fruit are prepared by herbalists as expectorant, anti-inflammatory and antitussive. Amygdalin, a substance in loquat leaves, is also found in apricot kernels and wild cherry bark and used in cough medicines. Herbalists also use loquat for bronchitis and lung congestion, vomiting and belching.

loranthus
(mistletoe, mulberry leaf, sang ji sheng)
A genus of flowering shrubs of the Loranthaceae family, such as *L. parasiticus* and *yadoriki,* that grow on host trees. Many legends are associated with mistletoe, including the Christmas tradition of kissing under a sprig of the shrub, possibly reflecting herbalists' prescriptions of mistletoe for infertility, sterility and unhappily single individuals. In traditional Chinese medicine, uses for loranthus include remedies for hypertension, threatened abortion, pain during pregnancy, bone and knee pain and excessive menstrual bleeding. Loranthus is also prescribed as a kidney and bone tonic and to induce lactation in women who have just given birth.

In Ayurvedic medicine, mistletoe (or *Viscum album,* of the Loranthaceae family) is used as a nervine, antispasmodic and emmenagogue.

Lorenzo's oil
Oleic and erucic acids administered as a dietary supplement to patients with adrenoleukodystrophy, or adrenomyeloneuropathy, a wasting disease caused by a severe deficiency or lack of these oils.

The supplement is named for a young boy whose father researched this rare disease and discovered the missing nutrients. A motion picture entitled *Lorenzo's Oil* (starring Nick Nolte and Susan Sarandon) and produced in 1992 is based on the true story.

lotus
(lian zi, lian xu, padma [Sanskrit])
A genus of leguminous herbs or subshrubs (also called sweet clover), such as *Nelumbo nucifera,* of the Nymphaeaceae family, considered India's most sacred plant whose blossom reflects and inspires spiritual unfoldment, hence, the lotus position during yoga and meditation in which one sits cross-legged with the right foot on the left thigh and the left foot on the right thigh. Lotus seeds and root are used by Ayurvedic practitioners as tonic, remedy and food. Indications include diarrhea, leukorrhea, bleeding disorders, venereal diseases, impotence and cardiac weakness. Lotus seeds are also thought to improve concentration, help stop stuttering and open the "heart center," one of the seven *chakras* (head, third eye, throat, heart, navel, sex and root centers of the body as references to function and spirit) described in Ayurvedic (Hindu) medicine.

According to Homer's *Odyssey,* people who ate lotus fruit became the dreamy, indolent and contented population of lotusland. The fruit allegedly came from the tree *Zizyphus lotus,* of the buckthorn family.

lovage
(lavose, sea parsley)
A European and Asian wild, aromatic perennial, *Levisticum officinale,* of the carrot family, cultivated as a potherb, flavoring agent and home remedy. Lovage rootstock is prepared for use as a stimulant, diuretic, carminative, expectorant and stomachic, although it is believed that large doses may cause kidney damage. However, lovage is

considered by herbalists to be effective against suppressed menstruation, flatulence and urinary problems.

luffa

(si gua, sponge gourd, smooth loofah)

An Old World tropical, annual herb, *Luffa aegyptiaca,* of the family Cucurbitaceae, whose seeds produce an edible oil and whose interior is used as a sponge commonly known as a loofah. Luffa's fruit juice is considered toxic, though it is known to be a strong purgative. In traditional Chinese medicine, luffa fruit fiber provides a remedy for pain, bleeding associated with dysentery and the uterus, testicular inflammation and piles. Ash from the fiber is prepared as treatment for jaundice, smallpox, internal bleeding and poor circulation.

lungwort

(Jerusalem cowslip, Jerusalem sage, spotted comfrey, maple lungwort)

A European and North American flowering perennial plant, *Pulmonaria officinalis,* of the Pulmonaceae family, whose leaves are used by Native American and other herbalists in preparations largely devoted to the treatment of pulmonary problems because of its anti-inflammatory, demulcent and mucilaginous properties. Lungwort reputedly contains vitamins C and B and iron, copper, silver, manganese, kerotin, nickel and other minerals. Lungwort tea is also prescribed as a diuretic and for external use for wounds.

lycium

(matrimony vine, box thorn, Chinese wolfberry, gou qi zi)

Tropical or temperate shrubs, *Lycium barbarum* and *chinense,* of the Solanaceae family, whose various uses in traditional Chinese medicine include treatment of impotence, backache, weakness, fever, diabetes, sore throat and pneumonia.

lygodium

(climbing fern, hai jin sha)

The fern of the Schizaeaceae family, named from the Greek word meaning flexible. *L. japonicum* leaves are used by Chinese herbalists to treat bloody sputum, gonorrhea, high fever and delirium. *L. flexuosum* leaves and spores are used to treat inflammation, fever and cystitis, among other complaints.

M

macrobiotic diet

Vegetarian diet originating from the late 19th century based on a philosophy that spiritual progress is made by restricting animal-derived foods. Initially, at the "lowest" stage, the diet consists of 10 percent cereal, 30 percent vegetable, 10 percent soup, 30 percent foods of animal origin, 15 percent fruits and salads and 5 percent dessert. As spiritualism progresses, every other food except cereal is reduced until the entire diet is cereal. This diet is seriously deficient in nutrition.

(See also VEGETARIAN DIETS.)

macrocytic anemia

See ANEMIA, MACROCYTIC.

macro minerals

Minerals such as calcium and phosphorus that are required in larger quantities than trace minerals. Macro minerals include calcium, chloride, magnesium, phosphorus, potassium, sodium and sulfur. (See MINERALS, ESSENTIAL.)

macrosupplementation

See MEGADOSE.

macular degeneration

Deterioration of the macular area of the retina of the eye, usually related to aging or growth of blood vessels under the retina, but the cause is unknown. Macular degeneration is a common cause of impaired central vision in individuals older than 50 years of age. There is some evidence that antioxidants, especially beta-carotene, play a role in the prevention of macular degeneration. Importantly, smokers develop this serious eye disease seven years before nonsmokers. Wearing sunglasses that block out destructive ultraviolet rays is also an important preventive measure.

magnesium

A metallic element whose salts are essential nutrients and required for more than 300 enzymatic reactions that are necessary for normal cell function. Magnesium functions in the conversion of carbohydrates, protein and fats to energy, and assists in the manufacture of proteins and genetic material within cells. The central nervous system is dependent on magnesium for the transmission of impulses. Muscles contract when calcium flows into muscle cells and relaxes when magnesium replaces calcium. Magnesium also aids in the removal of toxins such as ammonia from the body. Metabolic reactions involving thiamine (vitamin B_1) and biotin are dependent on magnesium.

Blood contains approximately 2 milliequivalents (milliequivalent or mEq is the number of grams of a solute contained in one milliliter of a normal solution) of magnesium per liter. Magnesium is found in both intracellular (in the cells) as well as extracellular (blood and lymph) fluids. Magnesium blood levels are regulated by the kidneys, and it is excreted in both urine and feces. Approximately 40 percent of the estimated 24 grams of magnesium present in the body is concentrated in muscle and soft tissues, 1 percent in the circulation and the balance in the skeleton.

There is some evidence that hard water containing high levels of magnesium may lead to a reduced risk of heart disease and lower blood pressure. Recent studies have failed to prove earlier reports that intravenous infusions of magnesium during the first 24 hours following a heart attack were beneficial.

Deficiency

Muscle tremors and spasms, depressed tendon reflexes, personality changes, anorexia, nausea and vomiting are signs of magnesium deficiency. Tetany, convulsions and coma may result if severe. The symptoms of hypercalcemia, or abnormally high levels of blood calcium, are similar to inadequate levels of magnesium.

Dietary magnesium deficiency is virtually unknown. However, malabsorption syndromes or other disorders in which there are significant losses of fluids and electrolytes, some kidney diseases that affect reabsorption of cations (ions carrying a positive charge because of a deficiency of electrons), states of malnutrition and alcoholism may result in magnesium deficiency. Medical therapies that can disturb electrolyte balance include nasogastric suctioning, magnesium-free intravenous feeding and some drugs, especially diuretics.

Primary idiopathic hypomagnesemia, a rare genetic disorder, is characterized by impaired ability to absorb magnesium from the intestinal tract.

Food Sources

Although all unprocessed foods contain magnesium to varying degrees, richest concentrations are found in nuts, legumes, unmilled grains, green vegetables and bananas. Removing the germ and outer layers of cereal grains results in an 80 percent loss of the mineral.

Recommended Daily Allowances

Magnesium interacts with other nutrients in complex ways making it difficult to establish a Recommended Daily Allowance (RDA). Nevertheless, the RDA has been established at 4.5 mg per kilogram (1 kilogram = 2.2 pounds) of body weight for adult men and women. A 20-mg daily increase is advised during pregnancy and 60 mg during lactation. Forty mg of magnesium for the first six months and 60 mg for the second six months are recommended, although there are no data on actual need for young children.

A daily intake of 6.0 mg per kilogram is sufficient for children and adolescents from one to 15 years of age.

Supplements

Magnesium supplementation may prevent the formation of oxalate kidney stones. The body seems to require a balance of calcium, magnesium and phosphorous. Therefore, some nutritionists advocate maintaining a ratio of two to one, calcium to magnesium when taking supplements. Phosphorous is plentiful in most diets and does not require supplements.

Toxicity

The large amounts of magnesium that occur in magnesium sulfate, or Epsom salts, have a laxative effect. Magnesium containing antacids cause diarrhea in some individuals. Magnesium is toxic only to people with abnormal kidney function. Early symptoms of magnesium excess are nausea, vomiting and a fall in blood pressure. Later, slow heart rate and other heart irregularities and central nervous system depression develop. Eventually coma, respiratory distress, cardiac arrest and death may occur.

magnolia

(swamp sassafras, beaver tree, Indian bark, white bay, hou po)

Evergreen or deciduous trees or shrubs, *Magnolia virginiana, M. glauca, M. acuminata* and *M. tripetata,* of the Magnoliaceae family, whose roots and trunk are used in herbal medicine. There are 35 to 40 species cultivated in the United States, especially in morasses from Massachusetts to the Gulf of Mexico, India, China and Japan.

In the past, magnolia has been listed in the United States Pharmacopoeia (USP) as a treatment for rheumatism because of its better action, greater safety and fewer side effects than quinine. Magnolia has also been used as a tonic to boost the system after chills, fever and stomachache. It is also known as a substitute for tobacco when it is desirous to break the tobacco-chewing habit.

In traditional Chinese medicine, *M. officinalis* bark is an antispasmodic and aphrodisiac, and it is given for malaria, respiratory complaints, cough, nausea, intestinal worms and other ailments.

mahabala
See MALLOW.

ma huang
(ephedra, somalata [Sanskrit])
The most popular of the ephedra shrubs, of the family Ephedraceae, a Chinese herb species prepared as medication to provide a boost for the immune system and a remedy for respiratory congestion. The drug ephedrine was first isolated from an ephedra shrub in 1887 by Nagai, although ancient Chinese practitioners have been using ma huang and other ephedra species for more than 5,000 years. Some ephedras work as diaphoretics and antipyretics. Once ephedra's action was studied and recognized by allopathic practitioners, ephedrine became known as a sympathomimetic drug that could be synthetically produced. The action of ephedrine is similar to that of epinephrine (also called adrenaline, one of the hormones produced by the adrenal medulla), a common ingredient in medications for asthma, local hemorrhage, constricted bronchioles and cardiac arrhythmias and for use in conjunction with anesthesia.

The effects of ephedrine, although less potent, last longer, especially when given orally, whereas epinephrine is effective only by injection. Orally or by injection, ephedrine dilates the bronchial muscles, contracts nasal mucosa, elevates blood pressure (and should be used cautiously by individuals with high blood pressure) and is mainly valued for its bronchodilating properties in the treatment of asthma and for its constricting effects on the nasal mucosa in hay fever. Ephedrine sulfate (USP) is marketed under the trade name Isofedrol.

Ephedra sinica, equisetina and *distachya* branches and roots are used by Chinese and other herbalists to treat influenza, whooping cough, lung fever, allergic rashes such as hives and many other ailments. Ma huang is a popular ingredient in supplemental preparations for women, possibly because it combats night sweats usually associated with menopause and general weakness, perhaps from loss of blood or change in hormone balance, that may be experienced during certain times of the menstrual cycle.

Ephedra is also considered medicinal according to the Vedas, the sacred scriptures of India. In Ayurvedic medicine, *E. vulgaris,* of the Gnetaceae family, works as a diaphoretic, antipyretic, antitussive, expectorant, analgesic and stimulant. Indications for the use of ephedra include arthritis, dropsy and facial edema as well as asthma, bronchitis and respiratory distress. Ayurvedic practitioners believe American ephedra (sometimes known as Mormon or Brigham tea) does not have the same diaphoretic and antitussive actions as ma huang and other Oriental species.

maidenhair
(common polypody, five-finger fern, rock fern)
A perennial plant, *Adiantum capillus-veneris,* of the family Filices, with about 80 species, some of which are found in the deep woods of Canada and the United States. The herb of the plant is considered by herbalists to be a supplement useful in the treatment of colds, nasal congestion, hoarseness, shortness of breath, asthma, pleurisy, influenza and other respiratory problems. Ayurvedic practitioners use maidenhair fern as a demulcent, refrigerant and tonic.

malabsorption
Impaired absorption of nutrients from the intestinal tract. Disorders characterized by chronic diarrhea such as celiac and Crohn's disease may cause vitamin deficiencies as well as disturbed electrolyte and fluid balance.

mallow
(malva, high mallow)

Plants of the family Malvaceae, whose herbs have been used by Native American, Ayurvedic and other herbalists as a remedy for respiratory irritation, coughs, kidney and bladder problems and other disorders. Malva leaves and flowers are claimed to soothe inflammation of the mouth and throat and help alleviate earaches.

Pliny the Elder, an Ancient Roman encyclopedist, known for his writings on scientific subjects including the medicinal power of spices and herbs, wrote "that anyone taking a spoonful of mallows will be free of disease." A good amount of Pliny's information has since been discredited as incorrect. However, mallow leaves are eaten raw or boiled by the Chinese, and Native Americans made poultices for skin eruptions from mallow leaves, stems and flowers. Russian folk medicine also includes malva as a tea or nastoika (with vodka). In Ayurvedic medicine, malva is considered a demulcent, emollient and astringent. Nutritionally, malva (*M. sylventris*) contains vitamin C, minerals and sugar.

malnutrition
Inadequate nutrition due to insufficient or unbalanced diet.

mandrake
A Mediterranean herb, *Mandragora officinarum,* of the nightshade family, said to have properties helpful in the case of chronic liver disorders and in regulating bowels. With a large forked root likened to human qualities, mandrake has been used as a cathartic, narcotic and soporific (sleep-inducer) and as a means of promoting conception. The Old Testament touts mandrake as a remedy for sterility. Mandrake is said to be highly effective and work best when combined with blackroot, senna leaves and other herbs.

American mandrake, or *Podophyllum pelatum,* of the family Berberidaceae, is also known as May or hog apple (see also BARBERRY), Indian apple, raccoon berry and wild lemon. Most parts of this plant, such as leaves, berries and seeds, are poisonous in the green state; ripening takes place during the fall in North American locations. The active substance in American mandrake is podophyllum or podophyllin, capable of treating chronic liver disease, according to homeopaths and herbalists. The dried rhizome (rootlike stem) and its roots are used in the topical treatment of certain papillomas (benign skin tumors) such as verruca acuminata and other varieties of warts, polyps and condylomas. Herbalists claim American mandrake is also therapeutic in treating cancerous skin growths. Other reported clinical uses of American mandrake are for chronic constipation, gallbladder problems and abnormal conditions of the lymphatic system, spleen and blood. In Ayurvedic medicine, mandrake is used as a cathartic, alterative and toxic. Both American and European mandrake are poisonous, and homeopaths use them cautiously for fever, colic and asthma, and sometimes to promote conception. An overdose of mandrake may cause death, and if taken by a pregnant woman, it may cause birth defects.

Nonetheless, mandrake enjoys a bit of literary fame in 17th-century poet John Donne's "Songs and Sonnets":

> Go, and catch a falling star,
> Get with child a mandrake root,
> Tell me, where all past years are,
> Or who cleft the Devil's foot,
> Teach me to hear mermaids singing.

manganese
Metallic element essential for synthesis of mucopolysacchaides and for a number of enzymes. Manganese is concentrated in the mitrochodria of pituitary, liver, pancreas, kidneys and bone. Manganese is plentiful in plant food sources; human deficiencies are virtually unknown. Toxicity has been seen only when workers were exposed to high concentrations of manganese dust or fumes. High dietary intake does not appear to be toxic.

maple

(sugar maple, swamp maple, red maple)
The tree of the Aceraceae, or maple, family, touted for its rich, flavorful syrup sought by bees and people. Cultivated in many regions of the United States, the maple's inner bark and leaves are used as a decoction (see DECOCTION) to strengthen the liver and spleen, soothe the nerves and provide a tonic boost for the entire body. While maple syrup continues to be a popular form of sugar, there is a pneumonitis called maple bark disease caused by inhalation of the mold *Cryptostroma corticale,* found in the bark of maple trees. Another disease, maple-syrup urine disease, has no link to the ingestion of maple syrup, but it is named for urine and sweat that smell like maple syrup. Maple-syrup urine disease is a metabolic disorder that involves defective metabolism of the amino acids leucine, isoleucine, baline and alloisoleucine (see AMINO ACIDS). In infants, the disease induces nervous-system deterioration and death.

Tea made from maple leaves is also claimed to be a muscle toner for new mothers and to help relieve pain in the liver or spleen.

marjoram

(mountain mint, wintersweet, knotted marjoram)
A native Portuguese perennial, *Origanum majorana* or *vulgare,* of the Labiatae family, used as an aromatic and fragrant cooking ingredient and thought to be effective against sour stomach, lack of appetite and general aches and pains. Marjoram, similar to oregano, is often combined with camomile and gentian when used medicinally.

In Ayurvedic medicine, marjoram is thought to be a stimulant, antispasmodic and diaphoretic. Ancient Romans prepared marjoram for calming the nerves, relieving menstrual and other pain, treating conjunctivitis and promoting urination. A European symbol of youth and beauty whose name in Greek means "joy of the mountains," the sedative marjoram was placed in closets and hope chests, made into a gargle for mouth infections or used as an inhalant or topical application for sinus congestion. Pregnant women should avoid marjoram, however, because it is a uterine irritant.

marshmallow

A European perennial herb, *Althaea officinalis,* of the Malvaceae family, bearing pink flowers and mucilaginous root that is used in the making of marshmallow candies. Its use in medicine is thought to help kidney and bladder function, including alleviating bladder infection, and to soothe inflammation. Ayurvedic and other herbal practitioners use marshmallow as a tonic, demulcent, diuretic and laxative.

(See also MALLOW.)

measles and vitamin A deficiency

This dangerous viral infection has an increased severity and potential for death in children with low levels of retinol (vitamin A). It is thought that the measles virus diminishes already low levels of vitamin A and that it may be advisable to give supplemental vitamin A to patients with severe cases.

(See also A, VITAMIN).

megadose

Doses of vitamin or mineral supplements that are 10 times or greater (five times with vitamin D) than the Recommended Dietary Allowance (RDA) dose.

megaloblastic anemia

See ANEMIA, MACROCYTIC.

megavitamin and megamineral therapy in childhood position statement from the Canadian Paediatric Society

(Société canadienne de pédiatrie)
Expresses an opinion that, ". . . as many as 10 percent of healthy children may be exposed to

vitamin polypharmacy and a substantial risk of accidental overdose. Among the chronically ill, unproven megavitamin regimens may be substituted for treatments of proven efficacy and established safety.

The administration of megavitamins and megaminerals to children involves special risks for various reasons. Parents concerned for their child's health may seek simplistic remedies for difficult behavioural and developmental problems or intractable disease. Children have difficulty expressing complaints that may arise from megavitamin use. Often the symptoms of chronic megavitamin use begin with nonspecific complaints such as malaise, anorexia and fatigability; these have led parents to increase their administration of megavitamins as a tonic."

Physicians are advised to counsel parents about a balanced diet and seek consultation with registered professional dietitians and nutritionists.

[Excerpted from the report of the Nutrition Committee of the Canadian Paediatric Society entitled, "Megavitamin and megamineral therapy in childhood." *Canadian Medical Association Journal* (1990) 143:10, with permission.]

megavitamins

Use of vitamins in doses exceeding the Recommended Daily Allowances (RDA). The importance of vitamins and minerals in amounts at least equivalent to the Recommended Dietary Allowance (RDA) is unquestioned. However, alternative medical practitioners often advocate vitamins to treat a variety of disorders, including cancer, heart disease, schizophrenia and the common cold. Often vitamins and other supplements are used to replace prescription drugs. Traditionalists are not only skeptical of the benefits of such doses but also worry about toxicity and the effects of discontinuing more conventional therapy that might be lifesaving or at least life-lengthening.

Studies with hyperactive, or attention-deficit, children initially seemed to indicate amazing improvements when given megavitamins. However, well-controlled studies fail to support this benefit. Improvement attributed to the vitamins by proponents of megavitamins are now thought by most pediatricians and psychiatrists to be the result of greater expectations placed on the children who were taking these substances.

It has been long been recognized that fat-souble vitamins accumulate in the liver and can be toxic. Most excessive amounts of the water-soluble vitamins are eliminated from the body by the kidneys, and therefore large doses are not toxic. However, niacin, pyridoxine, folic acid, ascorbic acid, and pantothenic acid are water-soluble and can cause adverse effects (see Table 20).

megavitamin study of the American Psychiatric Association

A task force led by American psychiatrist and biochemist Dr. Morris Lipton to review studies conducted by both proponents and protagonists for the use of large doses of vitamins (known as "orthomolecular " therapy) to treat psychiatric patients, espcially those with schizophrenia. They concluded that there was no evidence to support the orthomolecular theory.

(See also MEGADOSE.)

memory loss

See ALZHEIMER'S DISEASE.

Menkes' syndrome

Inherited defect in copper absorption characterized by poor and abnormal growth, defective skin pigmentation, kinky hair, mental impairment and usually premature death.

(See also COPPER.)

metabolism

Physical and chemical processes involved in the production, maintenance and utilization of energy in living organisms.

Table 20
THE MOST COMMON SERIOUS VITAMIN AND MINERAL ADVERSE AND TOXIC EFFECTS (USUALLY RELATED TO EXCESSIVE OR MEGADOSES)

Vitamin/Mineral*	Chief Toxic Effects**
Vitamin A (retinol) [There does not appear to be toxicity from the provitamin substance beta-carotene, which is converted to vitamin A in the body]	Birth defects if excessive maternal intake during pregnancy. Liver damage. Pseudotumor cerebri (increased pressure in the brain that acts like a brain tumor).
Vitamin D	Hypercalcemia and hypercalciuria (high blood and urine calcium) that could cause calcium deposits in soft tissues and irreversibly damage kidneys and the heart. Children are especially susceptible.
B-Complex Components Niacin	Liver damage. Worsen glucose control in diabetics.
Pyridoxine (vitamin B_6)	Irreversible nerve damage.
Pantothenic acid	Diarrhea.
Folic acid	May mask underlying B_{12} deficiency and result in irreversible nerve damage.
Ascorbic acid (vitamin C)	Kidney stones. Suppression of immune response.
Iron	Interferes with zinc absorption.
Zinc	Suppression of immune response.

*Vitamins/minerals most likely to pose a threat to health if taken to excess in normal persons.

**Individual vitamins for more complete list of adverse and toxic effects.

microcytic anemia
See ANEMIA, MICROCYTIC.

microgram (mcg)
Unit of measure equivalent to one millionth of a gram.

micro minerals
See MINERALS, TRACE.

milk, infant formula
Well-balanced cow's milk commercial products that also supply electrolytes, minerals and vitamins. These products are often more convenient than breast milk and, if consumed in adequate quantity, supply the Recommended Daily Allowances of those nutrients.

milk, human
Breastmilk, available without cost, safe, may strengthen resistance to infection, enhance intestinal development and bonding between mother and newborn. Although there seem to be insufficient amounts of calcium and phosphorus for bone development, this does not seem to be detrimental in otherwise normal infants. Although there is a possibility of the mother passing infection or toxins to her baby, the risk of infection is greater with improperly sterilized formula. Perhaps the most common problem with breast-feeding is assuring an adequate supply.

(See also MILK, INFANT FORMULA.)

milk thistle
See BLESSED THISTLE.

milkweed
(silkweed, swallowwort, Virginia silk)
A perennial herb, *Asclepias syriaca,* of the family Asclepiadaceae, that produces a milky juice (some

of the milkweed plants secrete latex) and umbellate flowers. Milkweed rootstock is claimed by herbalists to be a remedy for gallstones and bowel, kidney and gynecological problems. It is also said to increase the flow of urine.

minerals, essential

Inorganic elements required for a variety of functions including giving structure to the skeleton, muscle contractions, blood formation, the synthesis of protein and the production of energy. Minerals are found in red blood cells and cell membranes. They are components of hormones and enzymes. Major or "macro" minerals include calcium, phosphorous, sodium, potassium and others. Iodine, iron and zinc are among the "trace minerals" found in very minimal quantities. Some minerals found in even more minute concentrations possibly are necessary for health. (See Table 21.)

minerals, trace

Elements whose total body concentration does not exceed .005 percent are classified as trace minerals and include chromium, copper, iodine, iron, sele-nium and zinc. (See MINERALS, ESSENTIAL; MINERALS, ULTRATRACE.)

minerals, ultratrace

Minerals including arsenic, boron, bromine, cadmium, fluorine, lead, lithium, manganese, molybdenum, nickel, silicon, tin and vanadium that are found in the body in minute amounts even smaller than trace or macro minerals. Although they are poorly understood, since the early 1970s it has been theorized that these substances are essential for human nutrition and deficiencies of them contribute to a variety of diseases. (See MINERALS, ESSENTIAL; MINERALS, TRACE.)

mint

The herbs of the genus Mentha, of the Labiatae family, including peppermint, spearmint and pennyroyal (*M. piperita, M. spicata, M. pulegium*) used for their menthol, an alcohol derived from mint oils, in medicinal preparations and as a flavoring agent in chewing gum, candies and toothpaste. Many herbalists believe the leaves and stems of mint plants alleviate cramps and hiccoughs in children and adults, strengthen heart muscles, avert nausea and vomiting, particularly in motion sickness, and induce cleansing and relaxation. Mint preparations are also said to be useful for headaches, intestinal gas, toothache, lung inflammation and dizziness. Mentha arvensis, or field mint, is used in traditional Chinese medicine as an analgesic, a diaphoretic, a digestive stimulant, a cardiovascular medicine and an antiflatulent.

Menthol, also prepared synthetically and recognized by the United States Pharmacopoeia (USP), is an antipruritic (anti-itch agent).

(See also MOTHERWORT.)

Table 21
MINERALS ESSENTIAL TO HEALTH

Major or Macro Minerals

Calcium	Magnesium	Potassium	Sulfur
Chloride	Phosphorus	Sodium	

Trace or Micro Minerals

Chromium	Iodine	Selenium
Copper	Iron	Zinc

Ultratrace Minerals (Probably essential to health)

Arsenic	Lead	Nickel
Boron	Lithium	Silicon
Bromine	Manganese	Tin
Cobalt	Molybdenum	Vanadium
Fluorine		

mistletoe
See LORANTHUS.

molybdenum

An essential ultratrace mineral found in all body tissues but predominantly in the liver, kidney, bones and skin. A component of the important enzymes xanthine oxidase, aldehyde oxidase, sulfite oxidase and nitrate reductase. Xanthine oxidase is associated with the formation of uric acid as a metabolic breakdown product of purine (excessive amounts of purines in the diet increase the risk for gout). Molybdenum with riboflavin (vitamin B_2) helps convert food to energy. Molybdenum is also associated with the metabolism of iron.

Deficiency

Human deficiencies of molybdenum have been difficult to demonstrate. However, there is an inherited autosomal recessive metabolic disease resulting from a deficiency of molybdopterin, a molybdenum cofactor required for synthesis of certain enzymes. The deficiency of this cofactor interferes with the production of the enzymes sulfite oxidase and xanthine dehydrogenase, causing severe neurological abnormalities, mental retardation and dislocation of ocular lenses. There is also a possibility of increased incidence of esophageal cancer in molybdenum deficient individuals.

Dietary Sources

Hard tap water, milk, beans, breads and cereals are the principal dietary sources of molybdenum. The average American diet contains 180 mcg of the mineral daily but varies considerably, depending on where the food sources are grown. Plants grown in soils rich in the mineral may contain up to 500 times the amount found in molybdenum-poor soils. Excess copper in the diet may interfere with the absorption of molybdenum.

Recommended Daily Allowances

A recommended daily intake of 75 to 250 mcg of molybdenum for adults and older children is easily supplied in American diets. Requirements for infants and children is based on body weight.

Toxicity

Ingesting more than 10 mg of molybdenum daily may increase production of the enzyme xanthine oxidase (see above), leading to overproduction of uric acid. The presence of excessive uric acid may cause gout, a condition of exquisitely painful and swollen joints, or kidney stones.

motherwort

(lion's tail, lion's ear, throwwort, yi mu cao)

Perennial plants, *Leonurus cardiaca* and *heterophyllus,* of the Labiatae family, cultivated in Europe, Asia and North America, whose tops and leaves are said to have laxative, antispasmodic and nervine properties. Motherwort can be used as an infusion (tea made with boiling water), extract or tablet to relieve heart palpitations, stomach problems, mild goiter, epilepsy, cramps, high blood pressure, suppressed menstruation, hysteria, rheumatism, sciatica, neuritis, insomnia, chest colds, convulsions, worms and liver ailments. (See LEONURUS.)

mugwort

(moxa, ai ye)

A North American wild herb, *Artemisia vulgaris,* of the family Compositae, whose leaves are thought to have properties useful in the treatment of colds, colic, rheumatism, menstrual problems, kidney and bladder inflammations, gout, sciatica and fever. Some herbalists also claim that mugwort counteracts the effects of opium. Native Americans found mugwort juice effective as a topical treatment for poison oak rash and wounds. Mugwort also grows in Russia and is considered a home remedy for a number of conditions including wounds, nervousness, female reproductive disorders, tubercular lungs and epilepsy.

In traditional Chinese medicine, mugwort leaves are used to treat headache, asthma, bleeding and menstrual problems. Several other species of Artemisia are remedies for a host of ailments including malaria, dysentery, tuberculosis, indigestion, eye diseases and fungal infections.

mullein

(feltwort, Aaron's rod, candlewick, velvet dock, shepherd's club, flannel-flower, cow's lungwort, verbascum flowers)

A flowering biennial plant of 300 or more species that grow in North Africa, Europe, western and central Asia and the United States. An American species is *Verbascum thapsus,* of the Scrophulariaceae family. Mullein's leaves, flowers and sometimes the roots are prepared as a medicine to relieve ailments including lung congestion, lung hemorrhage, colds, hemorrhoids, constipation, asthma, epilepsy and headache in children, nervous disorders and heart, kidney and bladder conditions. Cows may be given fresh mullein leaves as a treatment for tapeworm. Mullein contains iron, magnesium and potassium. In Ayurvedic medicine, mullein is considered an expectorant, astringent, vulnerary and sedative.

Other species of mullein, such as orange mullein (*V. phlomoides*) and black mullein (*V. nigrum*), are also used medicinally.

multivitamin and mineral supplements

Proprietary products containing a variety of vitamins and minerals in varying quantities, less than, equal to or greater than Recommended Daily Allowances (RDA). In a 1986 survey of 11,775 adults and 1,877 children, approximately 3,400 different vitamin and mineral supplement products were identified. Vitamin C was found in 50 percent of these formulations, whereas calcium and iron were the most common minerals, being present in about 25 percent.

mustard

Annual plants, *Brassica nigra* and *hirta* (or *alba*), of the Cruciferae family, used by herbalists as a stimulant (especially of the appetite), expectorant and carminative. However, black mustard seed is mainly used as a poultice for rheumatism, back pain and inflammations. Internal use as a carminative is limited to small doses. White mustard seeds may be antiseptic and effective against pulmonary problems. A pungent, hot spice, mustard is also considered by Ayurvedic practitioners to be a painkiller.

myristica

See NUTMEG.

myrrh

An aromatic gum resin derived from the tree *Commiphora abyssinica* or *myrrha,* of the Burseraceae family, that grows in East Africa and Arabia. Myrrh is used as a spice, perhaps most famous as one of the gifts of the Three Wise Men to the infant Jesus in Bethlehem. Antiseptic myrrh is used medicinally as a colon cleanser and breath freshener. Herbalists may also offer myrrh to individuals suffering from sinus problems. Ayurvedic practitioners administer myrrh preparations as an alterative, analgesic, emmenagogue and rejuvenative.

(See also GUGGUL.)

myrtle

See PERIWINKLE.

N

nails and nutritional deficiencies

Difficulties or adverse reactions that are the result of a lack of a particular nutrient or combination of nutrients. For example, brittle, cracked, peeling, ridged, split or broken nails may indicate a deficiency of the minerals iron or copper or the vitamins B_6, B_{12}, C or folate. Spoon-shaped nails are found in persons with a long-standing iron-deficiency anemia. The deformity occurs because of an inadequate supply of oxygen-rich blood to the nail beds. Other causes of nail structural disorders include hypothyroidism and psoriasis.

National Academy of Sciences (NAS)

A private, nonprofit, self-perpetuating society of distinguished scholars engaged in scientific and engineering research, dedicated to the furtherance of science and technology and to their use for the general welfare. Although not a government agency, in 1863, during the Lincoln administration, the United States Congress granted a charter to the academy with a mandate that requires it to advise the federal government on scientific and technical matters.

The NAS is made up of approximately 1,200 scientists chosen in recognition of their achievements in research. The Academy elects a maximum 60 Americans and 15 foreign associates annually. There are three other organizations—the National Research Council, the National Academy of Engineering and the Institute of Medicine—created by the NAS that cooperate with the parent academy, but elect their own membership.

National Cancer Institute

See NATIONAL INSTITUTES OF HEALTH.

National Institutes of Health (NIH)

Federal agency that conducts or supports medical research. Part of the Public Health Service, under the direction of the Department of Health, Education and Welfare (HEW), the NIH is located in Bethesda, Maryland. Although formally named the National Institutes of Health in 1948, its roots date back to 1887, when it was established as the "Hygienic Laboratory" at the United States Marine Hospital on Staten Island.

The modern NIH is divided into 11 individual institutes: (1) aging; (2) allergy and infectious diseases; (3) arthritis, metabolism and digestive diseases; (4) cancer; (5) child health and human development; (6) dental research; (7) environmental health sciences; (8) eye; (9) general medical sciences; (10) heart, lung and blood; and (11) neurological and communicative disorders and stroke.

National Research Council

Organized in 1916 by the National Academy of Sciences to act conjointly with the National Academy of Engineering in furthering knowledge and advising the federal government. The Food and Nutrition Board is a committee of the council that oversees the establishment of the Recommended Dietary Allowances.

(See also NATIONAL ACADEMY OF SCIENCES; RECOMMENDED DIETARY ALLOWANCES.)

natural vitamins

Those vitamins obtained from nature, such as the vitamin C found in citrus fruits. With the exception of vitamin E, there is no significant difference chemically between natural or synthetic, or man-made, vitamins. (See E, VITAMIN; SYNTHETIC VITAMINS.)

naturopathy

An alternative method of health care whose practitioners advocate the use of natural foods and avoidance of drugs to allow the body to heal itself.

neem [Sanskrit]

An Ayurvedic herb, *Azadiracta indica,* of the Meliaceae family, used as a bitter tonic, antipyretic and alterative. In traditional Chinese medicine, the herb is known as *Melia azedarach,* or chinaberry, pride-of-India, Persian lilac, Indian lilac, bead tree and paradise tree. While the poisonous fruits (and probably the leaves, flowers and bark as well) of the plant have killed livestock and fish, the fruits, stem and bark are used in herbal medicine to treat angina pectoris, abdominal pain, intestinal worms and as an emetic.

nelumbo

See LOTUS.

nettle

Any herb of the genus *Urtica,* of the Urticaceae (or nettle) family, particularly *U. urens,* with prickly or stinging hairs. Also known as stinging nettle, the herb contains vitamins including C and A, potassium, protein, fiber, chlorophyll and other substances. The leaves may be used to make tea that is considered by herbalists to be a lung, stomach, urinary tract and general body tonic. Nettles are also prescribed to treat anemia, asthma, kidney and bladder inflammation, arthritis, urinary stones, rheumatism, dysentery, diarrhea, bleeding (especially caused by endometriosis) and other problems. It is said that deliberately allowing the leaf hairs to "sting" an area where there is arthritic pain will relieve the pain. Externally, the juice from heated and squeezed nettles may be applied to the scalp to stimulate hair growth, according to herbalists. A nettle powder applied to an open wound helps to stop bleeding.

Other reported uses of nettles include as a diuretic, tonic, astringent and for treating nosebleed and excessive phlegm. *U. dioica,* which grows in the United States, is often eaten as a vegetable, but one must handle nettles carefully so the bristly hairs do not sting skin or other body tissues. The roots and leaves are generally used in herbal preparations, but homeopaths prescribe tincture of the entire flowering plant for the treatment of sore throat, uremia, gout, gravel, vertigo and many other ailments.

neurologic diseases caused by vitamin deficiency

Wernicke's encephalopathy of alcoholism from insufficient thiamine (vitamin B_1) and degeneration of the spinal cord from a lack of vitamin B_{12} are the only two disorders involving the central nervous system proven to result from inadequate vitamins. Polyneuropathy, delirium tremens and cerebellar degeneration, which are also associated with chronic alcoholism, are possibly related to vitamin deficiencies, but this is unsubstantiated.

niacin

(nicotinic acid, vitamin B_3 or 3-pyridinecarboxylic acid)

A water-soluble member of the vitamin B-complex family. Although humans can synthesize small quantities of niacin, it is classified as a vitamin because the quantity made in the body is inadequate for normal function. Niacin is essential for the manufacture of the hormones cortisone, thyroxine and insulin, and the sex hormones estrogen, progesterone and testosterone. Niacin is also necessary for the normal function of the nervous system.

RECOMMENDED DIETARY ALLOWANCES

Birth to 6 months	5 mg NE*	
6 to 12 months	6 mg NE	
1 to 3 years	9 mg NE	
4 to 6 years	12 mg NE	
7 to 10 years	13 mg NE	

	Males	Females
11 to 14 years	17 mg NE	15 mg NE
15 to 18 years	20 mg NE	15 mg NE
19 to 24 years	19 mg NE	15 mg NE
25 to 50 years	19 mg NE	15 mg NE
51 and older	15 mg NE	13 mg NE
Pregnancy	—	17 mg NE
Lactating	—	20 mg NE

*NE = niacin equivalent (1 mg of niacin is equal to 60 mg of dietary tryptophan)

Dietary Sources and Supplements

Meat is high in niacin and tryptophan. Milk and eggs, although low in niacin, contain sufficient amounts of tryptophan, which is converted to niacin in the body. Cereal and many other foodstuffs contain forms of niacin bound to the food in a manner that prevents the utilization of the vitamin. To counter the poorly available niacin in those products, they are fortified with more bioavailable synthetic niacin.

Niacin causes an intolerable flushing in many persons, and therefore the niacinamide and nicotinamide forms of the vitamin, which are free of this annoying effect, are used in many multiple-vitamin preparations.

Other Uses

Niacin has been used as a drug for many years to treat various conditions unrelated to its vitamin properties. Doses much greater than required to satisfy its vitamin requirement are needed for these other uses.

Niacin decreases the production of low-density lipoproteins, or VLDL. This results in the production of less low-density, or LDL, cholesterol, the so-called "bad" cholesterol. Niacin also raises high-density cholesterol, or HDL, the "good, protective cholesterol." Studies have shown decreases of 15 to 30 percent in LDL and increases of 20 percent or more in HDL levels. In at least one study, heart attack survivors suffered 21 percent fewer repeat nonfatal heart attacks than a group not taking niacin. The same group had an 11 percent better long-term survival rate.

When the 1- to 3-gram doses of niacin required to significantly lower cholesterol are used, individuals should be monitored by a physician who can ascertain not only lipid (another name for the fats, cholesterol and triglycerides) but also blood-glucose and liver-function levels. High doses of the vitamin can aggravate diabetes mellitus in a patient previously controlled or can precipitate full-blown diabetes in a borderline individual. Niacin should also be avoided in patients with peptic ulcer disease and gout.

Although niacin is a very potent cholesterol-lowering drug, the huge doses required to lower cholesterol levels limit its usefulness, because only a few people can tolerate the adverse effects (see adverse and toxic effects below). There are claims that chromium combined with very small doses of niacin have a great ability to lower cholesterol, but this needs further study.

The most noticeable and common adverse efect of niacin is vasodilation, a severe flushing of the skin in which an individual feels an intense burning and itching sensation, the most common adverse effect of nicotinic acid. Often this discomfort can be prevented by taking an aspirin or ibuprofen tablets 30 minutes prior to ingesting the niacin. Starting with low doses, taking the drug with meals and avoiding alcoholic or hot beverages also lessens the "hot flashes." Less frequent but troubling side effects of niacin are diarrhea, nausea, vomiting and headaches.

Time-release niacin preparations, while reducing the flushing, may significantly increase liver complications of niacin therapy and should generally be avoided. Although rare, fatalities have

Table 22
ADVERSE EFFECTS
(Comparison of Regular Versus Long-Acting Niacin)

	Flushing	Gastric Distress	Liver Test Abnormalities	Liver Failure
Tablets	severe	minimal	minimal	minimal
Sustained Release	minimal	severe	moderate	moderate

occurred from niacin-induced liver problems. The sustained-release forms are considerably more expensive than niacin tablets, which are the least expensive cholesterol-lowering drug.

Niacin, and some older drugs derived from it, have the ability to dilate some peripheral blood vessels. These drugs have been used in hopes that they would increase blood flow to areas of the body compromised by acute or chronic arterial obstruction or vasospasm. However, despite their widespread promotion and use in the past, there is

Table 23
TOXIC EFFECTS OF NIACIN

Toxicity can occur from 100 mg to 10,000 mg (0.1 to 10 gram) oral dose or 20 mg to 750 mg intravenously.

Acute toxic symptoms	Itching or skin flushing
	Headache
	Heartburn, nausea, vomiting
Acute and chronic symptoms	Elevated glucose (diabetes)
	Elevated uric acid (gout)
	Duodenal ulcers
Chronic symptoms	Hepatitis and liver failure
	Heart rhythm irregularities
	Rare—hyperpigmentation of the skin
	Hypothyroidism
	Optic nerve disorder
	Inhibition of the effects of pyridoxine (vitamin B_6)
	Precipitation of underlying psychosis

(See also NIACINAMIDE.)

no acceptable scientific evidence that they are of value in the treatment of those conditions.

Niacinamide and nicotinamide, while providing the vitamin benefits of niacin, have no lipid-lowering or vasodilating properties.

niacinamide
(nicotinamide)

A form of vitamin B_3 converted from niacin or the amino acid tryptophan in small, but inadequate amounts to satisfy daily requirements. While supplemental niacinamide can satisfy the Recommended Dietary Allowance (RDA), it lacks the cholesterol-lowering or vasodilating properties of niacin. It also lacks the adverse itching or skin flushing of niacin.

(See also NIACIN.)

nicotiana
(tobacco)

The plant *Nicotiana tabacum,* of the Solanaceae family, named after Jean Nicot, French consul to Portugal (1530–1600), thought to be the first person to introduce tobacco to French and Portuguese courts. Cultivated by Native Americans and used in the West Indies in 1492, according to Columbus, nicotiana eventually became an addictive agent that could be smoked, snuffed or chewed. But herbal practitioners, including the traditional Chinese, used the plant to treat sore joints, rheumatism, numbness and snakebite.

nicotinic acid

Another term for the B-complex vitamin B_3 or niacin. (See NIACIN.)

nickel

Trace metal with no proven human need. Nickel deficiency has been shown to decrease growth and blood production in rats, sheep, cows and goats.

night blindness

A disease first recognized in Ancient Egypt in which a deficiency of vitamin A causes limited vision at night. The Papyrus Ebers recommended applying the juice squeezed from cooked liver to the eyes for a cure. The Ancient Greeks ate liver and also applied it to the eyes.

(See also A, VITAMIN.)

nightshade

(bittersweet, scarlet berry, violet bloom, woody, fever twig, felonwort)

Herbs of the Solanaceae family, including *Solanum dulcamara* and *nigrum,* whose root, bark and twigs, leaves and herb are used in herbal medicine as an emetic, diuretic and purgative, although the herbs are a mild poison and mainly used in topical applications for swellings, corns, skin diseases, herpes, gout, boils and other ailments.

(See also BELLADONNA.)

nutmeg

(jatiphala [Sanskrit])

The spice derived from the tree *Myristica fragrans,* a tropical evergreen of the Myristcaceae, or nutmeg, family. The nutmeg tree's aromatic seeds are ground into a powder, and herbalists believe small amounts may be taken to relieve cardiac and chronic nervous disorders. When added to other foods such as milk products or baked desserts, the relaxant nutmeg is said to relieve nausea and indigestion. Large doses must be avoided, however, because they can be toxic or even cause miscarriage. One of the world's major commercial nutmeg producers (and mace, a spice made from the dried covering of the nutmeg) is Grenada, an island in the western Caribbean Grenadines. Ayurvedic, Chinese and other herbal practitioners administer nutmeg for insomnia, sexual debility, gas, diarrhea, poor appetite, urinary incontinence and general weakness.

nutrition

The processes by which all living things, including human beings, animals, plants and microorganisms, obtain and use substances in their sources of food that are valuable and essential to their health. Nutrition is the end result of ingestion, absorption and metabolism—the utilization of nutrients. Studying nutrition involves identifying which nutrients create optimal well-being of the organism and which ingested substances may have harmful effects upon one's nutritional status. (See also NUTRITIONAL STATUS.) Scientists and researchers through the ages have isolated the vitamins, minerals and other substances necessary to human life and have approximated the quantities required for well-being, that is, growth, tissue repair and normal functioning, as well as therapy in the event that toxicity or deficiency of a nutrient exists. Essential inorganic nutrients that promote the growth and maintenance of living organisms are boron, calcium, chlorine, chromium, cobalt, copper, fluorine, iodine, iron, magnesium, manganese, molybdenum, nitrogen, phosphorus, potassium, selenium, silicon, sodium, sulfur, vanadium and zinc. Essential organic nutrients, the main sources of carbohydrates, proteins and fats that promote energy for living organisms requiring them are amino acids (the precursors of protein), fatty acids, glucose and other simple sugars, purine and pyrimidine and their derivatives (precursors of nucleic acids) and vitamins. Most of the essential organic nutrients for human beings must be obtained from other living organisms such as animals and plants.

All the nutrients required for human life work interdependently in order to metabolize and facilitate optimal functioning. For example, the intake of calcium also requires a certain complementary amount of magnesium so the calcium will be absorbed properly. An excess of calcium may be responsible for a magnesium deficiency; in sum, the nutrients must be balanced. The science of nutrition has not yet established irrefutable amounts of nutrients necessary to that balance, however, but has approximated amounts according to research studies and human experience. It is generally accepted that diets that do not provide adequate nutrition cause weakness possibly leading to illness and appear to impair immune defenses and psychological health.

As poor nutrition can induce disease, the state of disease can cause malnutrition. There are many factors that may adversely affect one's ability to obtain nutrients, including geographic, cultural, environmental and personal circumstances. Malnutrition is considered a world health problem.

Other adverse nutritional situations may include hospitalized patients. Practices such as prolonged infusion of intravenous fluids with glucose and/or salt solutions, failure to measure or monitor food intake, withholding meals while awaiting diagnostic tests, nutritionally inadequate meals and failure to recognize the need for increased nutritional support for some disease states or injuries or following surgery may predispose a patient to inadequate intake of nutrients.

nutritionist

(dietitian)

An individual with expertise in food and nutrition who instructs others in dietary matters. Registered dietitians (RD) are university-trained professionals.

nutrition therapy

Adjunctive treatment advocating the use of nutritious foods, vitamins, minerals and other supplements.

nutritional status

Assessment of adequacy of a person's intake of calories, fluids, proteins, carbohydrates, fats, vitamins and minerals. Chronic diseases or an acute illness may cause a change in the way you eat or make it hard for you to eat, putting your nutritional health at risk. Four out of five adults with chronic

diseases are affected by diet. In the elderly, confusion from memory loss may cause these individuals to forget to eat. Depression or anxiety often may cause loss of appetite. Poor dentition, alcoholism or not being able to afford a healthy diet may also be other causes of poor nutrition.

Nutritional status can be assessed using The Nutrition Checklist developed by the Nutrition Screening Initiative. Read the statements below. Circle the number in the yes column for those that apply to you or someone you know. For each yes answer, score the number in the box. Total your nutritional score.

	YES
I have an illness or condition that made me change the kind and/or amount of food I eat.	2
I eat fewer than two meals per day.	3
I eat few fruits or vegetables, or milk products.	2
I have three or more drinks of beer, liquor or wine almost every day.	2
I have tooth or mouth problems that make it hard for me to eat.	2
I don't have enough money to buy the food I need.	4
I eat alone most of the time.	1
I take three or more different prescribed or over-the-counter drugs a day.	1
Without wanting to, I have lost or gained 10 pounds in the last six months.	2
I am not physically able to shop, cook and/or feed myself.	2
	Total

If your score is:

0–2 | Good! Recheck your nutritional score in six months.

3–5 | You are at moderate nutritional risk. See what can be done to improve your eating habits and lifestyle.

| Consult a nutritionist, check out senior-citizen nutrition programs or your local health department. Recheck your score in three months.

6 or | You are at high nutritional risk. Speak
more with your doctor, see a nutritionist or social service professional.

—Adapted from The Nutrition Checklist of the Nutrition Screening Initiative.

nutrition and aging

Certain physiological changes that occur in the elderly make them more susceptible to malnutrition. Dental losses often make chewing difficult, resulting in reduced selection of foods, digestive problems or choking. Sensory losses may result in the inability to read labels, taste or smell food that may be spoiled or cause loss of interest in eating. Reduction in the quantity of gastric acid produced may reduce the absorption of vitamin B_{12} and other nutrients.

There is growing evidence that antioxidants can reduce death from heart disease and possibly other causes in the elderly. In a nine-year study conducted at the National Institute on Aging, researchers found that older persons taking both vitamins C and E had a 42 percent lower death rate from all causes than those who did not take the supplements. Death from heart disease was reduced by 53 percent in the vitamin takers.

Aging promotes changes in body composition with a relative increase in fat and loss of muscle and bone. The metabolic rate falls with advancing age and caloric requirements fall accordingly. In addition, some drugs cause nutritional deficiencies. The malnutrition that often accompanies alcoholism is magnified in the elderly.

Nutritional supplements are frequently taken by well-nourished individuals, but those who require them, such as elderly alcoholics, rarely do.

(See also NUTRITIONAL STATUS.)

O

oak

(tanner's bark, black oak, red oak, live oak, scrub oak, white oak)

Trees of the *Quercus* species and the Fagaceae family, found in the United States, England and other parts of the world, whose bark and acorns have long been significant to Native American herbalists and other practitioners as remedies for diarrhea and dysentery. In his book, *of Men and Plants: Autobiography of the World's Most Famous Plant Healer* (Macmillan, 1973), French herbal healer Maurice Méssegué wrote of the use of oak leaves and bark for ulcers, urinary incontinence, vaginal discharge, varicose veins, excessive menstrual flow, eczema and other ailments. A food staple of Native American tribes, acorns contain the astringent tannic acid, or tannin, a glucoside used in tanning, dyeing and the making of ink.

Homeopathic medicine employs tincture of acorns to treat alcoholism, bad breath, constipation, diarrhea, gout and other complaints. Folk medicine calls for an oak bark decoction for gastritis and tuberculosis, among other disorders. White-oak-bark infusion is also used as a treatment for goiter, sinus congestion and postnasal drip, inflammation and mucous discharges.

Also known for its strong wood for furniture, beams and other items, oak is celebrated by poet Robert Graves in *The White Goddess,* published in 1966: "Midsummer is the flowering season of the oak, which is the tree of endurance and triumph."

oats

(groats)

The cereal grass *Avena sativa,* of the Gramineae family, known throughout the world as a nutritive grain usually made into oatmeal. In various herbal medicine practices, oats (also oat straw) are prescribed as a nervine, tonic, stimulant and antispasmodic. Indications for oats include convalescence from illnesses such as gastroenteritis. Oatmeal and rolled oats are considered by Ayurvedic practitioners to be a food that creates heat in the body, a premise widely accepted by nutritionists who recognize oats as a source of carbohydrates and thus energy.

ocimum

See BASIL.

olive

The fruit of the tropical evergreen *Olea europaea,* of the Oleaceae family, used along with leaves and bark in herbal medicine to treat fever, nervous tension and constipation, and as a base ingredient for ointments and liniments. A popular dressing for salad and a cooking component, olive oil may be applied directly to insect bites and severely itching skin. Olives contain fat, calcium and vitamin A.

omega-3 polyunsaturated fatty acids (fish oil)

A group of polyunsaturated fatty oils, principally eicosapentaenoic acid (EPA) and docoshexaenoic acid (DHA), obtained from fatty fishes and plants. Capsules of these fish oils are promoted and sold for the prevention of cardiovascular disease. The highest concentrations of the oils are found in salmon, mackerel, sardines, herring, anchovies, whitefish and bluefish. Other seafoods containing these oils to a slightly lesser degree are striped bass, rainbow trout, swordfish, squid and Pacific oysters.

Plant sources of a fatty acid, linolenic acid, which can be converted in the human body to EPA and DHA, are linseed oils, walnuts and walnut oil, flaxseed, rapeseed, soybeans, spinach, mustard greens and purslane.

Benefits and Claims
At least two scientifically valid studies have shown a slight reduction in blood pressure in hypertensive but not normal individuals. Serum triglyceride levels are also lowered and blood-clotting times are increased, which suggests that claims for reducing heart-attack risk may be valid. However, there is evidence that ingesting excessive fish oil, whether from natural fish sources or in capsules, may increase the risk of cerebrovascular accidents (CVA), or hemorrhagic strokes.

In a study called Fish Oil Restenosis (FORT), 8 grams of fish oil were given to patients undergoing coronary angioplasty. The supplement, which was begun 12 days before the procedure and continued for six months, failed to demonstrate benefit in preventing restenosis, or reclosure, of the arteries following the procedure. (An earlier study had reported that fish oils seemed to prevent the reclosure of coronary blood vessels following coronary angioplasty.)

Omega-3 oils have also been shown to improve the inflammatory process that characterizes rheumatoid arthritis and psoriasis. These fatty acids are thought to be essential for good health and may be important for proper vision and brain development, but the manner in which this occurs has not been confirmed. A group of kidney-transplant patients were given daily fish-oil supplements during the first postoperative year. Although there were significantly lower episodes of transplant rejection, improved kidney function and better blood pressure in the treated group, survival at one year was not significantly different from the untreated control group.

Dosage
Nutritionists believe that ingestion of a one-to-one ratio of omega-3 oils to omega-6 oils, rather than the 10-to-one omega-6 to omega-3 ratio in most American diets, is important in preventing coronary artery disease. The omega-6 oils are found in some vegetable oils including corn and safflower. It is theorized that an excess of omega-6 causes substances called prostaglandins and leukotrienes to disrupt the immune system and promote the build-up of cholesterol-containing plaque on artery walls and blood clots. These changes may lead to heart disease manifested by angina pectoris (chest pain), heart attacks and irregular heart rhythms, or arrhythmias.

The recommended intake of omega-3 fatty acids is 0.8 to 1.1 grams per day. A diet containing bony fish or shellfish two or three times a week should provide a balanced level of omega-3 oils. The ratio can also be improved by reducing the use of fatty oils other than olive and canola oil.

Toxic Effects
In addition to the increased risks of strokes from excessive omega-3 fatty oils mentioned above, fish consumed eight or more times a week may supply an excess sufficient to weaken the immune system. And paradoxically, there is evidence that these oils may actually increase serum cholesterol.

Cold-water fish may be contaminated with mercury, and therefore pregnant women should consume them in moderation.

omega-6 fatty acids (evening primrose oil)
Group of fatty acids, of which gamma linoleic acid (GLA) is the most active, promoted to reduce cholesterol, thin the blood and reduce the inflammation in arthritis. There are also claims that capsules of evening primrose oil converts abnormal cancer cells to normal ones, relieves symptoms of premenstrual syndrome (PMS) and depression. Although there are no scientifically proven benefits to the supplements, they are probably nontoxic.

(See also OMEGA-3 FATTY ACIDS.)

Table 24
OMEGA-3 CONTENT OF VARIOUS FISHES
(Amount of omega-3 in a 3½-ounce serving of raw fish)

Highest (more than 1.0 gram)	Moderate (0.5 to 0.9 gram)	Lowest (less than 0.5 gram)	
Anchovies	Chum salmon	Carp	Mussels
Atlantic bluefish	Pacific oysters	Channel	Ocean
Atlantic salmon	Pompano	catfish	perch
Coho salmon	Rainbow trout	Clams	Roughy
Herring	Shark	Cod	Pike
Mackerel	Smelt	Crayfish	Pollock
Pink salmon	Spot	Eastern	Rockfish
Sablefish	Squid	oysters	Scallops
Sardines	Striped bass	Flounder	Sea bass
Sockeye salmon	Swordfish	Grouper	Shrimp
Spiny dogfish		Haddock	Snapper
Whitefish		Lobster	Tuna
		Mahi mahi	Whiting

onion

A biennial or perennial plant, *Allium cepa,* of the Liliaceae family, whose bulb is a popular raw or cooked vegetable throughout the world. Ayurvedic and other practitioners consider the onion a diaphoretic, tonic and aphrodisiac, with ammonia fumes that irritate eyes and mucous membranes. Onion juice mixed with honey is said to assuage asthmatic distress, cough, nausea, vomiting, intestinal worms and spasms. Onion can also be made into a poultice for joint pain and a nasal inhalant or eye drops for relieving epileptic seizure. Onions are also credited with the ability to lower the heart rate and cholesterol.

oral contraceptives

See CONTRACEPTIVES, ORAL.

orange peel

The rind of the fruit *Citrus aurantium,* of the Rutaceae family, used as a flavoring agent in baking recipes and marmalades and touted by Ayurvedic practitioners as a carminative, expectorant and stimulant. Oil of the rind alleviates flatulence and is also used in the treatment of chronic bronchitis. An infusion made with the flowers is used by herbalists as a nerve stimulant.

oregano

The bushy, perennial herb *Origanum vulgare,* of the Labiatae family, used widely as a pungent spice and an herbal stimulant, carminative and diaphoretic.

Oregon grape
(mountain grape)

A North American, flowering evergreen shrub, *Mahonia aquafolium,* or *Mahonia repens,* of the Berberidaceae family, whose root is used in Ayurvedic and other herbal medicine practices to treat liver disorders and liver-associated headache, indigestion, blood dyscrasias and coldness. Herbalists also report that the alkaloid berberine, found in the Oregon grape root, stimulates liver function. An infusion made of the berries is given to reduce fever.

organic

(natural or health foods)

Foods grown without synthetic fertilizers, insecticides or other contaminates. However, it may be virtually impossible to guarantee that soil has not been previously exposed to those substances. Foods grown with compost, manure or other natural fertilizers, as opposed to those grown in chemically fertilized soil, are considered healthier and better-tasting. Some foods erroneously labeled as "health foods" or "natural foods" have been found to be very high in fats, salt, additives, synthetic coloring or flavoring or preservatives.

orris

(Florentine iris)

A Mediterranean flowering herb, *Iris florentina*, of the Iradaceae family, whose fragrant rootstock has been used in the making of perfumes and remedies for water retention, dropsy, bronchitis, sore throat, colic and liver congestion, among other ailments. Orris root is commercially produced chiefly in Florence, Italy.

orthomolecular therapy

Theory of medical treatment utilizing doses of vitamins and minerals far exceeding the Recommended Daily Allowances. Studies have failed to demonstrate any long-term benefits to general health, cancer treatment or prevention or benefit to schizophrenia or other mental disorders. In addition, doses advocated may be toxic in some cases. (See MEGAVITAMIN STUDY OF THE AMERICAN PSYCHIATRIC ASSOCIATION; MEGAVITAMINS.)

oryza

(rice)

A flowering annual plant, *Oryza sativa*, of the Gramineae family, that provides the grain known throughout the world as a food staple. Named from the Arabic word *eruz*, rice has been cultivated since ancient times and used in traditional Chinese medicine as a tonic and remedy for stomach problems. Rice water is thought to be cooling to the body.

osha

The herb *Ligusticum porteri*, of the Umbelliferae family, used by Ayurvedic practitioners as a stimulant, antibacterial and expectorant.

(See also LIGUSTICUM.)

osteoporosis

A condition characterized by a reduction of the mass of bone per unit of volume, which can interfere with the strength and function of the bone, especially the lower vertebrae, hip and jaw. Supplemental calcium and vitamin D may help prevent or halt the rate of bone loss, but the nutrients do not seem to be effective in restoring porous, brittle bones.

It has been estimated that at least half of American women do not absorb sufficient calcium to maintain healthy bones. There are about 500,000 fractures attributed to osteoporosis yearly, and this is expected to increase to 1 million to 1.5 million by the year 2040 because of the aging population.

While osteoporosis is related to aging, more women, particularly postmenopausal women, and those who are extremely sedentary, are affected than men. Factors that appear to predispose women to osteoporosis also include low body weight, alcohol, smoking, the absence of pregnancy during child-bearing years, lack of previous use of oral contraceptives and lack of regular exercise. Only direct measurements of bone density are capable of determining which women should receive preventive treatment for postmenopausal osteoporosis.

An Australian study demonstrated lower than normal bone mass in otherwise healthy young adults whose older relatives had osteoporosis. In the study, bone mineral density was determined by computed tomographic scanning (CT-Scan) of the spine. Bone mineral content of the os calcis (the heel bone) by single-photon absorptiometry did not predict those at high risk.

(See also CALCIUM.)

oxalis
(yellow wood sorrel)

The creeping, herbaceous weed *Oxalis corniculata,* of the Oxalidaceae family, whose triple leaves so resemble the Irish shamrock that some people claim it was wood sorrel that St. Patrick used as a symbol of the Trinity in his attempt to convert pagans to Christianity. In traditional Chinese medicine, the oxalis plant treats intestinal worms, excessive body heat, scanty urine and copious bleeding.

oyster shell calcium
A source of calcium carbonate used as a supplement. (See CALCIUM.)

P

P, vitamin

A group of substances derived from plants that were originally thought to have vitamin properties. Now referred to as "bioflavonoids," they are widely promoted as a natural source of vitamin C. However, they are probably destroyed by the acidic gastric juices before they are absorbed. (See BIOFLAVONOIDS.)

PABA

(para-aminobenzoic acid)
A component of folic acid, it is found in brewer's yeast. It has no vitamin or other nutrient properties alone. The action of sulfonamide drugs is based on their structural relationship to PABA. The antibacterial drugs compete with PABA, preventing the normal metabolism of folic acid by bacteria. PABA-containing compounds, including procaine (Novocain), may interfere with the activity of the sulfonamide drugs.

The only proven therapeutic benefits of PABA are as sunscreen and local anesthetic in products for the relief of sunburn. PABA has been used to treat arthritis. There are no proven deficiencies of PABA in humans. Products containing PABA are a frequent cause of generalized or local allergic reactions. Allergic persons may develop severe skin rashes following sun exposure. Oral doses can cause nausea and vomiting.

pai shu

(bai zhu, atractylodes)
The plant *Atractylodes macrocephala,* of the Compositae family, whose root, according to Chinese traditional medicine, eliminates excess electrolytes (sodium and potassium, metabolic regulators pro-duced by the body) by inducing perspiration, thus energizing the body. Pai shu is also used as a spleen and pancreas tonic and for the treatment of diarrhea, indigestion, vomiting, edema, a feeling of tightness in the chest and other ailments.

panax

See GINSENG.

pangamic acid

(pangamate, vitamin B_{15})
A toxic substance obtained from apricot pits, without nutritional value and no scientifically proven use; by definition, pangamic acid is not a vitamin. Furthermore, it may cause genetic mutations.

pantothenic acid

(vitamin B_5, calcium pantothenate)
A water-soluble vitamin converted in the body to coenzyme A. Coenzyme A acts as a catalyst (see CATALYST) interacting with vitamin B_1, vitamin B_2, niacin, vitamin B_6, and biotin in various metabolic functions, including the breakdown of carbohydrates, proteins and fats for energy. Pantothenic acid is named from the Greek word *pantos,* meaning everywhere, consistent with its widespread occurrence in animals and plants.

This vitamin is also necessary for the synthesis, or manufacture, of vitamin D, steroids and other hormones, cholesterol and other fats, bile, red blood cells, porphyrins, neurotransmitters such as acetylcholine and other vital body biochemicals. Pantothenic acid may also be necessary for the normal function of the skin.

Pantothenic acid is absorbed with other B-complex vitamins from the gastrointestinal tract. It is found throughout the body tissues, usually as coenzyme A with the highest concentrations found in the liver, adrenal glands, heart and kidneys. There is little storage of the vitamin in the body and the vitamin is excreted unchanged by metabolic processes (70 percent in the urine and 30 percent in fecal waste).

History

Pantothenic acid was first synthesized by R. J. Williams and R. T. Major in 1940. However, it was not until 1947 that the vitamin's biological function in relationship with coenzyme A was demonstrated by F. Lipmann and others.

Deficiency

A deficiency of B_5 is virtually unknown. In an attempt to define the role of pantothenic acid, experiments have been performed with volunteers who were given a diet devoid of pantothenic acid and administered a medication that depletes tissue stores of the vitamin. These individuals exhibited many symptoms, including fatigue, heart irregularities, gastrointestinal effects, respiratory infections, skin rashes, burning sensations, lack of coordination, staggering gait, restlessness and muscle cramps.

Some researchers believe that pantothenic acid is important for normal adrenal gland function and therefore some claim the substance benefits those with Addison's disease. This research leads others to feel that B_5 is an "anti-stress" vitamin, and one study demonstrated that 10 mg daily allowed individuals to develop better tolerance to cold water stress. Since some who suffer from rheumatoid arthritis may have low levels of B_5, there is speculation that these patients may benefit from supplements.

There are as-yet-unproven claims for the role of pantothenic acid in the treatment of diabetic neuropathy, improved mental abilities, increasing gastrointestinal peristalsis, prevention of arthritis and allergies. Studies to prevent gray hair in humans based on the vitamin's ability to restore hair color in animals have been unsuccessful. Other uses, also not scientifically proven, include prevention of birth defects and some respiratory disorders; the topical use in creams, lotions or ointments to relieve itching and speed healing of minor rashes. Its value as a treatment for streptomycin and salicylate toxicities is questionable.

Recommended Daily Allowance (RDA)

Evidence to establish an RDA is lacking, since there is no proven need for pantothenic acid alone. The vitamin biotin appears to provide for any possible effects of a B_5 deficiency. The Food and Nutrition Board of the National Academy of Sciences suggests that 2 to 3 mg is appropriate for infants and 4 to 5 mg for children seven to 10 years of age. Four to 7 mg of the vitamin daily by age 11 and for adults is probably safe and adequate.

There is no demonstrated need for increased amounts of pantothenic acid during pregnancy, lactation or old age. However, there is probably an increased need in malabsorption disorders such as tropical sprue, celiac disease or regional enteritis (Crohn's disease).

Dietary Sources

A 2,500-calorie diet from plant and animal sources provides approximately 10 mg of pantothenic acid. Richest sources of vitamin B_5 include eggs, potatoes, salt-water fish, pork, beef, milk, whole wheat, peas, beans (except green beans) and fresh vegetables. There are very high levels of the vitamin in royal jelly of bees and in the ovaries of tuna fish and cod. Although cooking losses are minimal, milling of grains, canning or cooking after thawing frozen foods causes up to a 50 percent loss of the vitamin. Intestinal bacteria may also synthesize some of this vitamin.

Adverse Effects and Toxicity

Although there have not been reports of toxicity, occasionally diarrhea and water retention have occurred with megadoses of 10 to 20 grams of B_5 daily.

Supplements

Synthetic D-panthothenate is available as calcium or sodium salts but panthenol, an alcohol derivative, is widely used in multivitamin formulations because it is chemically more stable. Panthenol is easily converted to the active vitamin in humans.

Supplemental doses are usually up to 100 mg daily of panthothenic acid or calcium pantothenate tablets (each 10 mg of drug being equivalent to 9.2 mg of panthothenic acid).

papaver

(opium poppy)

A southeastern European and west Asian flowering herb, *Papaver somniferum,* of the Papaveraceae family, linked by name to Somnus, the Ancient Roman god of sleep (also called Morpheus, and in Greek mythology, Hypnus), who created the poppy for Ceres, the goddess of the harvest, so she could alleviate her exhaustion from tending the crops. Opium comes from the sap of the poppy fruit and contains alkaloids including morphine, a powerful hypnotic and analgesic. Highly addictive morphine sulfate (USP) acts on the central nervous system, and large or excessive doses may cause life-threatening morphine poisoning. One treatment for morphine poisoning is the drug naxolone, a narcotic antagonist.

In Chinese traditional medicine, opium is a sedative, analgesic and antispasmodic, and the poppy's empty fruits (that is, after the sap has run out) are used to treat headache, toothache, diarrhea, asthma and spasms.

papaya

(pawpaw, custard apple, melon tree)

The tropical American tree *Carica papaya,* of the Caricaceae family, whose fruit, leaves and seeds are used by herbalists to treat intestinal worms and digestive ailments. Papaya contains papain, an enzyme that digests proteins and is similar to pepsin produced in the stomach.

Paraguay copper tea

A stimulating beverage, also called yerba mate, made by steeping the leaves and stems of the *Ilex paraguariensis,* of the Aquifoliaceae family, in boiling water.

parsley

A Mediterranean, biennial herb, *Petroselinum sativum* or *crispum,* of the Umbelliferae family, whose leaves, roots and seeds are used by herbalists as a diuretic, laxative and expectorant. The essential oil of parsley, apiol, can substitute for quinia, given for intermittent fever, and ergot, as a parturient (administered after giving birth to stimulate contractions of the uterus). A popular kitchen herb that was once associated with Hercules, the Greek god of strength, because it seemed to give race-horses more stamina, parsley with its chlorophyll works as a breath-freshener and neutralizer of gastric juices. Parsley also contains vitamins A and C, niacin, riboflavin, thiamine, potassium and calcium. Psoralen in parsley may have some ability to fight cutaneous T-cell lymphoma (a type of skin cancer). Parsley is also thought to block histamine formation and therefore ward off allergy attacks, particularly of hives and hay fever. Apiol and another chemical, myristicin, in parsley produce laxative and diuretic effects.

While it may deplete the body's potassium supply, parsley's major fame lies in its role in the Passover Seder, the bitter herb eaten as a symbol of new beginnings. Native American and other herbalists prescribe parsley for kidney and bladder inflammation or stones, epilepsy, jaundice, venereal diseases and other ailments. Homeopathic uses include the treatment of intermittent fever and night blindness.

passion flower

(maypops, purple passion flower)

A flowering, climbing vine, *Passiflora incarnata,* of the Passifloraceae family, whose plant and flower are used by herbalists to treat nervous conditions such as headache, shingles, insomnia and hysteria. Passion flower is also considered an antispasmodic and diaphoretic.

patchouli
(pogostemon)
The fragrant southeast Asian plant *Pogostemon cablin,* of the Labiatae family, whose leaf oil is used in perfumery and in Chinese medicine to treat headache, gas, vomiting and diarrhea.

pau d'arco
(lapacho, tabebuia)
A Brazilian tree, lapacho (also grown in Argentina) or *Tabebuia haptaphylla,* of the Bignoniaceae family, whose inner bark is considered by herbalists to have antibacterial, antifungal, hypotensive, tonic, antidiabetic and antitumor properties. Prescribed for inhibiting the growth of cancers and tumors and for skin diseases, the immune system-supporting pau d'arco must be aged in order to be as potent as possible. Immature or outer bark is not believed to have the same effectiveness as the properly aged inner bark.

The Calaway tribe descended from the Incas had long used pau d'arco before it came to the attention of medical professionals in Brazil and Argentina. Allegedly, pau d'arco was responsible for curing cases of leukemia and other viral diseases in those countries. Other testimony has been given to the effectiveness of lapacho, but the substance has not yet been recognized or documented in allopathic literature.

pellagra
Syndrome caused by a deficiency of the vitamin niacin or a metabolic error in which the body is unable to convert tryptophan to niacin. The disorder is characterized by rashes, inflammation of the mucous membranes, diarrhea and mental symptoms including confusion, depression, anxiety, delusions and hallucinations. Supplemental niacin cures this disorder. (See NIACIN.)

pennyroyal
See MINT.

peony
(paeonia, white peony, bai shoa yao)
Eurasian and North American shrubs or herbs, including *Paeonia lactiflora* and *suffruticosa,* of the Ranunculeae family, known for their flowers and named after Paeon, the Greek physician who first used peony for medicinal purposes. Among the peony's history of uses are the peony-seed necklaces made by children of the Elizabethan era to ward off witches. According to Chinese practitioners, *P. lactiflora* roots are said to increase menstrual and urinary flow, work as an intestinal antiseptic and expectorant, and treat tuberculosis, stomach problems and other ailments. *P. suffruticosa* root bark is used as a remedy for convulsions, bloody vomitus related to fever, scarlet fever and other problems. An extract of the rootstock of *P. officinalis,* the common peony, is used by other herbalists as a sedative, diuretic and antispasmodic. A decoction made of the root is administered in minute doses for gout, asthma and other problems, although a tea is not to be made from the peony plant or flowers because they are poisonous and ingestion may be fatal.

peppermint
See MINT.

periwinkle
European, particularly British, and American creeping shrubs or perennial herbs, including *Vinca major* and *minor,* of the Apocynaceae family, utilized by herbalists for diarrhea, excessive

menstruation, nosebleed, bleeding in the mouth, toothache, seizures and other nervous conditions.

pernicious anemia
Potentially fatal anemia caused by vitamin B_{12} deficiency. (See B_{12}, VITAMIN.)

peyote
(mescal button, devil's root, dumpling cactus, sacred mushroom)
A southern Texan, Mexican and Central American spineless, succulent cactus, *Lophophora williamsii,* from which mescaline is derived. Mescaline is a poisonous alkaloid that causes hallucinations and an intoxication known as mescalism. In certain Native American tribes, peyote's flowering heads, called buttons, are used in religious ceremonies to produce altered states of consciousness, despite that peyote is classified as a narcotic whose use is restricted to scientific research.

phenylalanine
(α-amino-β-phenylpropionic acid)
An essential amino acid, most of which is converted by enzymatic reaction to tyrosine. When combined with aspartic acid it forms the artificial sweetener Aspartame. (See also AMINO ACIDS; PHENYLKETONURIA; TYROSINE).

Unproven Uses
Some claim that phenylalanine supplements can suppress the appetite, increase libido (sexual desire), improve memory, mental alertness, relieve depression and enhance the pain-killing ability of endorphins. Endorphins are narcoticlike hormones produced by the body in response to injury or disease.

Dietary Sources
Found in all protein-rich foods, phenylalanine content is also especially high in soy, cottage cheese, dry skim milk, almonds, peanuts, lima beans, pumpkin and sesame seeds.

Adverse Reactions and Toxicity
In the absence of the enzyme phenylalanine 4-monooxygenase, phenylalanine accumulates, causing the serious disorder phenylketonuria. Supplements should not be taken during pregnancy nor by those with skin cancer. This amino acid also may cause blood pressure elevation.

phenylketonuria
An inherited disease, expressed by an autosomal recessive trait, known as PKU, in which a defective enzyme, phenylalanine 4-monooygenase, causes the failure of the amino acid phenylalanine to oxidize to tyrosine. This reaction causes brain damage with severe mental retardation, convulsions, tremors and tumors. Other symptoms include hypopigmentation of the skin and hair, eczema, spasticity, contorted position of the hands and mousy odor in sweat and urine. If the disease is not detected at birth by a diagnostic test, brain damage may occur within the first three years of life.

If the disease is recognized at birth by a simple urine test, all symptoms of PKU are preventable by strict dietary restriction of phenylalanine. Therapy adherence in young children with PKU allows normal bone development. However, older patients with poor dietary compliance are at risk for low bone-mineral concentration.

phosphorus
Essential element in the diet found in all tissues and involved in almost all metabolic processes. Phosphorus is the second most abundant mineral in the body and the average adult contains 1 to 1½ pounds of the substance. It is a major component of bones and teeth occurring in a ratio of 1 part phosphorus to 2 parts calcium. Approximately 85 percent or 700 grams of the mineral are found in the adult skeleton. This mineral helps maintain the acid-base balance of blood, or pH.

Phosphorus is found in nearly all foods, and dietary deficiency is virtually unknown. One exception is a low-birth-weight infant fed exclusively breast milk in which supplementation is required to prevent rickets. Chronic users of antacids containing aluminum hydroxide may become deficient because aluminum interferes with phosphorus absorption. This deficiency causes bone loss, weakness, anorexia (loss of appetite) and pain.

Recommended Daily Allowances

For children one to 10 years and adults after age 24, 800 mg per day is recommended. For ages 11 to 24 years and during pregnancy and lactation, 1,200 mg is recommended. Phosphorus is adequate for full-term infants fed breast milk. Formula-fed infants should be given 300 mg through six months of age and 500 mg from six to 12 months.

Toxicity

In normal diets with adequate calcium and vitamin D, phosphorus is unlikely to have adverse effects. However, excess phosphorus may lower blood-calcium levels to unsafe levels.

pica

Compulsive eating of substances that lack nutrients including dirt, ice, gravel, flaking paint or plaster, clay, hair, wood, laundry starch. Pica is common in persons deficient in iron or zinc, but may also occur during pregnancy when there will frequently be craving for certain foods.

piper

(long pepper, bi ba, pippali [Sanskrit])
The pungent herbs *Piper longum, nigrum* and *sarmentosum,* of the Piperaceae family, used in Ayurvedic medicine as a stimulant, anthelmintic, expectorant and aphrodisiac, and in other herbal practices for various illnesses. *P. nigrum,* or black pepper (*maricha,* in Sanskrit), which is native to Sri Lanka and southern India and cultivated elsewhere in the tropics, is commonly used as a cooking and table spice. The fruits are used in Chinese medicine to treat colic, headache, gas,

scanty urine and menstrual pain. Other species are used whole or in part to aid digestion, treat stomach disorders and sunstroke.

(See also RED PEPPER.)

pipsissewa

(ground holly, prince's pine, wintergreen, zimolubka [Russian])
An evergreen of temperate zones whose herb bears fragrant, purple flowers, including *Chimaphila umbellata,* of the Ericaceae family. Roots and leaves of the plant are made into a tincture and prescribed by homeopaths and folk-medicine practitioners for cataracts, diabetes, fever, enlarged glands, gonorrhea, kidney, bladder and liver disorders, syphilis, malignant ulcers, scrofula and other ailments. Ayurvedic practitioners use the plant as a diuretic, astringent and alterative. Pipsissewa is not to be confused with *Gaultheria procumbens,* also called wintergreen.

PKU

See PHENYLKETONURIA.

plantain

(ribwort, Englishman's foot, greater plantain)
An herb of the Plantaginaceae family, particularly *Plantago* varieties of green-flowering plants such as *P. lanceolata* and *major.* Not to be confused with the plantain tree that produces a starchy fruit of the banana family, the plantain herb is prescribed by herbalists to treat bladder and kidney infections, hepatitis and bacillary dysentery. Externally, plantain is used on insect bites and stings and to promote the healing of wounds.

platycodon

(jie geng, balloon flower, Chinese bell flower)
A Chinese and Japanese flowering shrub, *Platycodon grandiflorus,* of the Campanulaceae family, whose roots are used in traditional Chinese medi-

cine for excess gas, congestion, tonsillitis, stomach ulcers, intestinal worms, influenza, sore throat, dysentery and other ailments.

pleurisy root
(butterfly weed, flux root, orange swallow-wort, tuber root, wind root, white root, Canada root)
A North American perennial plant, *Asclepias tuberosa,* of the Asclepiadaceae family, used by herbalists as a carminative, diuretic, diaphoretic and expectorant. Ayurvedic herbalists also use pleurisy root as a febrifuge. Native Americans either chewed the dried root or made tea from the root to treat respiratory infections and dysentery.

plumeria
(frangipani)
Fruit-bearing, flowering trees of the tropics, particularly *Plumeria rubra,* of the Apocynaceae family, named after Marquis Muzio Frangipani, who in the 16th century invented perfume for scenting gloves with this plant, and French botanist C. Plumier (1646–1706). While the plant's viscous white latex is toxic, the flowers are used by Chinese and other herbalists to treat diarrhea, dysentery and cough. Buddhist, Hindu and Muslim legend has it that even if the plumeria is uprooted, it continues to bear flowers and leaves and therefore is a symbol of immortality. In addition, planting a plumeria tree at a gravesite is a Malay custom.

PMS
See PREMENSTRUAL SYNDROME.

pogostemon
See PATCHOULI.

poke
(pokeroot, pokeweed)
An American perennial herb, *Phytolacca americana,* of the family Phytolaccaceae, used by herb-alists for blood and lymphatic purification, swollen glands, arthritis and rheumatism. Ayurvedic herbalists also use pokeroot as an emetic, alterative and cathartic.

polygonum
See KNOTWEED.

pomegranate
A southern Asian and tropical shrub, *Punica granatum,* of the Lythraceae family, that bears a thick-skinned fruit about the size of an orange. The fruit has many seeds and an acidic red pulp, and is used in Ayurvedic medicine as an astringent, tonic, alterative and anthelmintic. Tapeworm has been treated with pomegranate seeds since the Ancient Greeks, and the rind with its high tannin content makes both an internal and external astringent for skin conditions, a vaginal douche, a remedy for diarrhea and a gargle.

poppy
See PAPAVER.

potassium
Principal cation (ion carrying a positive charge) of muscle and most other cells. Adult bodies contain about 250 grams of potassium. It is essential in maintaining the fluid balance in our cells and is required for all cell reactions. Most of the potassium is concentrated in cells at a concentration more than 30 times greater than in the plasma and interstitial fluid. Cells contain 145 milliequivalents (mEq) of potassium per liter of fluid and plasma 3.8 to 5.0 mEq per liter (1 mEq of potassium equals 39 mg). Although the concentration of potassium in the blood is small, it is of great significance. Potassium is needed in the conversion of glucose into glycogen for storage, for the transmission of nerve impulses, for skeletal muscle contraction and the function of hormones. Potassium may

also play an important role in maintaining normal blood pressure. Populations that consume large amounts of dietary potassium have a lower incidence of hypertension. Animal studies have shown that potassium may have the ability to prevent strokes and protect the kidneys from the effects of hypertension even if the blood pressure itself is not lowered by potassium.

Potassium is absorbed from the gastrointestinal tract, and blood levels are kept in balance by kidney regulation. Although most potassium is lost in the urine, some is also lost in the stool and minimal amounts in the sweat.

Deficiency

Potassium deficiency can be caused by severe malnutrition, alcoholism, prolonged vomiting or chronic diarrhea. Diabetic acidosis, the most severe form of diabetes mellitus, and some forms of chronic kidney disease can also lead to severe deficiency. Low blood levels of potassium can also cause nausea and vomiting, which might in turn worsen the deficit. Anorexia, listlessness, apprehension, drowsiness and irrational behavior are signs of serious potassium depletion. Fatigue, muscle weakness, spasms and cramps, tachycardia, or rapid heat rate, and if severe, heart arrythmias, or irregular heart beat and eventually heart failure, potentially fatal, occur as potassium deficit progresses. Sudden death that can occur during prolonged fasting, such as occurs in persons with anorexia nervosa or starvation, may be a result from potassium deficiency.

Severe burns or trauma to large areas of the body and prolonged high fever deplete potassium. The beneficial action of diuretics, drugs used to treat high blood pressure and congestive heart failure, increases urine output and sodium excretion. Unfortunately, there is also a considerable loss of potassium. This loss is minimized by some diuretics such as amiloride, triamterene or spironolactone, called "potassium-sparing" diuretics.

Other drugs that can cause significant loss of potassium include laxatives, especially those containing phenolphthalein such as Ex-Lax and Feen-

A-Mint, bisacodyl (Dulcolax) and senna (Senokot), corticosteroids, the anti-Parkinson drug L-DOPA, salicylates, the antibiotic gentamicin and the antifungal drug amphotericin B.

Potassium deficiency may lessen a person's desire for water, worsening cases of dehydration.

Dietary Sources

Many dairy products, except for cheese; meats; poultry; fish; legumes; fruits; vegetables; and whole grains are rich in potassium. Although bananas, oranges and tomatoes are reputed to contain large quantities of potassium, ingesting them is not an efficient method of maintaining adequate potassium levels in the body.

Unfortunately, the processing of food has resulted in an increase in sodium and decrease of potassium in the diet of many persons. Potassium is also lost in cooking.

Supplemental Potassium

The average American diet contains 2 to 6 grams of potassium daily. A Recommended Daily Allowance (RDA) has not been established and normal individuals do not require supplemental potassium. However, most persons taking diuretics that are not potassium-sparing should take supplements if they have normal kidney function. Because of a potential for toxicity, potassium supplements should not be taken except under the direction of a physician. Supplements of potassium chloride require a prescription and come in tablet, capsule or liquid form. Potassium supplements must also be taken very cautiously with antihypertensives called "ace inhibitors," including captopril, enalapril and others. These drugs have potassium-sparing properties and may cause the potassium to rise to unsafe levels in patients who have compromised kidney function.

Toxicity

Daily intake of 18 grams of potassium or more can cause signs of toxicity. Blood levels can become elevated from excessive use of potassium-containing salt substitutes, kidney failure, acidosis, serious infections, gastrointestinal hemorrhages and severe muscle trauma. Signs of hyperkalemia (excessive levels of potassium) include muscle weakness, heart irregularities, heart failure and death by cardiac arrest. Toxicity can occur from smaller amounts of potassium, and may be fatal in persons with kidney failure.

pregnancy vitamin and mineral requirements

One of the most important times during life that normal women require vitamin and mineral supplements is during pregnancy. Over the past 150 years, the female reproductive span has increased to nearly 40 years, from menarche at about age 12.5 years to menopause after age 50. Unfortunately, the U.S. Department of Health and Human Services reports that between 25 and 30 percent of all pregnant patients do not enter into prenatal care before the second trimester of pregnancy. About 40 percent of pregnancies are followed in the public sector and average fewer than eight visits versus the recommended standard of 14 prenatal visits. There is a possibility that supplements taken by all women of child-bearing potential might reduce the risks for various pregnancy complications or birth defects. For instance, it is known that dietary iodine prevents cretinism (congenital hypothyroidism), and folic acid reduces the number of neural tube defects such as spina bifida. Some experts express concern that there will be a false sense of nutritional security in women relying too heavily on supplements rather than good dietary habits. There is also worry about excessive intake of some vitamins or minerals resulting in harm to either the women or her fetus (see Toxicity below).

At the first prenatal visit, the pregnant woman should have a total nutritional assessment, including a physical examination of the body and skin for evidence of nutritional deficiencies. A dietary food intake assessment should be made based on a dietary history of a three- to seven-day food intake. Measurements of height, weight and, if indicated, skin-fold thickness should be done.

Blood and urine tests to assess suspected deficiencies should be ordered. If even a minor deficiency is suspected, nutritional counseling from a professional trained in the special needs during pregnancy should be arranged immediately.

Additional dietary or supplemental calcium has been reported to reduce blood pressure and the development of pregnancy-induced toxemia. Added zinc has been associated with less incidence of abruptio placentae, fewer preterm deliveries and a lower rate of perinatal mortality.

Iron requirements of pregnancy are high. Loss of iron in the urine, stool and sweat amounts to an estimated 170 mg for the gestational period. The fetus requires about 270 mg and 90 mg are contained in the placenta and cord. Iron is needed for the increase in red blood cells that occurs during the last half of pregnancy. However, much of this is recovered when the red blood cell volume returns to normal after delivery.

Lactation contributes about 0.5 to 1 mg of iron per day. Therefore, the total iron loss for an uncomplicated pregnancy ranges from 420 to 1,030 mg or 1 to 2.5 mg per day over the 15 months of pregnancy and lactation. Iron lost by bleeding at delivery is approximately equal to that saved by not having menses during pregnancy.

Zinc requirement during pregnancy increases, and there are some reports that low zinc levels have been associated with congenital malformations, preterm birth and maternal complications in otherwise healthy women.

Pregnancy increases the demand for vitamin D, especially during the last trimester. Therefore, the Recommended Dietary Allowance is increased to 400 I.U. daily.

Folic acid is among the most important vitamins to be supplemented during the child-bearing years. Neural tube defects, including anencephaly, spina bifida and encephalocele are among the most common serious birth defects. They occur in approximately one of 1,000 births in the United States. The U.S. Public Health Service has recommended that all women of child-bearing age should consume at least 0.4 mg of folic acid daily. The evidence is so strong that these defects can be prevented by taking folic acid supplements before conception and through the first trimester, that the Food and Drug Administration has proposed requiring folic acid fortification of bread, rolls and buns, enriched flour and enriched self-rising flour, enriched cornmeal, enriched rice and enriched macaroni products. Since approximately half of all pregnancies are unplanned, this plan would lessen the dependence on behavioral changes to assure adequate folate levels in women.

During the last half of pregnancy, the fetus removes approximately 0.2 mcg of vitamin B_{12} daily. Therefore additional B_{12} is needed.

The fetus drains vitamin C from the mother as blood levels may be 50 percent higher in the fetus. An additional 10 mg of vitamin C daily to the recommended dietary allowance should suffice for this loss.

Toxicity

Vitamin/mineral supplements containing less than twice the RDA are presumed to be safe for both mother, fetus and breastfed newborn. However, vitamin A in doses only slightly higher have been shown to be teratogenic, or cause birth defects. Taken during early pregnancy, higher doses of vitamin A may cause permanent learning disabilities, spontaneous abortions and birth defects.

Although there is a serious need for adequate folic acid to prevent the birth defects mentioned above, daily intake in excess of 1,000 mg per day could mask pernicious anemia (associated with vitamin B_{12} deficiency) possibly resulting in irreversible nerve damage.

(See also B_{12}, VITAMIN; FOLIC ACID.)

premenstrual syndrome

(PMS)

An ill-defined variety of physical and emotional symptoms that occur on a regular basis starting a week or so prior to the onset of the menstrual period, or the luteal phase. For years women were told that the various symptoms were "all in their heads" and that they were "hysterical." But women consistently complained of more than 150 different symptoms. The most frequent complaints of PMS are bloating, headaches, mood changes, breast tenderness, weight gain and abdominal cramps. Despite the doubts of many, the myriad symptoms are probably legitimately explained by fluctuations in levels of the hormones estrogen and progesterone interacting with electrolytes and biochemicals called neurotransmitters that regulate the nervous system, and dietary factors such as poor nutrition, caffeine, smoking and alcohol. Reinforcing this theory, researchers in New Zealand reported that 15 of 21 women given fluoxetine (Prozac) experienced significant relief from their PMS symptoms. Prozac, an antidepressant, enhances levels of the neurotransmitter serotonin in the brain. When this drug was switched to a placebo for three months, only three of the group continued to show an improved response. However, similar symptoms that appear on and off throughout the month are probably not related to the menstrual cycle and should not be called "PMS."

There may be marginal vitamin deficiencies associated with the symptoms. A balanced diet may offer some improvement, and some advocate the use of various supplements. Magnesium, vitamin B_6, vitamin A and zinc have been reported to relieve PMS. Vitamin and mineral users must be cautioned that exceeding Recommended Dietary Allowances for some vitamins may be toxic. There have been studies in which placebo or sugar pills reduced symptoms as well as a diversity of supplements, reinforcing the possibility that psychological factors may indeed predominate in this syndrome.

Nutritionists recommend a well-balanced diet, with a vitamin-mineral supplement containing vitamin B_6; regular aerobic exercise; adequate sleep; and avoidance of caffeine, smoking and excessive alcohol. The symptoms can be so distressing in some women that hormonal suppression of ovulation may be necessary. However, Prozac and other antidepressants that affect the delicate chemical balance of the brain may provide a real breakthrough in the relief of this troublesome disorder.

preservatives
Substances added to foods or supplements to prevent them from spoiling. There are about 100 preservatives in common use. Antioxidant vitamins such as ascorbic acid, or vitamin C, are used to preserve frozen fruits, dry milk, beer and ale, flavoring oils, apple juice, soft drinks, candy, artificial sweeteners, canned mushrooms, processed meat products, jellies and preserves.

prickly ash
(yellow wood, toothache tree)
A North American shrub or tree, *Zanthoxylum americanum,* of the Rutaceae family, whose bark and fruit are used in herbal medicine. Native Americans believed the bark alleviated toothache. Ayurvedic practitioners use the pungent and bitter prickly ash as a stimulant, carminative and anthelmintic.

primrose
(butter rose, English cowslip)
A European perennial plant, *Primula vulgaris* and *officinalis,* of the Primulaceae family, whose flowers, herb and rootstock are used in herbal treatment of migraine, insomnia and other nervous problems, weakness, mucus congestion, respiratory infections, rheumatism, gout and blood dyscrasias, or diseases.

princes' pine
See PIPSISSEWA.

processing of foods
The preparation of the ingredients of food products, such as the milling of grains, that greatly reduces vitamin and mineral content. Processing wheat to make white flour results in the loss of up to 40 percent of vitamin C, 65 to 85 percent of B-complex vitamins, almost 60 percent of magnesium and 70 percent of zinc. In addition, fiber, protein and other vitamins for a total of 26 nutrients are reduced or removed. Only a trace of iron, calcium, niacin, thiamine and riboflavin are added to make "enriched" bread.

The addition of sodium bicarbonate to green beans and peas to preserve their green color or to dried beans to soften them alters the pH to greater than 8, inactivating thiamine. High temperatures in cooking and canning also destroy thiamine, but freezing does not affect levels. Thiamine is also destroyed by X-rays, ultraviolet irradiation and the addition of sulfite preservatives used for dehydrated fruits.

Heat reduces availability of pyridoxine. The presence of ascorbic acid increases the loss of pyridoxine and vitamin B_{12} in processes requiring heat.

(See also COOKING METHODS.)

prostate cancer
Malignancy of the walnut-sized gland present at the base of the male bladder. Although 13 percent of all men will eventually be diagnosed with this cancer, as many as 50 percent have microscopic evidence of the malignancy at autopsy. High-fat diets, especially those rich in the types of fat found in meat, have been blamed for increasing the risk for prostate as well as many other cancers. There is an almost 50 percent lower rate of prostate cancer in Florida when compared with Maine. It has been theorized that the difference is caused by an as-yet-unexplained protective effect of vitamin D that is present in warmer climates with more

sun exposure. Sunlight produces vitamin D in human skin.

protein

A nitrogenous compound found in plants and animals that, when hydrolyzed, converts to amino acids required for the development and repair of body tissues and the source of heat and energy. The word protein is derived from the Greek word *protos,* meaning first—a particularly apt definition in view of the necessity of protein to human and animal life.

Different food protein sources influence the utilization and possibly the requirements for other nutrients. Therefore, it is very difficult to determine rational and safe dietary requirements for individuals or different populations.

Deficiency

Protein deficiency is usually linked to a lack of adequate calories and results in malnutrition. This condition, called kwashiorkor, is usually seen in infants and children as a result of poor diet, infections, intestinal parasites and other factors. Protein deficiencies are rare in the United States.

Toxicity

There is no strong evidence that ingestion of excessive protein up to twice the Recommended Daily Allowance (RDA) is harmful in persons with normal kidney function. However, there may be significant risk to persons with kidney disease in even normal quantities of proteins.

(See also AMINO ACIDS.)

provitamin

Any compound that can be converted, or metabolized, to a vitamin in the body. An example is the carotenoid beta-carotene, a fat-soluble pigment in orange, dark-yellow and dark-green vegetables and fruits. When ingested, it can be converted to vitamin A. Other provitamins are vitamin D_2, ergosterol and D_3, 7-dehydrocholesterol, which are converted to vitamin D.

(See A, VITAMIN, D, VITAMIN.)

prunella

(heal-all, self-heal)

A Eurasian perennial, flowering herb, *Prunella vulgaris,* of the Labiatae family, whose stem, leaves and flowers are used in Chinese medicine to treat lymphatic tuberculosis and fever, and whose fruits are made into remedies for eye inflammation, headache, vertigo, nervousness and other ailments.

pseudotumor cerebri

An uncommon cause of increased intracranial pressure that may result in severe headaches and visual disturbances. Among the many causes of this rare condition are very high and prolonged doses of vitamin A.

(See also A, VITAMIN.)

pseudovitamins

A group of compounds that do not satisfy requirements for classification as vitamins but are nevertheless promoted as vitamins by some. These substances include orotic acid (vitamin B_{13}), inositol, choline, methione, para-aminobenzoic acid (PABA), carnitine (vitamin B_4), amygdalin or laetrile (vitamin B_{17}), bioflavonoids (vitamin P), pangamic acid or pangamate (vitamin B_{15}) and gerovital (vitamin H_3).

psoriasis

Common, chronic, inflammatory skin disorder characterized by reddened, dry, scaling patches of various sizes, covered by grayish-white or silvery-white scales. There may be small areas of bleeding under the lesions, which are most commonly found on the extensor surfaces of the extremities, such as the elbows and knees, scalp, genitalia and lumbosacral region. The nails may become pitted and a particularly severe form of arthritis may accompany the rash.

Various dietary measures and vitamin supplements have been promoted for psoriasis, but it is very difficult to assess the results because the disorder waxes and wanes. Some report that a very low-fat and modified-protein diet is successful in a limited number of patients. Dr. Kempner's Rice Diet was popular in the 1940s, but adherence is difficult. Two articles published in 1986 reported disappearance of psoriatic lesions on the rice diet. The rice diet has severe limitations nutritionally and must be supplemented with at least the Recommended Daily Allowance (RDA) for vitamins and minerals. The diet also is deficient in protein and must be closely monitored by a physician or nutritionist. Vitamin A has been promoted for the treatment of psoriasis, but it is safer to use the provitamin form, beta-carotene, which is nontoxic. Vitamin D taken by mouth or applied topically seems to have some benefit, as reported in the British medical literature. However, large oral doses of vitamin D are toxic.

A diet deficient in the essential fatty acid linoleic acid may contribute to the occurrence or severity of psoriasis. This nutrient is found in safflower and other vegetable oils, nuts and seeds. An inadequate supply of zinc, required for absorption of linoleic acid, may play a role by limiting the availability of the essential fatty acid.

Leukotrienes are biochemicals in the body that contribute to the inflammatory process of psoriasis. The omega-3 fatty acids found in fish oils seem to limit production of leukotrienes, and there have been reports of improvement in the skin disorder with the use of fish-oil supplements.

Capsaicin, a substance derived from chili peppers, has been used as a cream to relieve the pain and itching of psoriasis. For severe cases of psoriasis, a chemotherapeutic drug called methotrexate may be helpful. Methotrexate is chemically related to the vitamin folic acid. However, while its chemical structure is similar enough to fool cells to take up this substance, it lacks the vitamin's ability to promote cell growth and therefore may have a limiting effect on the skin disorder and some cancerous tumors.

A well-balanced diet, regular exercise, stress reduction and a multivitamin-mineral supplement may be beneficial for those who have psoriasis.

psyllium
(isaphgul)
A laxative, demulcent and astringent derived from *Plantago psyllium,* of the Plantaginaceae family. See FIBER.

pyridoxine
(pyridoxal, pyridoxamine or vitamin B_6)
A group of chemically related structures that are converted in the liver to the active form of the vitamin. The Council on Pharmacy and Chemistry has assigned the name *pyridoxine* to the vitamin. B_6 acts as a coenzyme (see COENZYME) by participating in more than 60 enzymatic reactions involving amino acids and essential fatty acids. Amino acids are the building blocks of proteins, and therefore B_6 is essential for the growth and maintenance of almost all of our body functions.

The vitamin stimulates the conversion of amino acids to carbohydrate or fat to be utilized for energy or stored for later use. It is also essential for the enzymatic reaction that releases sugar from storage in the liver. B_6 is essential in the conversion of tryptophan to niacin (see TRYPTOPHAN). B_6 is also involved in the synthesis of hormones, the red-blood-cell protein hemoglobin and formation and maintenance of the nervous system. It helps in the manufacture of some neurotransmitters that regulate nerve impulses and prostaglandins that help regulate blood pressure, muscle contractions and the heart and other processes.

History

Vitamin B_6 was first discovered in 1926 in rats fed a diet deficient in vitamin B_2, which caused a rash. However, it was not until 1936, when György recognized that it was another substance that caused the rash, that it was named vitamin B_6. The chemical structure was determined in 1939.

Deficiency

Rarely seen alone, B_6 deficiency usually occurs in individuals also lacking other B-complex vitamins. Skin rashes, seizures, carpel tunnel syndrome and, rarely, anemia are the most characteristic features of pyridoxine deficiency.

Some infants who are born with a defect in B_6 metabolism develop mental retardation and seizures, or convulsions. B_6 levels may be low during pregnancy, and in the past the vitamin has been used to treat the nausea and vomiting of pregnancy. It has also been used to treat the depression that accompanies the use of oral contraceptives by some women.

Recommended Daily Allowances

The RDA for adult men is 2.0 mg and 1.6 mg for women. These values are based on the anticipated average quantities of protein consumed of 100 grams. However, if a person eats huge amounts of protein, these allowances may need to be increased.

Dietary Sources

The highest concentrations of vitamin B_6 are found in chicken, fish, kidney, liver, pork and eggs. Unmilled rice, soy beans, oats, whole-wheat products, peanuts and walnuts are also good sources of the vitamin. Up to 70 percent is lost during freezing and processing luncheon meats, and up to 90 percent in milling cereal.

Drug Interactions

Up to 40 drugs are known to affect the availability or metabolism of vitamin B_6. Foremost among these are prolonged use of the antituberculosis drug isoniazid; penicillamine, a chelating agent used in the treatment of copper, mercury and lead poisoning and rheumatoid arthritis; cycloserine, an immunosuppressant drug; and hydralazine, an antihypertensive. The administration of vitamin B_6 may alleviate some adverse effects of those drugs. B_6 speeds up the metabolism of levodopa and thus lessens the effectiveness of the drug used in the treatment of Parkinson's disease.

Toxicity

Chronic toxicity from vitamin B_6 to the central nervous system may result in ataxia, or an unsteady gait, and muscle weakness. Some have had withdrawal symptoms of dependency after chronic use of as little as 200 mg.

Doses of 200 mg intravenously or 200 to 600 mg orally may result in adverse drug interactions with the anti-Parkinson drug levodopa, the heart drug quinidine and penillamine, a chelating agent used to treat Wilson's disease, a potentially fatal inherited disorder in which copper accumulates in the liver, and severe rheumatoid arthritis.

(See also COPPER.)

pueraria
See KUDZU.

pumpkin

The roundish, usually bright-orange fruit of the *Cucurbita pepo* vine, of the Cucurbitaceae or gourd family, whose pulp is eaten as a vegetable or made into pies and other foods, and whose seeds are considered of medicinal value by herbalists. Ayurvedic practitioners, as do most herbalists, prescribe them as a diuretic and anthelmintic. The seed oil is also used for chapped skin, wounds and burns.

pyrola
See WINTERGREEN.

Q

quassia
(bitter ash, bitter wood)
A tropical American and West Indian tree, *Picraena excelsa,* of the ailanthus family, named after Quassi, an 18th-century Surinam slave who discovered the quassia heartwood's use as a remedy for roundworms in children and its value as an insecticide. Herbalists also use quassia-wood infusion for fever, indigestion and rheumatism. If the infusion is used as an enema, it is effective against pinworms.

queen of the meadow
See GRAVELROOT.

quercus
(daimyo oak)
A Korean, Japanese and Chinese tree, *Quercus dentata,* of the Fagaceae family, named from the Latin word for tree. Its acorns are used by Chinese practitioners as a remedy for diarrhea and excessive menstrual flow; leaves are used to stop bleeding, quench thirst and treat hemorrhoids and dysentery; its bark is thought to expel intestinal worms.

quick weight-loss programs
Drastic and prolonged reduction of caloric intake to stimulate weight loss. Diets below 800 calories per day have many shortcomings, and they may cause potassium deficiency, which may lead to heart irregularities. Diets of less than 1,200 calories may be deficient in thiamine, pyridoxine, vitamin B_{12}, iron, magnesium and zinc. Very low-calorie diets use protein as a source of energy. In fact, diets of less than 1,000 calories, with protein content greater than carbohydrate, are actually deficient in protein. These diets may also contain excessive fat and cholesterol.

The safest and most sensible weight-reducing diet is based on a balanced intake of the Four Food Groups. Four servings of whole grains and four of fruits and vegetables, two milk and two meat or legume will provide about 1,600 calories. The high-fiber content of this diet probably reduces drastic fluctuations in blood-sugar levels and in turn usually reduces hunger.

Weight loss should be slow and gradual, averaging 1 to 2 pounds per week. Weight loss that exceeds 2 pounds results in loss of water and lean body tissue rather than fat. A multiple vitamin-mineral supplement and exercise, of at least 30 minutes of aerobic activity (treadmill is best) every other day, should be an integral part of all diet programs. If weight loss does not occur, then exercise time should be increased instead of further reducing calories. Supplements should not exceed two or three times the Recommended Dietary Allowances to avoid toxicity.

Group diet programs such as Weight Watchers offer emotional support and behavioral modification. However, once the desired goal has been reached it is important to stay on a maintenance program. The majority of patients in these programs regain lost weight after dropping out of the program. An individual's weight gain may even exceed what was lost within a short time of going off a diet.

quisqualis
(rangoon creeper)

A Burmese, Malaysian Filipino and New Guinean climbing shrub, *Quisqualis indica,* of the Combretaceae family, whose name in Latin means "What is this?" Chinese practitioners use the fruits and seeds as a roundworm remedy, and the seeds in oil for skin diseases and eruptions.

R

radish
(raphanus, lai fu zi)
An annual or biennial Eurasian plant, *Raphanus sativa,* of the family Cruciferae, with a pungent, fleshy root that is eaten as a vegetable and used in herbal medicine to aid digestion and treat cough, rheumatism and gallbladder disturbances. The leaves are used for headache, and the whole plant treats diarrhea, dysentery and intestinal worms. Radishes contain small amounts of calcium and vitamin C.

rasayana
The Sanskrit word roughly meaning "give life," referring to certain herbal nutritional supplements used to rejuvenate, strengthen, balance, restore and purify the body. In Ayurvedic medicine, herbs and minerals are used separately or in combination as rasayanas. Amla (Indian gooseberry, the highest natural source of vitamin C), guggul, ashwaghanda, ginseng, licorice, aloe vera, saffron, gotu kola, elecampane and honey are examples of rasayanas, which are more closely associated with Indian food than medicine. One brand of rasayana preparation is Biochavan, either as a jam or tablets made by Ageless Body, Timeless Mind products (Quantum Publications).

raspberry
A European and North American prickly perennial or biennial plant, *Rubus idaeus* and *strigosus,* of the Rosaceae family, whose fruit (not true berries but aggregates with several drupelets) and leaves are used in Native American, Ayurvedic and other herbalist practices as an astringent, stimulant, laxative, tonic and emmenagogue. Raspberry leaf tea is said to prevent miscarriage. Raspberry is also a remedy for diarrhea and dysentery and irritation of the urinary tract, and widely utilized as a flavoring agent for syrups and other preparations. Nutritionally, raspberry contains vitamins A and C, calcium and traces of other minerals.

RDA
Abbreviation for Recommended Dietary Allowance. (See RECOMMENDED DIETARY ALLOWANCE.)

recommended dietary allowance (RDA)
The levels of intake of essential nutrients that, on the basis of scientific knowledge, are judged by the Food and Nutrition Board to be adequate to meet the known nutrient needs of practically all healthy persons (see Appendix 5, Recommended Dietary Allowances).

The Food and Nutrition Board is a subcommittee of the National Research Committee and has developed RDAs since 1941. The Board has offered 10 revisions of its recommendations since their first publication in 1943.

The RDAs are not minimal requirements but are published to set standards for good nutrition. The RDA serves as the basis for the United States Recommended Daily Allowances (USRDA) established by the Food and Drug Administration (FDA) for labeling purposes.

red pepper
(cayenne, chili pepper, capsicum, Spanish pepper, Zanzibar pepper, la jiao)
A tropical perennial plant, *Capsicum frutescens* or *anuum,* of the family Solanaceae, whose fruit is

used in herbal-medicine practices as an appetizer, digestive, stimulant, irritant and tonic. It is prescribed to build up the body's resistance for a cold that is just beginning, and it can be made into an infusion to treat stomach or intestinal cramps. Large amounts of cayenne can cause damage to the gastrointestinal tract and kidneys. As a spice used on foods, cayenne is thought to stimulate the appetite.

rehmannia

A northern Chinese perennial herb, *Rehmannia glutinosa,* of the family Scrophulariaceae, named after Russian physician Joseph Rehmann (1779–1831). Rehmannia root is an herbal Chinese remedy for bleeding, fever, anemia, sore throat, mouth ulcers, bloody vomitus, vertigo, irregular menses and premature ejaculation.

retinaldehyde, retinoic acid, retinol

Substances found in animal fats that are active forms of vitamin A. (See A, VITAMIN.)

rheumatoid arthritis (RA)

Chronic, crippling form of arthritis, characterized by inflammation of the lining, or synovial tissue, of the joints. All joints may be affected, but the small joints of the fingers and feet are the most commonly involved. Inflammatory changes can involve the heart, lungs and other vital organs. The cause of RA is undetermined, but probably involves an impairment of the immune system. RA differs from osteo- or degenerative arthritis in that the latter is a degeneration of cartilage.

Many supplements have been promoted as treatments or cures for RA; however, symptoms of this disease come and go, and it is difficult to prove benefits for supplements as well as for traditional treatments. Selenium has antioxidant properties and is involved in the production of prostaglandins, hormonelike compounds that regulate the inflammatory process. Blood levels of selenium, as well as pantothenic acid, have been found to be lower than normal in some patients with RA. While preliminary studies have suggested some improvement in joint pain in those given supplements, benefits have been inconsistent. Pantothenic acid alone has never been proven to be of value in treating any disease. Vitamin E alone or in combination with selenium has also been reputed to have benefits for RA.

Although cooper bracelets have been promoted for the relief of arthritis, high copper levels have been seen in some persons with RA and other inflammatory disorders. Paradoxically, drug compounds containing copper may be effective in treating some of these disorders. Omega-3 fatty acids, or fish oils, have been found to improve some patients with RA. Penicillamine, a drug used to treat rheumatoid arthritis, increases the elimination of pyridoxine (vitamin B_6) in the urine.

rhubarb

(rheum, da huang)

Asian plant, *Rheum tanguticum, palmatum* and *officinale,* of the Polygonaceae family, named from the Greek word, *rha,* meaning rhubarb. In herbal medicine, the roots are used to treat constipation, jaundice, fever, infectious hepatitis, diarrhea, amenorrhea related to blood clotting, internal bleeding, dysentery, worms and menstrual pain.

rhus

(sumach)

East Asian temperate-zone trees or shrubs of the *Rhus* genus, including *R. verniciflua* (varnish tree or Japanese lacquer tree) and *R. succedanea* (wax tree). In Chinese traditional medicine, rhus is used to treat bleeding, diarrhea, dysentery, intestinal worms and tuberculosis. Lacquer is a product of the wax tree.

riboflavin

(vitamin B$_2$)

Formerly called vitamin G, water-soluble component of the vitamin B-complex. Riboflavin is converted by the body to two coenzymes, flavin mononucleotide (FMN) and flavin dinucleotide (FAD), which are necessary for normal tissue respiration (transport of oxygen to the cells) and the metabolism of lipids such as fatty acids. This vitamin is also required for the activation of pyridoxine (vitamin B$_6$) and the conversion of tryptophan to niacin. Riboflavin may also play an important role in maintaining the stability of erythrocytes (red blood cells).

In healthy individuals, the B vitamins including riboflavin are readily absorbed from the gastrointestinal tract, mainly in the duodenum. However, this is not the case for those suffering from malabsorption disorders or alcoholism. Vitamin B$_2$ is metabolized or broken down by the liver, and its metabolites are eliminated by the kidneys. The vitamin or its breakdown products are found in all body tissues, especially the liver, spleen, kidneys and heart, and in breast milk. Excess B$_2$, beyond the body's requirements, is excreted mostly unchanged in the urine and feces. Riboflavin is found in retinal pigment and appears to be essential in the eye's ability to adjust to light.

Deficiency

Ariboflavinosis, or vitamin B$_2$ deficiency, is a rare form of malnutrition or malabsorption that causes angular stomatitis and cheilosis (soreness in the mouth and tongue and cracks in the corners of the mouth), corneal vascularization and dermatosis (rashes in the genital area and dryness of the skin on the face). Severe deficiency may interfere with the production or premature death of red blood cells, resulting in anemia and neuropathy. Animal studies suggest that a lack of riboflavin may inhibit the production of antibodies to protect against infections and increase susceptibility to esophageal cancer. Persons highly sensitive to light and those with cataracts may have B$_2$ deficiency, and increasing intake may improve or prevent these troublesome problems.

Supplementation

Riboflavin may be of value in physical stress situations and tissue repair including burns, following gastrectomy, hepatic-biliary tract disease (alcoholism and cirrhosis or obstructive jaundice), phototherapy by blue light in the treatment for hyperbilirubinemia in newborns that causes photodecompensation of the vitamin, hyperthyroidism, prolonged infection, chronic fever, diseases including celiac, tropical sprue and Crohn's, in which there is severe diarrhea, malignancy and prolonged emotional stress.

Studies in China conducted by the collaborative efforts of the National Eye Institute and the Chinese Academy of Medical Sciences have demonstrated the protective effects of riboflavin and niacin in preventing a type of common cataract. Riboflavin is part of the enzyme system that maintains a supply of the antioxidant glutathione in the eye (See also EYE DISEASES.)

Other Possible Uses

Claims of riboflavin's benefit in the following disorders or situations are unsubstantiated: acne, burning foot syndrome, migraine headaches or muscle cramps. Higher than RDA doses of vitamin B$_2$ and other vitamins and minerals have been reported to strengthen the immune system. A combination of vitamins B$_2$ and B$_6$ may improve carpal tunnel syndrome. Depression and anxiety have been attributed to inadequate B$_2$.

Precautions

There have been no confirmed abnormalities or other problems during pregnancy or breast-feeding with normal daily requirements.

Adverse Effects/Toxicity

There is no known toxicity or other side effects of large doses of riboflavin, although the urine may turn dark yellow or orange with very high doses. However, in some animals high doses of riboflavin have increased the growth of some tumors.

The United States Pharmacopeia (USP) maintains that cooking generally does not alter the availability of riboflavin. Some authors dispute this, claiming that cooking meat causes a 25 percent loss, and milk loses 10 to 12 percent of vitamin B_2 following pasteurization and irradiation for vitamin D.

Storing milk in clear glass bottles increases loss of riboflavin up to 75 percent in three and one-half hours. Blanching of vegetables before they are canned or frozen can destroy up to 40 percent of this vitamin. Milling of grains destroys a large percentage of the B vitamins, but many of the

Table 25
RECOMMENDED DIETARY REQUIREMENTS (RDA) FOR RIBOFLAVIN[1,2]

Infants and children	
birth to 6 months	0.4 mg
6 to 12 months	0.5 mg
1 to 3 years	0.8 mg
4 to 6 years	1.1 mg
7 to 10 years	1.2 mg
Adolescent and adult females	
11 to 50 years	1.3 mg
51 years and older	1.2 mg
Pregnant females	1.8 mg
Lactating females	
first 6 months	1.6 mg
second 6 months	1.7 mg
Adolescent and adult males	
11 to 14 years	1.5 mg
15 to 18 years	1.8 mg
19 to 50 years	1.7 mg
51 years and older	1.4 mg

[1] Adequate diet generally provides sufficient riboflavin without need for supplementation
[2] Use of the following drugs may increase the requirement for vitamin B_2: phenothiazines, tricyclic antidepressants and probenecid.

Table 26
BEST FOOD SOURCES OF RIBOFLAVIN

Milk and dairy products	Fish
Meats	Green leafy vegetables
Whole grain and enriched cereals and bread	

processed products are enriched by replacing riboflavin and other vitamins and minerals.

Supplements
There are no studies available in geriatric patients to determine their increased need for riboflavin. See Table 25 for dosage to treat vitamin B_2 deficiency.

rice
See ORYZA.

rickets
Disruption in the growth plate of bone caused by vitamin D deficiency. Called osteomalacia in adults, children with rickets have poor appetite and grow slowly. They have weak muscles, deformed bones that buckle or appear "bowlegged" or "knock-kneed," a bulging forehead and may have pelvic and spinal deformities. Misshapen breastbones can cause "sunken" chests that can lead to breathing difficulties. In addition there may be bone pain, fatigability, growth retardation and convulsions and tetany in its most severe form. These children have delayed dentition and are especially susceptible to tooth decay.

Vitamin D is synthesized by the skin upon exposure to sunlight. It is essential for the utilization of calcium and phosphorus to make normal bone. Rickets has been recognized for thousands of years and was first described scientifically in the mid-1600s. In the early 1800s, air pollution from the industrial revolution reduced sun exposure, and rickets become a serious health problem in northern Europe and England. However, it was not until the 1930s that vitamin D was demonstrated to be the cure.

(See also D, VITAMIN.)

rose hips
The ripe accessory fruit or seed pods of the *Rosa* species of the Rosaceae family, recognized as a rich source of vitamin C. In addition to widespread popularity as a vitamin supplement, usually in tablet or capsule form, rose hips are used in Ayurvedic medicine as a stimulant, carminative and astringent. Flowers and hips of roses are of medicinal value, especially *Rosa californica, centifolia, damascena, eglanteria, gallica, laevigata* and *roxburghii.*

rosemary
Originally a Mediterranean evergreen shrub, *Rosmarinus officinalis,* of the family Labiatae, cultivated throughout the world as an aromatic seasoning. The leaves and flowering tops are useful in herbal remedies for indigestion, headache, arthritis, nervous stomach, insomnia, colds, suppressed menses, hypotension, poor circulation and, externally, for wounds, eczema, sores and baldness. Excessive amounts of rosemary may be toxic.

rue
(herb-of-grace, German rue)
A southern European, North American and northern African flowering, perennial plant, *Ruta graveolens,* of the Rutaceae family, whose herb is valued by herbalists for the treatment of palpitations related to menopause, painful gas and colic, gout and rheumatic pain. Because it is also prescribed to promote the onset of menstruation, rue should not be used by pregnant women. Ayurvedic practitioners use rue as a nervine and anthelmintic as well.

rutin
A bioflavonoid obtained from buckwheat and other plants. (See BIOFLAVONOIDS.)

S

safe and adequate intakes

Levels that are considered nontoxic for nutrients and for which there is inadequate knowledge to establish RDAs. Prior to the 10th edition in 1989 of the book *Recommended Dietary Allowances,* the Food and Nutrition Board of the National Research Council listed vitamin K, biotin and pantothenic acid; trace elements, copper, chromium, fluoride, manganese, molybdenum and selenium; and electrolytes sodium, potassium and chloride in that category. By the 10th edition of the publication, RDAs have been established for vitamin K and selenium, and minimal requirements have been given for electrolytes.

safflower

(dyers' saffron, false saffron)
A European, especially Mediterranean, and North American annual plant, *Carthamus tinctorius,* of the Compositae family, whose flowers can be made into a tea that induces perspiration, considered effective against colds and certain cases of hysteria. In Ayurvedic medicine, pungent safflower is prescribed as an alterative, emmenagogue and carminative. An edible oil is made from the seeds of the safflower; it is high in linoleic acid and low in saturated fatty acids. The flower heads yield a red or orange dye.

saffron

(autumn crocus, Spanish saffron)
A perennial flowering plant cultivated largely in France, Spain, Sicily and Iran, *Crocus sativus,* of the Iridaceae family, used as a perfume and dye by the Ancient Greeks and Romans. From the 14th to 18th centuries, spice dealers were called "saffron grocers," because saffron was an important commodity. The plant's dried flower stigmas serve as antispasmodic, aphrodisiac, expectorant, sedative and emmenagogue in herbal medicine. Ayurvedic practitioners also use saffron as a carminative. A food flavoring and coloring agent (Spanish rice is typically yellow because of the saffron), saffron is used as a remedy for cough, stomach gas, gastrointestinal disturbances, whooping cough and insomnia, although its high price prohibits its accessibility, and it takes some 40,000 flowers to produce one pound of saffron. Furthermore, it contains a toxic substance that affects the central nervous system and may cause kidney problems.

sage

(salvia, dan shen, sauge [French])
A wild and cultivated perennial shrub, *Salvia officinalis,* of the Labiatae family, named from the Latin *salveo,* meaning "I heal" and *salvus,* to save. Sage leaves in herbal medicine are believed to be capable of arresting perspiration (such as night sweats related to tuberculosis), stopping the flow of breast milk, soothing nervousness, counteracting diarrhea and inflammations of the stomach and intestines, relieving mucus congestion and assuaging menstrual difficulties. Overdose or prolonged use of sage may be toxic. With their legend that they tempered grief when laid on graves and served as a fortune-telling device for single girls in medieval England, sage's grayish-green, aromatic leaves are also a meat flavoring. According to an old English proverb, "He that would live for aye must eat sage in May." And 17th-century English author John Evelyn wrote that proper intake of sage could make a man immortal, following the

prehistoric and ancient use of sage as a means of promoting longevity.

The leaves, flowers and dried roots of the Asian species *Salvia militorrhiza* and *japonica* are recognized by traditional Chinese practitioners as treatment for menstrual and uterine problems; liver and gastrointestinal ulcers; stomach pain; internal abscesses; insomnia; inflamed kidney, bone or breast; parasitic worms; enlarged organs; and malarial fever.

While Chinese herbalists believe sage increases mental alertness and physical strength, the English surgeon and herbalist John Gerard wrote in 1597: "Sage is singularly good for the head and brain, it quickeneth the senses and memory, strengtheneth the sinews, restoreth health to those that have the palsy, and taketh away shakey trembling of the members."

St. Benedict thistle
See BLESSED THISTLE.

St. John's wort
(amber, goatweed, Klamath weed, Tipton weed)
An eastern North American and Pacific coastal shrubby perennial, *Hypericum perforatum,* of the Hypericaceae family, used by Ayurvedic and other herbalists as an antispasmodic, astringent, nervine and expectorant. During the medieval, customary St. John's Eve (June 23) fires—to "purify the air" of evil spirits and thereby protect people, animals and crops—St. John's wort, along with ivy, mugwort, figwort, vervain, lavender and others, was smoked and hung in homes and other buildings to ward off evil powers. Some people even wore the smoked herbs around their necks.

With an odor like turpentine, St. John's wort is believed to have medicinal use for nervousness, bedwetting, insomnia, depression and other ailments. Oil extract from the herb treats stomachache, intestinal distress and lung congestion, while St. John's wort tea is prescribed for menstrual

cramps. The herb may be toxic to animals and may cause photosensitivity of the skin.

salt, table, versus sea salt
Sea salt is proclaimed in health food stores to be beneficial; however there is no significant benefit, although sea salt may contain small quantities of other minerals such as magnesium and calcium. Sodium chloride is the basic ingredient in both, and the negligible quantities of other minerals are not worth the additional cost. Ordinary table salt is fortified with the mineral iodine. Iodized salt has resulted in the reduction in cases of goiter (enlarged thyroid glands) from areas of the United States formerly called the "goiter belt," caused by iodine deficiency (see IODINE).

sandalwood
(white saunders)
A tree native to India, *Santalum album,* of the Santalaceae family, whose wood is used in herbal medicine preparations for the treatment of bronchitis, indigestion, fever and nervousness. In ancient Burma, India and China, Hindus and Buddhists burned sandalwood in funeral pyres and as incense, and used it also as a perfume and an embalming substance. After sandalwood trees were cut down and the branches removed, they were left to the termites who devoured the superfluous outer layer of wood. The valuable, aromatic heartwood was then available for commercial use.

sanicle
(pool root, wood sanicle, black snakeroot)
An American perennial plant, *Sanicula marilandica,* of the carrot family, long thought to have healing powers as an anodyne or astringent. The rootstock is prepared as a remedy for sore throat, mouth sores, ulcers, hemorrhage, intermittent fever, chorea and excessive menstrual bleeding. Leaves of *S. europaea* yield an astringent, styptic

and expectorant, especially for chest congestion and, used externally, treatment for wounds and skin eruptions.

Homeopaths prescribe sanicle also for such problems as night terrors, foot sweat, crusted nose, neuralgia, diabetes, sore coccyx, ulcerated cornea, potbellied children, itching, emaciation and premature ossification.

sarsaparilla
(smilax, greenbrier, spignet, quay, quill, zarzaparilla [Spanish])
A Central American, Mexican, northern South American and West Indian perennial, *Smilax officinalis,* of the Liliaceae family, whose rootstock is used by herbalists as a carminative, diaphoretic, diuretic and tonic, particularly in treating gout, rheumatism, colds and gas. In Chinese medicine, the *S. glabra* species yields a cooling tonic and purgative, as well as an insecticide and an external preparation for boils and abscesses.

Following Swedish anthropologist Alfred Metraus's discovery that Amazon Indians took sarsaparilla as a cure for general weakness, the plant—named from two Spanish words, *zarza,* bush, and *parilla,* little vine—became a sensation in the United States in the mid-1800s. Sarsaparilla was known as a spring tonic that purified the body, especially after various winter infections and ailments. Today, sarsaparilla is a sweet, carbonated beverage flavored with sassafras oil and distilled European birch oil.

sassafras
(saxifrax, saloop, ague tree, cinnamon wood)
A North American deciduous tree, *Sassafras albidum* or *Laurus sassafras,* of the Lauraceae family. A tea made from sassafras bark is used in herbal medicine as a blood-purifier and promoter of perspiration and urination. Native Americans drank sassafras tea to reduce fevers and relieve pain.

saw palmetto
(fan palm, sabal)
A North American, fruit-bearing shrub, *Serenoa serrulata,* of the Palmae family, with berries of medicinal value. Herbalists use either an infusion or a tincture made with the berries as remedies for respiratory irritation such as bronchitis, kidney and prostatic problems and diabetes. Ayurvedic practitioners also prescribe saw palmetto as an aphrodisiac.

savory
(bean herb)
A Mediterranean annual, aromatic plant, *Satureja* or *Satureia hortensis,* of the Labiatae family, whose herb serves as a seasoning, and an astringent, expectorant, carminative, stimulant and stomachic. Savory tea is the most popular form of the herb as a medicinal supplement.

schizophrenia, vitamin therapy in
There have been reports for many years that large amounts of niacin were beneficial in the treatment of mental illness, especially schizophrenia. There have been attacks and counterattacks by proponents of megadoses (doses exceeding by 10 times or more the Recommended Dietary Allowances) of vitamins, especially niacin, and by traditional psychiatrists, most of whom are adamant about its detriments. Each side in this controversy claims the other is being either narrow-minded or "unscientific."

There is no question that niacin has marked pharmacologic (druglike) effects that differ from its vitamin activity. However, most of the benefits demonstrated by proponents of the supplements were observed on patients who also required the use of tranquilizers.

(See also MEGAVITAMINS; ORTHOMOLECULAR THERAPY.)

scullcap

(scutellaria, hoodwort, mad dog weed, side flower, blue pimpernel, helmet flower, huang qin) An East Asian bitter herb, *Scutellaria baicalensis,* of the Labiatae family, whose root is utilized by Chinese, Ayurvedic and other herbalists as treatment for high blood pressure, bloody vomitus, constipation or diarrhea, dry cough, high fever, jaundice and breast inflammation. Scullcap is also considered useful in preventing miscarriage.

scurvy

Nutritional disease caused by an ascorbic acid, or vitamin C, deficiency and it can be cured by vitamin C supplementation. Symptoms have been described since ancient times by the Egyptians, Greeks and Romans. In children, scurvy causes poor bone and tooth structure. However, the human toll of suffering and death was probably greatest among the sea explorers of the 16th to 18th centuries, A.D. Within months of departing for journeys across the seas, sailors experienced symptoms including bleeding and rotting gums and the bad breath that accompanies it, loosening of teeth, painful swelling of joints, dark blotches on the skin from bleeding under the skin, muscle weakness and loss of energy. From 1740 to 1744, six British ships set out to circle the globe. On these expeditions 1,051 men died, most from scurvy, and only Admiral Anson's flagship returned. Although James Lind, a Scottish surgeon, is credited with discovering in 1747 that citrus fruits can prevent or cure scurvy, it was probably recognized by others much before this time. However, Lind's nutritional experiments led to the dramatic cure of the disorder. Lind gave six different diet supplements to six pairs of sailors suffering from scurvy. Those sailors given oranges, lemons, limes and apple cider improved. Lind incorrectly reasoned that the citrus fruits counteracted the poisonous and noxious "putrid humors" resulting from blocked perspiration from the damp,

salty sea air. Unfortunately, it was not until 40 years later that the British made lemon or lime juice a routine part of sailors' diets.

Captain James Cook should be credited with first proving that long sea voyages could be completed without the dread of scurvy. During his voyages from 1768 to 1775, he insisted that his crew eat local greens and other available foods when on land and maintain good hygienic practices.

Despite the findings that led to the prevention of scurvy at sea, scurvy continued to plague the 19th-century populations on land. Scurvy was ever-present in soldiers of the United States Civil War and other conflicts, found in miners during the California gold rush and was widespread during the potato famine in Europe.

It was not until almost 1930 that vitamin C was isolated as the factor that cured scurvy, by Albert Szent-György and Glen King.

(See also ASCORBIC ACID.)

seawrack

(bladderwrack) A type of seaweed, *Fucus vesiculosus,* used by herbalists as an antirheumatic, a weight-reduction aid and a thyroid regulator. It is also used in the preparation of kelp and as a manure.

selenium

Nonmetallic element principally obtained as a by-product in the refining of copper, named from the Greek word *selene,* meaning moon. Selenium is an essential mineral required as a constituent of the enzyme glutathione peroxidase and may be vital to the functions of the antioxidant vitamin E. Current research is identifying other evidence of important functions.

Deficiency

It was not until 1979 that Chinese scientists associated selenium deficiency with a fatal cardiomyopathy called Keshan disease (named for Keshan, one of the provinces of China where the disease was studied in relation to selenium deficiency) that occurs most frequently in children and in women of child-bearing age. Dietary deficiencies occur in areas with soil poor in selenium, such as parts of China, New Zealand and Finland. A study in which several thousand Chinese children were given selenium supplements seemed to support this conclusion. However, some scientists feel that selenium-deficient persons are more susceptible to a virus, not selenium deficiency itself, that actually causes Keshan disease.

Patients intravenously fed total parenteral nutrition (TPN), which is deficient in selenium, have occasionally experienced muscular discomfort or weakness that responded to supplements. Rarely, those on TPN developed a cardiomyopathy suggesting a human requirement for this mineral.

Dietary Sources

Meats, especially kidney and liver, and seafoods are the most consistent sources of selenium. Grains and other seeds are dependent on the soil for selenium content. Drinking water and fruits and vegetables contain minimal amounts of the mineral. Although organically bound forms of selenium seem to be more bioavailable, this form did not significantly change glutathione peroxidase activity tests when compared to the activation by inorganic sources. American adult diets provide on average 83 to 129 mcg of selenium per day.

Requirements

By studying the amount of selenium needed to prevent Keshan disease in Chinese people and New Zealanders, it has been estimated that North American adult males require 70 mcg based on 79 kilograms (174 pounds) of body weight and females weighing 63 kilograms (139 pounds), 55 mcg.

By accounting for weight changes, dietary absorption factors and milk production, it has been estimated that an average increase of 10 mcg during pregnancy and 20 mcg of dietary selenium during lactation would be needed to assure adequate levels of the mineral in the mother and breast milk.

Ten mcg of selenium allow for 5 mcg as calculated from adult values with an additional 5 mcg to allow for growth in the first six months of life. This need for selenium increases to 15 mcg from six to 12 months of age. These amounts provide a level of safety from deficiency when compared to the lower and average levels available to breast-fed infants in New Zealand and Finland who do not seem to suffer ill effects from those levels. Recommended selenium levels for older children is based on adult values because insufficient information is available to determine needs.

Toxicity

In a selenium-rich soil of one Chinese region, approximately 5 mg per day of dietary selenium causes hair loss and changes in fingernails. Thirteen Americans developed nausea, abdominal pain, diarrhea, nail and hair abnormalities, peripheral neuropathy (pain, numbness or weakness in one or more peripheral nerves), fatigue and irritability when they were accidentally poisoned by taking nonstandardized tablets containing more than 27 mg of selenium per tablet. Some plants accumulate levels toxic to grazing animals from the soil rich in this substance.

self-heal

See PRUNELLA.

senna

(sana [Arabic])

Dried leaves, leaflets or pods of various senna plants, such as *Cassia acutifolia* and *angustifolia,* of the Leguminosae family, widely used in allopathic and herbal medicine as a cathartic.

sesame seeds

Seeds of the tropical and subtropical annual herb *Sesamum indicum,* of the Pedaliaceae family, used as a source of an edible oil, a flavoring agent and a nutritive tonic, demulcent and rejuvenative.

shark cartilage

Gristle, or dense connective tissue, obtained from sharks, powdered and marketed as a natural anti-cancer substance that allegedly reduces tumors. Shark cartilage is one of the various alternative treatments for cancer patients whose conditions have not responded to other treatments and who are considered to be in the final stage of the disease. Only scant data exist on the effectiveness of shark cartilage. It was popularized by Dr. I. William Lane, a biochemist and head of Cartilage Consultants, in Short Hills, New Jersey, and author of the book *Sharks Don't Get Cancer.* Other scientists and cancer researchers claim sharks do get cancer and that Lane's book exaggerates the substance's effects.

However, the unadulterated shark cartilage products (that is, *not* cartilage derivatives filled with sugar) available in stores have gained popularity and have been approved for study by the federal Food and Drug Administration (FDA).

shatavari

(Indian asparagus)

The Ayurvedic herb *Asparagus racemosus,* of the Liliaceae family, used as a nutritive tonic, demulcent, emmenagogue and rejuvenative. Chinese traditional practitioners use the roots of *A. cochinchinensis,* or shiny asparagus, as a treatment of phlegm in the respiratory passages, scanty urine, chronic cough, bloody sputum and fever.

shepherd's purse

(cocowort, St. James' weed, mother's heart, case wort, toywort, pickpocket)

A common annual, malodorous plant, *Capsella bursa-pastoris,* of the Cruciferae family, that tastes like cabbage, although it has not been used as food since American pioneer roasted the seeds and ate the herb. Herbalists and folk-medicine practitioners believe shepherd's purse effective against stomach and intestinal disturbances, venereal disease, pulmonary disease, internal bleeding, diarrhea, intermittent fever and bedwetting.

shiitake

(black mushroom, xiang gu)

The Oriental mushroom *Lentinus edodes,* of the family Agaricaceae, eaten as a vegetable and considered by Chinese and other herbalists to enhance the immune system, promote circulation, lubricate the intestinal tract and thereby relieve constipation.

Siberian ginseng

The herb *Eleutherococcus senticosus,* of the Araliaceae family, prescribed by herbalists for increasing energy and endurance. (See GINSENG.)

silicon

Non-metallic element essential for normal development of long bones and skulls in chickens. Although no human deficiency has been identified, some scientists feel that silicon and other trace minerals (see TRACE ELEMENTS) may play a role in human enzyme systems, specifically in the development and maintenance of bone and in the formation of connective tissue.

Elevated levels of silicon have been found in persons with atherosclerosis but evidence of a role in its development has not been found. Whole grain products, vegetables, dried beans and peas provide adequate silicon and supplements are not recommended.

skin

The integument, or outer covering of the body, that is a major body organ and essential to life, composed of the epidermis, or outer layer, and the thicker dermis, which rests against the subcutaneous tissues. The skin's main functions are to protect the body against injury and parasites, regulate body temperature, help in eliminating bodily waste (perspiration), prevent dehydration, serve as facilitator of the cutaneous senses (such as heat, cold, pain, etc.) and provide a reservoir for water and nutrients, such as vitamin D that emerges when the skin is exposed to the sun.

A wide variety of skin disorders occur from deficiencies of several nutrients, such as vitamin A, essential for growth and maintenance of the skin. Vitamin A deficiency can cause a condition known as follicular keratosis, hyperkeratosis or xeroderma, in which there is excessive production of keratin, a hard protein. The excess keratin causes keratin deposits to form around hair follicles, resulting in a rough texture to the skin suggestive of "goose-flesh" or "toad-skin." Niacin deficiency causes cracked, scaly, deeply pigmented skin. These changes are especially seen in areas of the skin exposed to sunlight. Riboflavin deficiency (vitamin B_2) and protein-energy malnutrition (PEM, that includes kwashiorkor, marasmus or a combination of the two) may also cause rough, scaly, spotty, "sandpaper" and sore skin.

Facial skin that is scaly, off-color, cracked or dry to the point of flaking may be attributable to PEM, lack of vitamin A and iron deficiency. A skin rash may occur in persons taking high doses of pyridoxine (vitamin B_6) when they are exposed to the sun. The skin also gives rise to nails that should be firm and pink and hair that should be shiny and firmly attached to the scalp. Dull, loose, brittle hair may be caused by PEM, and irregularly shaped, brittle or ridged nails may indicate poor iron status. Paleness may be caused by anemia (severe anemia can cause ashy skin) or general malnutrition. Bronzing of the skin may indicate the early stages of pellagra, a niacin-deficiency disease. Some anemias and gastrointestinal disorders induce a sallowness in the skin. Jaundiced, or yellow, skin may be caused by excessive intake of carotene or by liver disease.

(See also NIACIN.)

slippery elm
(moose elm, red elm, Indian elm)
A Central and North American and Asian deciduous tree, *Ulmus fulva,* of the Ulmaceae family, whose inner bark is used as a demulcent, emollient and nutritive by herbalists, particularly Native American practitioners. The fresh or dried bark is usually powdered and prepared as an emulsive drink for any inflammatory, gynecological, digestive, catarrhal and cancerous diseases. Slippery elm is also made into lozenges for sore throat and laryngitis. Tincture of the bark prescribed by homeopaths treats constipation, hemorrhoids, pain, syphilis, herpes and other ailments.

smokers
See CIGARETTE SMOKING EFFECTS ON VITAMINS AND MINERALS.

sodium
Alkaline metallic element that is the chief cation (an ion—an atom or group of atoms—with a positive charge) of the extracellular body fluids and the primary regulator of body-fluid volume. Sodium regulates the osmolarity, or concentration of body fluids, as well as its acid-base balance. Sodium is involved in an active transport across cell membranes and must be pumped out in exchange for potassium (called the "sodium pump") in order to maintain a proper balance of fluids and other substances within body cells. Sodium homeostasis, or balance, is controlled primarily by the hormone aldosterone's action on the tubules in the kidneys. Aldosterone levels increase when sodium levels are low and urinary levels are practically zero. The hormone is decreased when sodium levels are excessive, increasing the excretion of sodium in the urine. Despite the kidneys' ability to conserve sodium, some of this electrolyte is lost in sweat and fecal waste.

Table 27
SODIUM BALANCE IN THE BODY

Consumption of a fatty meal → sodium concentration in the blood increases → stimulates thirst → consumption of water is increased → blood sodium is diluted back to normal → kidneys excrete excess water and sodium in the urine

Sodium is very active and chemically combines with many substances and is widely found in nature. Salts of sodium are widely used in medicine.

Deficiency

If blood concentration of sodium becomes too low and water is replaced without sodium, water moves from the blood into the cells and symptoms of water intoxication may develop. These symptoms include headaches and muscle weakness. Despite losses of sodium in sweat, depletion is rare, except in disorders such as chronic diarrhea, severe trauma or some kidney diseases. Deficiency is rare in persons on salt-restricted diets.

(See also WATER INTOXICATION.)

Requirements

The minimum average adult requirement is 5 milliequivalents, or 115 mg of sodium or 300 mg of sodium chloride (table salt) per day. To accommodate various levels of physical activity, a safe minimum intake is probably about 500 mg per day. Most American diets exceed this amount easily, even in the absence of "added" salt. Since there is no benefit to the consumption of high levels of sodium, the Food and Nutrition Board recommends a limit of 6 grams of sodium chloride per day.

Toxicity

Excessive salt intake increases the extracellular space pulling water from cells to maintain sodium concentration. This process can lead to edema, congestive heart failure and hypertension. Increasing water intake in many cases will allow the kidneys to remove the excess sodium.

sodium ascorbate

A soluble salt of ascorbic acid, or vitamin C, used for injectible forms of the vitamin.

(See also ASCORBIC ACID.)

soft drinks

(soda water)

Popular beverages that contain large amounts of phosphorous in the form of phosphoric acid. High phosphorus intake impairs the absorption of calcium, increases the loss of calcium in the urine and reduces the calcium in bones. These changes may result in osteoporosis.

(See also CALCIUM; PHOSPHORUS.)

solanum

See NIGHTSHADE.

Solomon's seal

(sealwort, drop berry, yu zhu)

Various *Polygonatum* species of the perennial herbs of the Liliaceae family, especially *P. odoratum, multiforum, biflorum* and *commutatum,* found in the north temperate zone. The name refers to various folklore, such as a description of the cut rootstock: "Scars" on that inner surface resemble Hebrew characters. Sixteenth-century herbalist Gerard said the herb "sealed up" wounds and fractures. The flower inked and pressed onto paper yields a Star of David (a six-pointed star) that is also called the Seal of Solomon.

The rhizome has medicinal value as an astringent, demulcent and tonic in herbal medicine. Treatments include gastrointestinal inflammations, hemorrhoids, erysipelas, neuralgia, ruptures and gynecological problems and pain.

sophera

Trees of the *Sophera* genus, of the Leguminosae family, such as *S. japonica* (Japanese pagoda tree, Chinese scholar tree) and *S. subprostrata,* whose flower buds, fruits, seeds and root are prepared by Chinese traditional practitioners as remedies for ailments including many types of bleeding, high blood pressure, intestinal worms, sore throat and tumors.

sorrel
(sourgrass, meadow sorrow, red top sorrel)
A European and North American plant, *Rumex acetosa,* of the Polygonaceae family, characterized by sour or acid sap or juice, whose leaves are used in Native American, homeopathic and other herbal medicine practices as a diuretic, antiscorbutic, refrigerant and vermifuge. Sorrel may be eaten in salad or as a pot herb. Fever, thirst, cardiac weakness, jaundice, kidney and bladder stones, scurvy, excessive menstruation, convulsions and other ailments are treated with sorrel preparations.

spearmint
See MINT.

spikenard
(old man's root, wild licorice, petty morrel, life-of-man)
A Himalayan aromatic plant, *Nardostachys jatamansi,* of the valerian family, and an American herb, *Aralia racemosa,* of the ginseng family. The American perennial herb root and rhizome were used by North American Indians as a food, and herbalists use them as an alterative, diaphoretic and expectorant. Spikenard is also believed to strengthen and purify the blood, alleviate pain of childbirth and alter the course of uric acid disorders. Homeopaths prescribe spikenard for asthma, cough, diarrhea, hay fever and other ailments.

sprue
See MALABSORPTION.

squaw vine
(partridgeberry)
The herb *Mitchella repens,* of the Rubiaceae family, used by herbalists as a treatment for menstrual problems and to strengthen the uterus for childbirth.

sticklewort
See AGRIMONY.

stress
The body's response to emotional disturbances, or physical injuries caused by severe burns, illness, starvation, surgery, or exercise. Stress often initiates changes in metabolism, including the metabolic rate itself, hormone levels, energy reserves, immune response, blood-glucose levels, negative nitrogen balance, fluid and sodium retention and increased elimination of potassium. Stressful situations have also been linked to low levels of vitamins A, B-complex and vitamin C and the minerals selenium, zinc and magnesium. Deficiencies of vitamins B_1, B_6 and B_{12} can cause symptoms including depression, confusion and mental disturbances, but they have no bearing on the psychological stresses of everyday life. In New York State the attorney general took action to force a major vitamin producer to stop advertising the vitamins for relief of emotional stress. However, the metabolic alterations caused by stress serve, importantly, to signal the body against further depletion, damage or diminished organ function. The better a person's nutritional status, the better chance he or she has to recover as quickly as possible from the many forms of stress. Some nutritionists and health professionals refer to this as a "bank account" for good health, with vitamins and minerals in adequate supply to be drawn upon when necessary.

Nutrition counseling to assure a well-balanced diet is important but especially essential in those under stress. Unfortunately, some situations inhibit adequate nutrition, e.g., malabsorption disorders such as ulcerative colitis or Crohn's disease, in which diarrhea prevents the absorption of vitamins and minerals, and nutrient imbalances may prevail. When food and nutrient intake becomes altered by illness—loss of appetite, dry mouth, difficulty swallowing, nausea or the like—an individual is at risk of malnutrition. The illness may extend into problems with digestion and absorption of nutrients; surgery involving the stomach or intestines, radiation enteritis or diseases characterized by diarrhea can intensify nutrient loss. Metabolic changes, such as a loss of energy, and changes in the excretion of nutrients, such as loss of fat-soluble vitamins and calcium in the feces of persons with certain cancers that affect enzyme secretion, may contribute to malnutrition and malabsorption. Malnutrition in the elderly may involve a combination of mental or physical illness and deteriorating motor skills and senses, especially an impaired sense of taste and smell that often leads a person to eat less or eat only foods with strong flavor. In general, illness may lead to malnutrition, and malnutrition may lead to illness.

sugar
(saccharum, sugarcane)
An Old World tropical perennial grass, *Saccharum officinarum,* of the family Graminae, named from the Greek word *saccharum.* Sugarcane was brought by Columbus to America, where the crop thrived and became a major industry, especially in the West Indies and other Caribbean islands. Sugar is known throughout the world as a sweetener and energizing nutrient. Chinese herbalists use sugarcane juice to treat excess phlegm in the respiratory tract, to stimulate the stomach and, externally, for wounds, ulcers and other skin conditions.

sulfur
Nonmetallic element found in all body tissues especially those high in protein content. Sulfur is a constituent of the amino acids cystine, cysteine and methionine, building blocks of protein. It is also found in the B-complex vitamins thiamine, pantothenic acid and biotin. Sulfur is an important component of hair, muscle, skin, the connective tissue that holds cells together, bones and teeth. This mineral is involved in the clotting of blood and the activation of some enzymes and is a component of insulin.

A sulfur deficiency is unknown. Dietary protein supplies adequate sulfur. There are no recognized toxic effects of dietary sulfur.

suma
(Brazilian ginseng, para toda)
The plant *Pfaffia paniculata,* of the Amaranthaceae family, whose root is considered by herbalists to be a nutrient, demulcent, and energy tonic adaptogen similar in effect to other ginsengs. Suma preparations are prescribed by homeopaths and other herbal practitioners for chronic fatigue and low energy level. It has also been given to cancer patients, but there is insufficient research to assume the herb an effective anticancer agent.

sumach
See RHUS.

sunflower
A tall, common plant, *Helianthus annuus,* of the family Compositae, said to have been cultivated in pre-Columbian America, with large, yellow flowers and black or brownish disk, and bearing nutritious seeds. Sunflower—the state flower of Kansas and a symbol of Peru—contains phosphorus, calcium, iron, fluorine, iodine, potassium, magnesium, sodium, protein, thiamine, niacin and vitamin D. Herbalists use sunflower preparations as a diuretic and expectorant, as a decoction for the treatment of jaundice, heart conditions, diarrhea, malaria and in various topical preparations such

as ointments and liniment for pain associated with rheumatism.

sunlight and vitamin D
See D, VITAMIN.

supplements, vitamin and mineral
In a 1986 survey, the United States Health and Nutrition Examination Survey (NHANES II) reported that about 35 percent of adult Americans took vitamin-mineral supplements regularly. In 1987, the National Health Interview Survey showed that 51.1 percent of adult Americans from 18 to 99 years took a vitamin-mineral supplement in the previous year. However, only 23.1 percent took them daily. Whites, women and the elderly were more likely than blacks, men and younger persons to do so. Most took multivitamin products, with vitamin C, calcium, vitamin E and vitamin A supplements the next most commonly consumed. Users took a mean of 2.15 supplements in 1980, but only 1.77 in 1986. Interestingly, and unfortunately, the most likely people to take the supplements were also the most likely to be well nourished, those with higher income and education levels. It was also determined that the vast majority of persons taking supplements take them in quantities considered to be safe.

The American Dietetic Association estimates that 60 million Americans spent $4 billion on supplements in 1993. These figures were basically unchanged since earlier studies in the 1970s, when the first National Health and Nutrition Examination Survey (1971 to 1975) was conducted. A follow-up survey approximately 10 years later indicated no statistically significant increase in longevity among vitamin-users in the United States.

sweet flag
See CALAMUS.

synthetic vitamins
Supplemental products manufactured rather than obtained from natural sources. Studies conducted by the United States Department of Agriculture (USDA) demonstrated that equal blood levels of vitamin C were obtained when comparing the vitamin obtained from oranges, orange juice, cooked broccoli or vitamin C tablets.

The only naturally occurring vitamin that may be somewhat more potent than a similar dose of the synthetic vitamin is E. Probably of greater importance is the dissolution time of the product, which determines its ability to be absorbed into the blood stream.

(See also ABSORPTION; E, VITAMIN.)

T

tamarind

A tropical, flowering evergreen, *Tamarindus indica,* of the Leguminosae family, whose fruit is eaten and made into beverages, and whose fruit and leaves are used by herbalists as a laxative, anthelmintic and refrigerant.

tansy

(bitter buttons, parsley fern, hindheal)

A European and North American perennial, aromatic herb, *Tanacetum vulgare,* of the Compositae family, considered by Ayurvedic and other herbal medicine practitioners to be an anthelmintic, emmenagogue and tonic. Tansy leaf tea, also prescribed for nervousness and anxiety, may be toxic if taken in large doses.

tarragon

(estragon)

A perennial North American, southern Asian, European and Siberian shrub, *Artemisia dracunculus,* of the Compositae family, named from the Latin *dracunculus,* or little dragon. A seasoning with a slight licorice flavor, especially popular in French cuisine, tarragon has healing properties, according to herbal practitioners, effective against pain (it acts like a local anesthetic, such as on toothaches), intestinal gas, irregular menses, arthritis, rheumatism and gout and worms. Tarragon tea is said to stimulate the appetite and help alleviate insomnia.

Other *Artemisia* species, including mugwort, are used in Chinese traditional medicine.

(See also MUGWORT.)

tea

A beverage made by steeping the leaves or other parts of various herbs or plants in boiling water. Many teas contain caffeine, tannin and a volatile oil that gives the tea its flavor and aroma. Caffeine is a stimulant also used in the manufacture of painkillers. Green tea, prepared by heating the leaves in an open tray, has nearly twice the amount of the element fluoride as black tea, which is made from fermented, then dried, leaves. Herbal teas, made from herbs, barks, grasses, flowers and other plant parts, are widely used throughout the world as remedies for any number of ailments or symptoms. Some herbal teas may be harmful.

(See CAMOMILE; PARAGUAY COPPER TEA.)

thiamine

(vitamin B$_1$)

Water-soluble member of the B-complex vitamins whose deficiency is the cause of beriberi. Thiamine is an important coenzyme required for the intermediary metabolism of carbohydrates and some amino acids. It is especially vital for a normally functioning central nervous system. Thiamine also is vitally involved in the conversion of fatty acids into steroids and is essential for normal growth and skin integrity. Thiamine may also exhibit antioxidant properties (see ANTIOXIDANTS). Vitamin B$_1$ deficiency causes beriberi.

Historical Background

Beriberi was first described in 2697 B.C. by the ancient Chinese in the Neiching, a medical book. A Japanese surgeon, Tomoe Takaki, attributed the disorder to an improper diet in 1884. In 1912, chemist Casimir Funk isolated an extract from rice bran which he called "vitamine," but despite claims that it would cure beriberi, it did not. However, Dutch chemists Pierre Janssen and Willem Donath, again working with rice bran extracts, did isolate the factor effective against the disease. In 1934, American scientist Robert Runnels Williams isolated and determined the structure of thiamine, and in 1936 it was synthesized. The active coenzyme form of thiamine was determined in 1937.

Deficiency

The characteristic manifestations of beriberi change with age and systems of the body involved. The disease is most common in infants between the ages of two and three months. Afflicted babies exhibit a distinctive cry that varies from a loud piercing cry to hoarseness or aphonia (a total loss of voice). They become cyanotic, short of breath, vomit, have tachycardia (a rapid heart rate), develop an enlarged heart and may convulse. Death may result in a matter of hours, unless thiamine is administered.

Older children and adults may have the dry, paralytic or nervous form of beriberi; the wet or cardiac type; the cerebral type; or subclinical, with minimal or no apparent symptoms.

In dry beriberi there is a symmetrical, or bilateral, peripheral neuropathy (a wasting of the nerves) in which the distal, or lower, segments of limbs are affected more severely than the proximal, or upper, ones, with calf tenderness and difficulty raising from a squatting position. These symptoms also are found in wet beriberi, as well as congestive heart failure, with an enlarged, poorly functioning heart muscle that causes fluid retention in the lungs and extremities.

Thiamine and vitamin B_{12} are the only vitamins whose deficiencies have proven causes of neurologic disease. It takes only three weeks of total dietary lack of thiamine to see the first signs of deficiency. Malnourished patients, especially those with severe alcoholism, are likely to develop the Wernicke-Korsakoff syndrome, or "cerebral beriberi." Wenrnicke's syndrome is characterized by ocular abnormalities such as paralysis of the muscles controlling the movements of the eyes; dysfunction of the cerebellar or vestibular regions of the brain causing ataxia, or a staggering gait; and generalized confusion, with the patient appearing listless and spatially disoriented. Lethargy is common but stupor and coma are rare.

COLLOQUIAL DESCRIPTION OF SEVERE THIA-
MINE DEFICIENCY:
"HOT AS A HARE; BLIND AS A BAT; DRY AS A
BONE;
RED AS A BEET; MAD AS A HATTER"

If the patient survives Wernicke's syndrome, symptoms of Korsakoff's psychosis may develop. The state of amnesia that denotes this condition may be recognized by confabulation, in which the patient relates imaginary stories to fill in gaps in memory.

Although anyone deficient in thiamine may develop this serious disorder, alcoholics have both a diminished dietary vitamin supply and decreased ability to absorb thiamine in the gastrointestinal tract. Furthermore, alcoholic liver disease impairs the conversion of thiamine to its active form, thiamine pyrophosphate, and the ability of the liver to store thiamine. It is critical to administer thiamine before glucose is given in any alcoholic or malnourished patient, since carbohydrate loading may trigger the Wernicke-Korsakoff syndrome.

Even persons with a subclinical or minimal thiamine deficiency may exhibit behavioral changes such as irritability, frequent headaches and fatigue. (See also BERIBERI.) Oral thiamine has been reported to have mosquito-repellant properties.

Recommended Dietary Allowances

One mg of thiamine daily is recommended for adults. Maximum absorption is 8 to 15 mg daily, and absorption is enhanced by taking supplements in divided doses with food. An additional 400 mcg, or 1.4 mg, is recommended during pregnancy to allow for increased maternal caloric intake and fetal growth. During lactation, 1.5 mg is recommended to allow for increased energy consumption and the 200 mcg of thiamine secreted daily in breast milk. There is only limited information on thiamine requirements for infants and children (see Table 28).

Dietary Sources

Thiamine is widely found in plant and animal food sources but there are significant amounts in only a few. Meat, especially liver and pork; dried beans; peas; soybeans; peanuts; whole grains; egg yolk; poultry; and fish are the richest dietary sources of thiamine.

Food processing destroys much of the thiamine in foods (see PROCESSING OF FOODS). Alcoholics not only have a vitamin-deficient diet but alcohol actually interferes with the absorption of thiamine.

There are factors in the diet that may interfere with the bioavailability (ability of the body to utilize dietary substances or drugs) of thiamine. These are called antithiamine factors (ATF) (see ANTITHIAMINE FACTORS). Tea, coffee (both caffeinated and decaffinated) and the chewing of betel nuts or tea leaves deplete thiamine. Citrus fruits high in ascorbic acid, or vitamin C, have a protective effect on thiamine. Thiamine is also poorly absorbed by persons with folic acid or protein deficiencies.

Table 28
RECOMMENDED DIETARY ALLOWANCES FOR THIAMINE (VITAMIN B₁)*

	Age	Dosage
Infants	birth to 6 months	0.3 mg
	6 to 12 months	0.4 mg
Toddlers	1 to 3 years	0.7 mg
Children	4 to 6 years	0.9 mg
	7 to 10 years	1.0 mg
Males	11 to 14 years	1.3 mg
	15 to 50 years	1.5 mg
	over 50 years	1.2 mg
Females	11 to 50 years	1.1 mg
	over 50 years	1.0 mg

(*Food and Nutrition Board, National Academy of Sciences-National Research Council, 1989)

Adverse Effects and Toxicity

Oral doses of thiamine up to 500 mg daily are easily eliminated by the kidneys, and there are no reports of oral toxicity in adults. However, one study has reported toxic effects of large doses in infants. There have also been reports of allergic reactions from intravenous administration of thiamine, ranging in severity from itching and hives to deaths from anaphylactic shock (the most severe form of an allergic reaction).

thuja

(arborvitae, tree of life, yellow or white cedar)

A North American evergreen pine tree, *Thuja occidentalis,* of the family Cupressaceae, whose branchlets, leaves and bark are used in herbal medicine as a diaphoretic and emmenagogue. Thuja is also said to be effective against muscular and joint pain, headache and pain in the heart. Thuja is a dangerous herb, however, because it contains a toxic oil, and its use is restricted to medical supervision.

thyme

Eurasian herbs of the Labiatae family, such as *Thymus vulgaris,* with pungent, aromatic leaves that are used as a seasoning and as herbal-medicine preparations for cough, colds, intestinal gas, indigestion, diarrhea and, as a tea, for nightmares.

tin

A metallic element whose organic compounds exhibit varying levels of toxicity. It is unknown if traces of this mineral are essential in human nutrition. If it is required, it is sufficiently plentiful in food, water and air to satisfy human needs.

tincture

A basic, medicinal, alcohol solution to which can be added powdered or liquid herbs. Homeopaths prescribe a certain number of drops of tinctures of various herbs for the treatment of ailments.

tocoferols
See E, VITAMIN.

tooth development
See DENTES.

total parenteral nutrition (TPN)
Nutritional support given intravenously to individuals unable to eat, be fed or absorb nutrients through the gastrointestinal route. Amino acids must be supplied in adequate amounts for protein synthesis as well as glucose and fats. Vitamin supplements are essential in these patients, although excessive amounts of vitamins A and D should be avoided. In addition to a daily multivitamin formula, additional supplemental folic acid must be given initially and weekly and vitamins K and B_{12} every three weeks. A biotin deficiency may occur in infants on TPN characterized by acidosis, rash and hair loss.

The electrolytes sodium, chloride, potassium, magnesium, calcium and phosphorus are essential components for TPN. If TPN exceeds one to two weeks, zinc, copper and chromium should be supplemented.

toxicity
Ability to cause poisonous effects, such as damage to tissues or disturbance of body function, that may cause illness or death. All nutrients at some level become toxic. Some adverse effects result from a pharmacologic, or drug type, of activity. High amounts of water or salt can be fatal. The fat-soluble vitamins A and D may cause significant and well-recognized toxicity if taken to excess. However, water-soluble vitamins such as niacin and pyridoxine (vitamin B_6) can cause adverse effects in large amounts.

TPN
See TOTAL PARENTERAL NUTRITION.

trace minerals
See MINERALS, TRACE.

tryptophan
(L-tryptophan, α-amino-β-3-indole propionic acid, proteinochromagen [obsolete term])
One of nine amino acids essential in the human diet. In the presence of thiamine (vitamin B_1), riboflavin (vitamin B_2), and pyridoxine (vitamin B_6), tryptophan is converted to niacin in the body (approximately 1 mg of niacin is formed from 60 mg of dietary tryptophan). Tryptophan is also required for growth in infants and for nitrogen balance in adults. It is also necessary for the formation of the neurotransmitter serotonin.

Uses
In the absence of adequate niacin, tryptophan may lessen the symptoms of pellegra. Tryptophan has questionable therapeutic value as a supplement for the relief of insomnia and depression and in reducing sensitivity to pain (including migraine) and premenstrual tension (PMS). There are also unproven claims of its ability to reduce dependency on alcohol.

Deficiency
Tryptophan deficiency is rare. However, an inherited disturbance in tryptophan metabolism interferes with the conversion of this amino acid to niacin in the body. This disturbance may result in the symptoms of pellegra despite the presence of adequate niacin. Abnormal metabolic breakdown of trpytophan may result in carcinoid syndrome (a group of symptoms characterized by cyanotic flushing of the skin, diarrhea, wheezing, sudden drops in blood pressure and edema caused by the secretion of chemically active substances from a tumor in the stomach or intestines). The drug isoniazid used in the treatment of tuberculosis causes a deficiency in the coenzyme pyridoxal

phosphate required for the conversion of tryptophan to niacin.

Dietary Sources

A 3-ounce serving of fish or meat will satisfy the 200-mg minimum daily adult requirement. Dairy products, turkey, bananas, dates, peanuts and other protein-rich foods are good sources of tryptophan.

Supplements

L-tryptophan supplements have been withdrawn in the United States and Canada because of toxicity resulting from contaminated batches (see below).

Toxicity

Eosinophilia-myalgia syndrome (EMS) is a serious and life-threatening adverse effect caused by impure L-tryptophan supplements. In 1989 physicians in New Mexico reported three cases of severe muscle pain and very high blood eosinophil (white blood cells that are elevated in allergic and some other disorders) counts linked to L-tryptophan. After many other cases were reported, on November 17, 1989 the Food and Drug Administration (FDA) recalled most products containing this substance, and on March 22, 1990 a second recall was ordered.

The Center for Disease Control (CDC) defines EMS as a patient having an eosinophil count of at least 1,000 cells/cubic millimeter; generalized myalgia (muscle pain) severe enough to interfere with patient's daily activities; and the absence of any infection or tumor that could account for the first two points.

There have been many milder cases with "flu-like" symptoms that would not satisfy all three points. By September 1, 1991, 1,507 cases of EMS and 31 deaths from EMS had been reported to the CDC. It has been estimated that as many as 5,000 persons have probably been afflicted, with most of these not being reported.

The real cause of EMS is thought to be a contaminant of the L-tryptophan made by a single Japanese manufacturer. However, until that contaminant can be identified and eliminated from the manufacturing process, all brands of this drug should be avoided. Some cases of EMS respond to stopping the drug and taking corticosteroids (derivatives of cortisone).

turmeric

See CURCUMA.

tussilago

See COLTS FOOT.

tyrosine

(oxyphenylaminopropionic acid
p-hydroxyphenylalanine)

A nonessential amino acid, synthesized from the essential amino acid phenylalanine, which is found in most proteins.

Uses

Tyrosine is required for the formation of thyroid hormones, catecholamines (biochemicals such as the neurotransmitters dopamine, norepinephrine and epinephrine, or adrenaline) and melanin (dark skin pigment). Tyrosine seems to aid cocaine and amphetamine ("speed") users to withdraw from these drugs.

Deficiency

A dietary lack of phenylalanine for conversion to tyrosine or a problem with the enzyme needed for this reaction to occur may result in a deficit of norepinephrine. An inadequacy of this important neurotransmitter may cause depression.

Phenylketonuria, or PKU, is an inherited disorder in which a defective enzyme fails to convert the phenylalanine to tyrosine. This disease causes brain damage, mental retardation, tremors, spasticity, convulsions, eczema, contorted position of the hands and malodorous sweat and urine. If the disease is not detected at birth by a diagnostic test of the newborn's urine, brain damage may occur within the first three years of life. Expression of the disease may be prevented by rigid dietary restriction. (See PHENYLKETONURIA.)

U

ubiquinone

(coenzyme Q-10 [CoQ])

A substance synthesized by cells throughout the body, or ubiquitous, hence its name "ubiquinone." CoQ acts as a catalyst in the series of chemical reactions called the respiratory chain that create energy from carbohydrates. It is not classified as a vitamin and no deficiencies have been identified. However, levels of CoQ generally decrease with age and have been found to be low in patients with heart disease. CoQ also has antioxidant properties and is structurally similar to vitamin E.

Some studies suggest that CoQ has the potential to protect the myocardium, or heart muscle, during open-heart surgery. CoQ is used in Japan to treat congestive heart failure and has resulted in less shortness of breath and stamina. Exercise tolerance also improved following the compound's use in a group of patients with chronic stable angina.

Dosage

The National Research Council does not consider CoQ an essential nutrient since it is synthesized in the cells, and therefore there is no Recommended Dietary Allowance (RDA). Doses of supplements range from 10 to 300 mg but doses up to 600 mg have been used in clinical trials.

Dietary Sources

Good sources of CoQ include beef heart, sardines, peanuts and spinach. A similar compound is found in plants but does not have the same beneficial properties.

Toxicity

Adverse effects include loss of appetite, nausea and diarrhea, but are unusual.

ulmus

See SLIPPERY ELM.

usnea

(beard lichen)

Common lichens (algae and fungus in symbiotic growth resembling moss) of the *Usnea* genus, such as *U. barbata,* that thrive on tree branches. Usnea is considered by herbalists to be a remedy for fungal, viral and bacterial infections.

uva ursi

(bearberry)

A trailing evergreen plant, *Arctostaphylos uva-ursi,* of the Ericaceae family, whose leaves are used in herbal medicine as a diuretic, urinary antiseptic and astringent, especially for the treatment of bladder, urethra and kidney inflammation and blood in the urine.

V

valerian
Perennial herbs of the Valerianaceae family long believed to have medicinal properties, such as *Valeriana officinalis,* named after the Roman province Valeria. In Ayurvedic practice, valerian serves as a nervine, antispasmodic, carminative and sedative. The herb's rhizome is the medicinal part used in preparations for insomnia, stress and anxiety, pain and cramps.

vanadium
A rare metallic element. Although the human body stores about 29 mg, very little is known about requirements for this mineral. If it is essential, it is sufficiently plentiful in food, water and air to satisfy human needs.

There are some reports that vanadium plays a role in cholesterol metabolism and hormone production. Animal studies suggest that vanadium may also play a role in slowing the growth of tumors and protect against breast cancer. Sources of vanadium include whole-grain breads and cereals, nuts, root vegetables, liver, fish and vegetable oils.

Chronic inhalation of vanadium compounds (vanadiumism) may cause pneumonitis, an inflammatory lung condition. It may also cause anemia and inflammation of the eyes.

varnish tree
See RHUS.

vegetarian diets
The daily intake of foods and liquids partially or totally devoid of animal sources. Because dietary fats are essential for the absorption of some nutrients, these diets are at risk of being deficient in protein, vitamins B_{12}, D and riboflavin and the minerals iron, selenium, copper, manganese and zinc. Modifications such as lactovegetarian or lacto-ovo vegetarian diets include dairy products in the former, and dairy and eggs in the latter. Essential nutrients including vitamin B_{12} can be obtained in the diet that includes dairy products or eggs.

vervain
See BLUE VERVAIN.

vetiverian
The plant *Andropogon muricatus,* of the Graminaceae family, whose root is used in herbal medicine as an antipyretic and astringent.

vidari-kanda
See GINSENG.

viola
(violet, sweet violet)
The flowering plant *Viola odorata,* of the Violaceae family, made into a syrup for sore throat, cough and dry airways and prepared as an herbal medicine for high blood pressure, tumors and cancerous growths. Violet is also a pot herb. Ayurvedic practitioners use it as an alterative, antiseptic and expectorant.

vision and vitamin A
See A, VITAMIN; EYE DISEASES.

vitamin

An organic compound that is required in small amounts for normal health, growth and well-being of the organism. Vitamins are not utilized primarily as a source of energy or as a source of structural tissue components, but rather as catalysts. Vitamins are micronutrients that promote physiologic processes necessary for continued life of the organism. There are 13 vitamins; only three of these, vitamins D, biotin and pantothenic acid, are manufactured by the body, and even these may not be sufficient for good heath. Therefore vitamins must be supplied by exogenous, or from outside, sources. Vitamin deficiency results in a well-defined disease that is prevented or cured by replacement of that vitamin.

vitamin deficiency

A syndrome or disease caused by a lack or an inadequate supply of a substance required by the body for optimal functioning and health. A deficiency is often curable with adequate supplementation of the missing or inadequate substance. According to the American Dietetic Association, most Americans can get adequate nutrition from the United States food supply. However, because of social, cultural or economic factors, several groups may have diets deficient in recommended nutrients. Surveys identify adolescent girls, individuals on limited incomes, pregnant and lactating women and the elderly as the groups most likely to have inadequate intake of the vitamins A, C and folic acid and the minerals calcium, iron and zinc.

Table 29
CAUSES OF DIETARY VITAMIN DEFICIENCY

- Crop failure
- Improperly stored or prepared foods
- Inadequate oral intake because of poverty, eating disorders, anorexia due to disease or depression, fad and weight-loss diets, nausea of pregnancy or alcoholism
- Decreased absorption (malabsorption) from diseases, malignancies and parasitic infestations
- Increased requirements by increased physical activity, infections, pregnancy and lactation, some drugs, rapid growth, vitamin imbalance
- Increased losses due to excessive sweating or diuresis.

---

vitamin-like substances
See PSEUDOVITAMINS.

vitamin metabolism

The intake, processing and elimination of vitamins by the human body. Vitamins are ingested orally (or by injection directly into the bloodstream), then absorbed through the intestinal wall into the bloodstream. They are metabolized, or processed, by the liver and then transported through the blood to tissues. Once the vitamin or its metabolites (breakdown products) enter tissue cells, they convert to coenzymes, couple to enzymes, perform metabolic tasks or break down to other metabolites. Finally, the vitamin and in some cases its by-products are excreted in urine or feces.

vitis
(grape)

Vines of the Vitaceae family, found in the northern hemisphere, such as *V. vinifera, thunbergii, amurensis, bryoniaefolia, flexuosa* and *lambrusca,* whose fruit is eaten or made into juice, jellies, jams and wine. As the oldest cultivated fruit of the Ancient Greeks and Romans, grapes and grape root, root bark, and leaf sap also have medicinal value, according to herbalists. Various preparations are made for the treatment of wounds, cancer, lymphatic tuberculosis and urinary problems.

W

wahoo

(spindle tree, arrow wood, bitter ash, burning bush)
A North American deciduous, fruit-bearing shrub
or tree, *Euonymous atropurpureus,* of the Celastra-
ceae family, with bark of medicinal value in the
treatment of chest and lung congestion, cardiac
irregularities, and other ailments. Other herbalists
use wahoo as a purgative, antipyretic and diuretic.
Wahoo may cause symptoms of poisoning.

walnut

See JUGLANS.

water

The combination of hydrogen and oxygen that
forms a generally tasteless, colorless, odorless
fluid. Constituting about 65 percent of male body
weight and 55 percent of female body weight,
water is necessary for cellular metabolism and
as the agent that transports various substances
including nutrients throughout the body. In addition, water is considered the universal solvent and
the basis for all body fluids, including blood,
lymph, tissue fluid, secretions such as saliva, bile,
sweat and stomach juices, and excretory fluids
such as urine.

An excessive intake of water results in water
intoxication; an excessive loss or lack of water
results in dehydration, which can be life-threatening especially in infants with severe diarrhea.
Symptoms of water intoxication are sodium retention, abdominal cramps, dizziness, lethargy, nausea, vomiting, convulsions and coma. Although a
certain amount of moisture may be derived from
food, the human body cannot survive very long
without water, also responsible for regulating and
maintaining a constant body temperature and for
providing the base solution for the electrolytes
sodium and potassium.

(See also WATER INTOXICATION; WATER, HARD;
WATER SOFT.)

water, hard

Water containing the dissolved salts of the minerals calcium and magnesium.

water intoxication

Results when excessive water is ingested, dis-
turbing the electrolyte balance. As intoxication
worsens there are subtle changes in mental status,
lethargy, confusion and diminished urine output.
With progression the individual may lapse into a
coma and die. This disorder is rare, but seen
occasionally in psychotic individuals.

water, mineral or spring

Water that contains dissolved mineral salts sufficient to impart a particular taste or other properties.
There is no standardization of commercially available brands.

water, potable

Safe drinking water, that is, water free of harmful
microorganisms and minerals.

water, purified

According to the U.S. Pharmacopeia (USP), min-
eral-free water as a result of distillation or deion-
ization.

water, pyrogen-free
Water free of proteins (specifically, bacteria and their metabolic products) that cause fevers. Sterilized, pyrogen-free water is suitable for hypodermic injection.

water, soft
Water containing only a small amount of dissolved magnesium and calcium salts.

watercress
(scurvy grass, nasturtium)
A European and American perennial, *Nasturtium officinale* or *Rorippa nasturtium,* of the Cruciferae family, that flourishes in clear, cold water. Fresh watercress is eaten as a salad green and has herbal medicinal value in its leaves, roots and young shoots. It is used as a diuretic, purgative, expectorant, stomachic and stimulant. Watercress is rich in vitamin C, hence the name scurvy grass, and contains minerals including iodine and iron.

Wernicke-Korsakoff syndrome
See BERIBERI; THIAMINE.

wheat
Varieties of grasses cultivated for their grains, which are hulled and ground into flour to make bread that contains minerals, fat, protein and starch. Cereals and pastas are also made from wheat. The milling process removes the bran and germ of the wheat, which results in the loss of B-complex vitamins, vitamin E and phosphorus and iron.

wheat germ
Embryo of the wheat kernal separated during the milling process. It is a source of vitamin E.
   (See also E, VITAMIN; PROCESSING OF FOODS; WHEAT.)

wild Oregon grape
See OREGON GRAPE.

Wilson's disease
(hepatolenticular degeneration)
An inherited disorder of autosomal recessive expression in which copper accumulates in the body tissues, especially the red blood cells, kidneys, liver and brain. Treatment with D-penicillamine is usually successful. However, if untreated, this disorder is fatal, with death resulting from liver failure or infection.
   (See also COPPER.)

wintergreen
(pyrola, wild lily-of-the-valley)
The plant *Pyrola rotundifolia,* of the Pyrolaceae family, named from the Greek word *pyrus,* or pear, found in Eurasia, Greenland and parts of North America including Quebec, Nova Scotia, and Newfoundland. In Chinese medicine, the fermented plant is used to treat weakness, tuberculosis, anxiety, bloody sputum and rheumatism.

wintersweet
See CHIMONANTHUS.

wormwood
An alternate name for species of Artemisia. See MUGWORT.

X

xanthium

(cocklebur)

A Japanese, Chinese, Korean, Taiwanese and European herb, *Xanthium strumarium,* of the Compositae family, whose fruits, stems, roots and hairy leaves are used in Chinese traditional medicine as remedies for the common cold, headache, German measles and other ailments.

xanthosis

The yellowing of the skin as a result of eating foods containing excessive amounts of carotenoids, such as carrots, squash, egg yolk, etc. While xanthosis may increase lipochromes in the blood of individuals with thyroid or pancreatic disease, it is usually harmless and reversible by reducing the quantities of yellow or orange foods eaten.

Y

yam
See DIOSCOREA.

yarrow
(nosebleed, soldier's woundwort, milfoil)
The aromatic, flowering herb *Achillea millefolium,* of the Compositae family, found in Eurasia, with herbal medicinal use as an anti-inflammatory, antipyretic, astringent, antispasmodic, hemostatic, diaphoretic, carminative and stomachic. Ailments including influenza, the common cold, menstrual cramps, bleeding and hemorrhoids may be treated with yarrow infusion or other preparation.

yeast, brewer's
A yeast (of the fungus family), resulting from the brewing process of beer, that may be dried and used as a source of proteins and B-complex vitamins. Brewer's yeast, usually sold as a powder in health food stores, can be an ingredient in breads, pancakes, milkshakes and a wide variety of foods.

yellowdock
(rumex, garden patience, sour dock, narrow dock)
A European, American and southern Canadian perennial, *Rumex crispus,* of the Polygonaceae family, whose root serves as an astringent and tonic in herbal medicine. Considered a "blood purifier" in the 19th century, yellowdock has also been used as a laxative and cholagogue, or agent that promotes the flow and discharge of bile into the small intestine. Yellowdock is a source of organic iron.

yellow wood sorrel
See OXALIS.

yerba mate
See PARAGUAY COPPER TEA.

yerba santa
(bearsweed, holy herb, mountain balm, tarweed, consumptive's weed)
A western American evergreen shrub, *Eriodictyon califoricum* or *glutinosum,* of the Hydrophyllaceae family, whose leaves were chewed or smoked by Native Americans with asthma. In contemporary herbal medicine, the aromatic leaves are considered a good expectorant as well as an antispasmodic and tonic. Yerba santa reduces fever and has been prescribed for tuberculosis and rheumatism.

yogurt
A milk product with a puddinglike consistency that has been curdled by the *Lactobacillus bulgaricus* and claimed to be nutritive and therapeutic, particularly for bowel disorders, when added to the daily diet.
(See ACIDOPHILUS.)

yohimbe
The extract of the bark of the mature African Coryanthe Yohimbe tree, claimed to be an aphrodisiac and remedy for sexual problems.

yucca
(Spanish bayonet)

Mostly western American plants of the *Yucca* genus and Liliaceae family. Yuccas have a woody base and rigid, swordlike leaves, and they bear large white flowers. Yucca root is used by herbalists as a remedy for arthritic and rheumatic pain and intestinal cramps.

Z

zea
See CORN.

zein
The maize or corn protein that is lacking in two of the amino acids, lysine and tryptophan.

(See AMINO ACIDS.)

zinc
A bluish-white metallic element whose salts are often used in pharmaceuticals. First recognized as an element in the early 1500s, it was not considered necessary for animals until 1934 or recognized that human deficiency could occur until 1956. In trace amounts, zinc is an essential (required in the diet) mineral as a component of many enzymes, playing a role in protein synthesis and cell division. While not an antioxidant alone, zinc works in conjunction with antioxidant enzymes and is included in many antioxidant vitamin and mineral supplements.

Large amounts of zinc are deposited in muscle and bone, but these supplies are not readily available. The freely available zinc pool is small, and deficiencies may become apparent (demonstrated in laboratory animals) despite the total body zinc content.

Small amounts of dietary zinc are absorbed more efficiently than larger amounts. Individuals who are zinc-poor seem to more readily absorb the mineral. The amount of zinc excreted in the feces is approximately proportional to that ingested in the diet.

Deficiency
Loss of appetite, anemia, growth retardation resulting in short stature and hypogonadism, impaired wound-healing and other signs of impaired immunity, diminished sense of taste and geographia, hair loss, night blindness and photophobia (difficulty tolerating light) and behavioral changes are signs of zinc deficiency. Hypogonadism, a deficiency in sexual growth and development, in the Middle East has been attributed to zinc deficiency. Male infants seem to be more sensitive to zinc deficiency since increasing zinc supplementation results in increased growth rate in male but not female babies.

There may be problems with the metabolism of zinc in diabetics with increased losses of zinc in the urine. Both insulin and non-insulin dependent diabetics might benefit from zinc supplements. Alcoholics, those with malabsorption disorders with chronic diarrhea, pregnant and elderly persons and those with chronic infections and AIDS may also benefit from additional zinc in their diets or by supplements.

Dietary Sources
Meat is the principal source of zinc in American diets, supplying approximately 70 percent of intake. Cereals supply most of the balance. The amount in drinking water is negligible. The bioavailability of zinc from meat, especially liver, eggs and seafood such as oysters, is greater than that from whole-grain foods. Zinc in American diets may interact with protein, phosphorus and iron, thereby increasing zinc requirements. But no strong evidence of any clinical significance of suspected interactions exists. In some parts of the world, high dietary fiber and phytate may impair zinc absorption.

Average North American diets supply from 5.5 mg daily for infants to 10 to 15 mg for adults. However, the elderly may only take in 7 to 10 mg.

Recommended Daily Allowances

The Food and Nutrition Board of the National Research Council estimates that the at least 12 mg of zinc is required to maintain normal zinc status in healthy young men. To allow for a margin of safety, the RDA has been set at 15 mg for adult males and for females during pregnancy, and 12 mg for nonpregnant women. During lactation, mothers require an additional 7 mg for the first six months and 4 mg per day from six through 12 months of age for infants. These RDAs take into account that some individuals may consume diets low in bioavailable zinc on a routine basis. Studies have demonstrated that formula-fed infants supplemented with zinc had better growth rates than those who did not receive the supplements. The zinc RDA established, then, for formula-fed infants is 5 mg per day. Preadolescent children require 10 mg per day.

Toxicity

While as little as 2 mg of zinc as sulfate can cause gastric upset and vomiting, 18.5 to 25 mg have been shown to reduce copper levels, resulting in microcytosis (smaller than normal red blood cells) and neutropenia (diminished number of neutrophillic white blood cells). Megadoses of zinc equivalent to 20 times the RDA for six weeks caused impaired immune responses in a group of healthy adults. Furthermore, doses of 80 to 150 mg daily for as little as several weeks reduced high-density lipoproteins (the so-called "good" cholesterol) levels.

In vitro (test tube) experiments with zinc and human A-beta, a substance found in the human brain and other body tissues, suggest that zinc may be instrumental in forming plaques in the brains of Alzheimer's patients. Therefore Boston researchers caution against megadoses of zinc.

The chronic ingestion of greater than 15 mg per day of zinc on a daily basis is not recommended without careful medical scrutiny.

zingiber

See GINGER.

ziziphus

(Chinese jujube, Chinese date, hong zao, suan ao ren)

A southern Chinese and Indian spiny shrub or tree, *Ziziphus jujuba* and *spinosa,* of the Rhamnaceae family, whose fruits, seeds, bark, root and leaves are used in Chinese traditional medicine to treat anxiety, insomnia, alopecia, night sweats, vertigo, scorpion stings, fever and diarrhea.

APPENDIX 1: FOOD PYRAMID

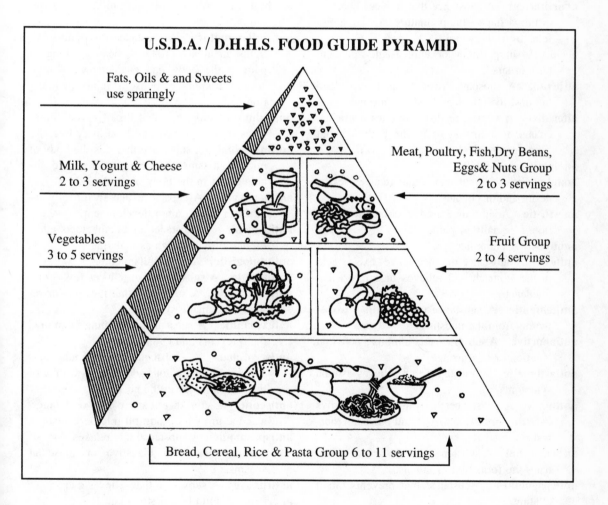

U.S.D.A. / D.H.H.S. FOOD GUIDE PYRAMID

Fats, Oils & and Sweets
use sparingly

Milk, Yogurt & Cheese
2 to 3 servings

Vegetables
3 to 5 servings

Meat, Poultry, Fish,Dry Beans,
Eggs& Nuts Group
2 to 3 servings

Fruit Group
2 to 4 servings

Bread, Cereal, Rice & Pasta Group 6 to 11 servings

APPENDIX 2: GLOSSARY

abortifacient A substance that induces abortion or miscarriage—the premature expulsion of a fetus from the womb.

acrid A sharp, bitter or unpleasantly pungent taste or smell.

adjuvant A substance (usually an herb) added to boost the effect of another substance.

alterative A substance that promotes a gradual change in nutrition or in the body without creating a particular effect of its own.

analgesic A painkiller.

anaphrodisiac A substance that reduces sexual desire and/or potency.

anesthetic A substance used to obliterate sensation, especially of pain.

anodyne A painkiller.

antacid A substance that neutralizes excess acid in the stomach and relieves discomfort and flatulence.

anthelmintic A substance used to kill or expel worms from the intestines.

antiabortive A substance that inhibits a potential abortion or miscarriage.

antiasthmatic A substance that relieves asthma symptoms.

antibiotic A substance that inhibits or destroys bacteria, viruses, amoebas and other microorganisms.

anticatarrhal A substance that thwarts or eliminates the formation of mucus.

anticoagulant A substance that prevents blood clotting.

antiemetic A substance that prevents or alleviates nausea and vomiting.

antihydrotic A substance used to inhibit perspiration.

anti-inflammatory A substance that reduces or fights an area of redness, heat, swelling or pain in the body that characterizes a non-specific immune response to injury or infection.

antilithic A substance that dissolves or diminishes stones or gravel in the urinary tract.

antimicrobial A substance that rids the body of microorganisms that have caused an undesirable effect in the body or on the skin.

antineoplastic A substance that specifically inhibits or fights tumor development.

antiperiodic A substance that counteracts intermittent diseases such as malaria.

antiphilogistic An anti-inflammatory.

antipyretic A substance that reduces fever.

antirheumatic A substance that prevents or relieves rheumatic symptoms.

antiscorbutic A substance containing vitamin C that prevents and cures scurvy.

antiscrofulous A substance that counteracts scrofula, a tuberculous adenitis or swelling of the lymph nodes in the neck.

antiseptic A substance that prevents or counteracts the growth of harmful microorganisms.

antispasmodic A substance that relaxes nervous tension related to digestive or muscular spasms.

antitussive A substance that relieves coughing.

aperient A mild bowel stimulant.

aphrodisiac A substance that stimulates or increases sexual desire and/or potency.

appetizer   A substance that stimulates the desire to eat.

aromatic   A substance whose fragrance or agreeable odor acts as a relaxant or stimulant.

astringent   A substance that reduces secretion or discharges from bodily tissues; a drying agent.

Ayurveda   The 6,000 year-old holistic medical science of India, named from two Sanskrit words, "life" and "knowledge."

balsam   A resinous substance from trees that has soothing and healing action.

bitter   One of the characteristic taste sensations (along with salt, sour and sweet) that may be acrid, astringent or disagreeable; a substance that increases appetite and promotes digestion.

botany   The study, or science, of plant life.

calmative   A substance used as a tranquilizer or sedative.

cardiac   A substance that has an effect on the heart.

carminative   A substance that relieves griping (severe bowel pains) and intestinal gas.

cathartic   A laxative.

caustic   A substance capable of corroding or burning bodily tissue.

chologogue   A substance that increases the flow of bile into the intestinal tract.

coagulant   A substance that promotes the formation of clots, such as blood clots.

counterirritant   A substance that irritates one part of the body to counteract irritation in another part.

decongestant   A substance that relieves mucus build-up in the respiratory tract.

demulcent   A substance that soothes irritated membranes and other tissues.

deodorant   A substance that masks or destroys undesirable odors.

depressant   A substance that reduces nervous stimulation.

depurative   A purifying, cleansing substance, especially for the bloodstream.

detergent   A substance that cleanses wounds and removes diseased or necrotic material.

diaphoretic   A substance that promotes perspiration.

digestive   A substance that promotes the digestion of foods throughout the alimentary tract.

disinfectant   An antiseptic.

diuretic   A substance that promotes urination.

dysmenorrhea   Menstrual pain or disorder.

emetic   A substance that induces vomiting.

emmenagogue   A substance that encourages menstrual flow.

emollient   A softening, soothing agent used externally.

errhine   A substance that induces sneezing and nasal discharge.

euphoriant, euphorigen   A substance that induces an extraordinary or abnormal sense of happiness, "floating," etc.

expectorant   A substance that promotes the expulsion of mucus from the lungs and other respiratory structures.

family   The biological reference to a group of related plants or animals; a family is a category above a genus and below an order (e.g., Brassica, the crucifer family).

febrifuge   An antipyretic, or fever-reducer.

galactagogue   A substance that promotes and increases the secretion of mother's milk.

genus   A biological classification, in Latin, between family and species.

hallucinogen   A substance that induces bizarre visions, apparitions, sounds or other visual or auditory hallucinations.

hemostatic   A substance that arrests bleeding.

herb   An annual, biennial or perennial plant used for its aromatic, flavoring or medicinal properties.

hepatic   A substance that affects the liver.

hydragogue   A laxative that promotes copious watery discharge.

hypnotic   A sleep-producing agent.

irritant   A substance that produces adverse reaction.

laxative   A substance that promotes the evacuation of fecal material from the intestines.

lithotriptic   A substance that dissolves or eliminates urinary, kidney or biliary gravel and stones.

mucilaginous   Gummy or having the consistency of gelatin.

narcotic   Therapeutically, a substance that kills pain and induces sleep.

nauseant   A substance that creates the desire to vomit.

nephritic   A substance that affects the kidneys.

nervine   A tranquilizer or sedative.

oxytocic   A substance that promotes uterine contraction to aid in childbirth.

parasiticide   A substance that kills parasites that have invaded the digestive tract or the skin.

pectoral   A remedial substance for chest and lung diseases.

poison   A substance that can harm or destroy living tissue.

purgative   A substance that promotes a dramatic expulsion of waste materials from the intestines; a strong laxative.

refrigerant   A cooling agent; a substance capable of lowering body heat.

restorative   A substance capable of reviving consciousness or normal bodily functions.

rubefacient   A mild irritant that creates redness of the skin.

sedative   A substance that reduces nervous tension.

sialagogue   A substance that promotes salivation.

species   A biological classification, in Latin, of related organisms under the category of genus.

specific   A substance used to affect a particular disease or problem.

stimulant   A substance that excites or activates a bodily (including physical and mental) process.

stomachic   A substance that fortifies the stomach or promotes healthy stomach activity.

styptic   An astringent or hemostatic; a substance that arrests bleeding.

sudorific   A diaphoretic, or substance that promotes perspiration.

taeniacide   A vermifuge, or agent that destroys tapeworms.

tonic   A strengthening agent.

vasoconstrictor   A substance that causes blood vessels to narrow and increases blood pressure.

vasodilator   A substance that causes blood vessels to expand and lowers blood pressure.

vermicide   An anthelmintic; a substance that kills worms in the intestines.

vermifuge   A substance that induces the expulsion of intestinal worms.

vesicant   A substance that causes blisters.

vulnerary   A substance that promotes cell growth and repair in the case of wounds.

APPENDIX 3: NUTRITION CHRONOLOGY

The Garden of Eden, in the Old Testament, is the archetypal garden, with a central tree as the life-nourisher.

In Tibetan mythology, the goddess of healing introduced fragrant healing plants and planted gardens of them, called the paradise gardens. The Buddha is also associated with "a cosmic tree" and legendary gardens.

5000 B.C. A Chinese herbal lists rhubarb, poppy and ephedra among the medicinal plants.

About 4,500 years ago, the Ancient Hindu text, the *Rig Veda,* listed more than 1,000 medicinal herbs, including senna and cinnamon.

2700 B.C. Chinese medicine expands to acupuncture and a system of polypharmacy.

c. 2697 B.C. Chinese Emperor Shen Nung becomes known as "the divine farmer" and the father of agriculture and herbal medicine.

c. 2697–2595 B.C. Chinese Emperor Huang Ti wrote *The Nei Ching,* or *Yellow Emperor's Classic of Internal Medicine.* The book is still used as a medical text in China. The Chinese combined acupuncture, herbs, massage, exercise and diet as therapeutic modalities.

2000 B.C. "Oracle bones," i.e., bones that had the names of plants and diseases etched on them,

are considered part of China's prehistoric evidence of herbal medicine.

1500 B.C. The Ancient Egyptian Ebers papyrus listed plants, including garlic and the opium poppy, and medicinal formulas made from them. The Arabs were considered the first modern pharmacists. Among their accomplishments, they distilled the first pure alcohol (*al-kohl,* in Arabic, meaning quintessence) in which to soak medicinal plants. These concentrated extracts are known today as tinctures. Ancient Egyptians are also credited with knowledge of what came to be known as vitamins.

By 1000 B.C., Ayurveda, the Hindu "science of life," is thought to be already highly developed.

c. 600 B.C., King Nebuchadnezzar of Babylon created The Hanging Gardens, one of the seven wonders of the world, for his homesick wife. In the three-acre gardens the king ordered the cultivation of shrubs, trees and flowers that were both beautiful and medicinal.

460–377 B.C. Hippocrates, Ancient Greek physician called "the father of medicine," listed 350 plants, including thyme and mint, as useful for cooking and medicine.

In Greek mythology, famous gardens include the Blessed Isles. There the Hesperides guarded and cultivated golden apples of the sun.

c. 1000 A.D. Europe emerges from the Dark Ages, during which Greek and Roman medicine languished. Renewed trade between Arab countries and Europe brought Arab medical knowledge to the Benedictine monks, who were enthusiastic herbalists praised by Charlemagne. He encouraged the monks' "physic gardens" and their prowess as physicians. In their tinctures, they substituted wine for pure alcohol and invented liqueurs (meant to settle the stomach after dinner).

In the 1st century A.D., the *Charaka Samhita,* an Indian Vedic medical text, is written based on the oral tradition since preliterate times. The text lists 500 herbal drugs.

Also in the 1st century A.D., Roman physicians Galen and Dioscorides set forth books on medicine that included information on animal, vegetable and mineral therapies and a system of classifying herbs for medicinal use.

For about 500 years following the 6th century A.D., Anglo-Saxon medicine relied on *The Leech Book of Bald,* authored by a 10th-century monk. The book included many Greek and Roman medical therapies.

11th, 12th, and 13th centuries The Crusades sparked Europe's desire for Asian spices for cooking, perfumes and medicines. The Crusades also introduced Europeans to a new manner of gardening, and eating and celebrating in open, fragrant and lush gardens. In the 1400s, Christopher Columbus reached the West Indies and returned with *kian* (cayenne) pepper from the Caribbean peoples.

Paracelsus, a Swiss-born alchemist and physician (1493–1541), catalyzed the movement toward mineral medicines and predicted that there were therapeutic substances in plants and minerals.

1497 Portuguese navigator Vasco da Gama lost 100 of his 160 men to scurvy, a disease caused by the lack of vitamin C, during the voyage around the Cape of Good Hope.

1542 German physician and botanist Leonhard Fuchs wrote a book citing 400 medicinal plants, including American corn and pumpkin. The fuschia was named after him.

1597 Surgeon John Gerard published *Herbal,* a book on herbs and their uses.

Also during the Renaissance, "wise women," as they were called, handed down herbal recipes, cosmetics and medicines to younger generations after a great many years of practice. These women contributed significantly to the survival of herbal knowledge.

1640 John Parkinson published his book on herbs.

1649 Nicholas Culpeper, a British astrologer/physician, educated at Cambridge University, published *The Complete Herbal.* One of the most revered herbalists of all time, Culpeper refused to participate in other physicians' snobbery evidenced by their much-inflated medical mystique. Rather, he wrote in vernacular (as did Paracelsus) and treated the poor of London with herbal preparations they could afford. Culpeper could aptly be called a grassroots caregiver. More than 41 editions of his book have been published, the latest by Sterling Publishing Company, Inc., New York, in 1983: *Culpeper's Color Herbal,* edited by David Potterson.

1754 Scottish naval surgeon James Lind discovered that scurvy could be prevented and cured by lemon and orange juice.

1773 The Boston Tea Party: Outraged North American colonists dumped tons of tea into Boston harbor when Parliament threatened a tax. Originally a Chinese stimulant, tea became the "item" that led to the American Revolution.

Concurrently, colonists learned Native American herbalism from the Plains Indians. Old World herbalism blended with Native American practices, among them the use of cascara sagrada (a tree bark) as a laxative, and echinacea to fight colds, flu and infections.

1775 Dr. William Withering discovered the benefits of digitalis, from the foxglove plant, in treating angina pectoris (chest pain related to heart disease).

Also during the 18th century, French chemist Antoine Laurent Lavoisier described the relationship between respiration (the intake of oxygen and output of carbon dioxide) and food metabolism. Lavoisier, known as "the father of nutrition," investigated the calorie and energy values of carbohydrates, proteins and fats.

1896 W. O. Atwater, known as "the father of American nutrition," published the first comprehensive table of food values in America, where it was heretofore believed only protein and calories were important.

1897 Christiann Eijkman described a beriberi-like disease in pigeons and chickens, which led to the modern concept of vitamins.

1906 The federal Food and Drug Administration was established.

1909 The American Home Economics Association was established.

1912 The original term "vitamine," referring to "vital amine," was coined by Casimir Funk, a chemist of the Lister Institute in London. Funk designated the accessory food factors required for human life. The final "e" was eventually dropped when it was discovered that most vitamins were not amines.

1916 Nutritionist E. V. McCollum, who specialized in the field of accessory food factors, gave the public the idea of "protective foods," the best sources of vitamins and minerals. As a result, milk, citrus fruit and green leafy vegetables became more popular in the American diet. Around the same time, calorie-expert Graham Lusk emphasized that adolescents required as much food as adults.

1917 The American Dietetic Association was established.

1929 Sir Alexander Fleming (1881–1955), a British bacteriologist, discovered penicillin in mold.

1933 The American Institute of Nutrition was established.

1940 The Food and Nutrition Board of the National Research Council was established. As precursor to a new international approach to nutrition, the council began to study nutrition throughout the world.

1941 The first recommended daily dietary allowances were published by the League of Nations as a result of the studies by the National Research Council. Also in 1941 the Nutrition Foundation, which published the monthly *Nutrition Reviews,* was established.

1947 Reserpine, an antihypertensive drug, was isolated from the rauwolfia plant by Ciba, a Swiss chemical company. Rauwolfia had been used in Asian Indian folk medicine.

1952 The Committee on Therapeutic Nutrition published the amounts of extra nutrients necessary in the event of disease and injury.

1954 American chemist Linus Pauling (1901–1994) won the Nobel Prize in chemistry for his research on DNA molecules and the structure of antibodies, proteins and other complex substances.

1962 Linus Pauling won the Nobel Prize for peace for his campaign against nuclear weapons.

1966 The International Education and Health Act (along with the Foreign Aid Program and the Food for Freedom Program) was established to fight malnutrition. These programs were associated with the Food and Agriculture Organization (FAO), the World Health Organization (WHO) and the United Nations International Children's Emergency Fund, later known as the United Nations children's fund, but still called UNICEF.

1968 The first set of dietary guidelines in the world appeared in Scandinavia.

1969 A White House Conference on Food, Nutrition and Health was held. The purpose of the conference was to improve the nutritional status of pregnant and nursing mothers, children, adolescents, the elderly and the very poor; to develop new technologies for food production; to improve education on nutrition in schools, including nursing and medical schools; and to improve federal programs—school lunches, food stamps and others—that affect nutritional status.

During the 1970s, hearings were held by the Senate's Poverty Subcommittee and the Select Committee on Nutrition and Human Needs. Hunger and malnutrition in the United States thus became a political issue.

1970 American chemist Linus Pauling, of the Linus Pauling Institute of Science and Medicine in Palo Alto, California, published a best-selling book, *Vitamin C and the Common Cold,* which advocated large doses of the vitamin as a preventive and therapeutic measure against colds, cancer and cardiovascular diseases. Although Pauling's theories had many detractors, he enjoyed many awards—the National Medal of Science in 1975 and the Priestly Medal from the American Chemical Society in 1984, among them.

1974 Four private nutrition agencies, the American Institute of Nutrition, the American Society for Clinical Nutrition, the American Dietetic Association and the Institute of Food Technology, formed the National Nutrition Consortium, Inc. Also in 1974, the first meeting of the United Nations World Food Council was held in Rome.

1977 *Dietary Goals for the United States* was published by the government.

1987–1988 Nutrition survey conducted by the Health and Nutrition Examination Survey (HANES) and the Nationwide Food Consumption survey. One of the factors the survey indicated was that overweight and obesity were not so much caused by overeating as by inactivity.

1988 *The Surgeon General's Report on Nutrition and Health* was published.

1989 The National Research Council published *Diet and Health: Implications for Reducing Chronic Disease Risk.*

1990 *The Dietary Guidelines for Americans* was published.

1991 The Nutrition Labeling and Education Act of 1990 was passed into law by Congress and signed by President George Bush.

1994 Public Law 103-417, Dietary Supplement Health and Education Act of 1994, was enacted.

APPENDIX 4: DRUG AND NUTRIENT INTERACTIONS

[Many of the interactions listed below are dose-related and some may be clinically important and some are not. If you are taking prescription medications, always ask your physician before adding any supplements to your regimen. Furthermore, the authors make no claims for the completeness of this list.]

Drug causing vitamin deficiency	Deficient fat-soluble vitamin
cholestyramine (Questran) colestipol (Colestid) mineral oil neomycin antacids	A

cholestyramine (Questran)
colestipol (Colestid)
mineral oil
neomycin
antibacterials:
  sulfonamides (Bactrim,
  Septa, etc.)
  naldixic acid (NegGram)
  tetracyclines
antacids
antituberculars:
  isoniazid (INH)
  rifampin
major tranquilizers:
  thioridazine (Mellaril)
  chlorpromazine (Thorazine)	

Drug causing vitamin deficiency	Deficient fat-soluble vitamin
trifluoperazine (Stelazine) haloperidol (Haldol) anticonvulsants: phenytoin (Dilantin) primadone (Mysoline) phenobarbital thiazide diuretics corticosteroids: prednisone (Deltasone) dexamethasone (Decadron) methyprednisolone (Medrol)	D
cholestyramine (Questran) colestipol E (Colestid) mineral oil	E
cholestyramine (Questran) colestipol (Colestid) mineral oil neomycin antibacterials (see above) anticonvulsants (see above) laxatives	K

Drug causing vitamin deficiency	Deficient water-soluble vitamin
antibacterials (see above) oral contraceptives salicylates such as aspirin indomethacin (Indocin) acetominophern (Tylenol) nicotine (smokers) corticosteroids (see above)	ascorbic acid (vitamin C)
antacids antibacterials (see above) oral contraceptives alcohol to excess	thiamine (vitamin B_1)
neomycin oral contraceptives	riboflavin (vitamin B_2)

Drug causing vitamin deficiency	Deficient water-soluble vitamin
major tranquilizers (see above) tetracycline estrogens (Premarin)	
antitubercular drugs (see above) tetracycline	niacin
neomycin oral contraceptives antitubercular drugs (see above) hydralazine (Apresoline) anticonvulsants (see above) penicillamine estrogens (Premarin) corticosteroids (see above)	pyridoxine
cholestyramine (Questran) colestipol (Colestid) neomycin oral contraceptives major tranquilizers (see above) ascorbic acid (megadoses) methyldopa (Aldomet) estrogens (Premarin)	vitamin B_{12}
cholestyramine (Questran) colestipol (Colestid) antacids antibacterials (see above) anticonvulsants (see above) antitubercular drugs (see above) oral contraceptives salicylates, e.g., aspirin alcohol excess methotrexate tetracycline methyldopa (Aldomet) estrogens (Premarin) corticosteroids (see above)	folic acid

Drug causing mineral deficiency	Deficient mineral
cholestyramine (Questran) colestipol (Colestid) neomycin oral contraceptives anticonvulsants (see above) tetracycline furosemide (Lasix) digoxin (Lanoxin) corticosteroids (see above)	calcium
penicillamine	copper
cholestyramine (Questran) colestipol (Colestid) neomycin antacids salicylates, e.g. aspirin indomethacin (Indocin)	iron
oral contraceptives anticonvulsants (see above) tetracycline thiazide diuretics cisplatinum loop diuretics e.g., furosamide (Lasix) digoxin (Lanoxin) estrogens (Premarin)	magnesium
hydralazine (Apresoline)	manganese
antacids	phosphate
neomycin thiazide diuretics loop diuretics corticosteroids (see above)	potassium
thiazide diuretics	sodium
penicillamine thiazide diuretics	zinc

Vitamin or mineral causing toxicity	Drug toxicity
vitamin D	magnesium-containing antacids (may cause toxicity in kidney dialysis patients)
vitamin D + calcium	digitalis products (Lanoxin and others) High calcium levels may cause heart rhythm disturbances verapamil (Isoptin, Calan, Veralan) atrial fibrillation
vitamin E niacinamide (in doses larger than those found in multivitamin formulas) potassium digitalis products (see above) may cause heart rhythm disturbances A.C.E. inhibitors, e.g., captopril (Capoten), enalapril (Vasotec) others	warfarin (Coumadin) carbamazapine (Tegretol) primidone (Mysoline)
oral contraceptives	vitamin A

thiazide diuretics
    + vit D in patients
    with hypoparathyroidism
	calcium

phenytoin and barbiturates	vitamin D
A.C.E. inhibitors (SEE ABOVE)	potassium

Vitamin-mineral causing diminished effectiveness of drug	Drug

ascorbic acid
niacin
pyridoxine (vitamin B_6)
	warfarin (Coumadin) [rare]
	sulfinpyrazone or probenecid
	anticonvulsants (moniter blood levels):
	    phenobarbital
	    phenytoin
	levodopa

Vitamin-mineral causing diminished effectiveness of drug	Drug
folic acid	anticonvulsants (moniter blood levels) (see above)
vitamin K	warfarin (Coumadin)
calcium salts	iron salts
	atenolol (Tenormin)
	tetracyclines
	verapamil (Calan, Isoptin, Veralan)
calcium carbonate	norfloxacin (Norloxin)
iron salts	doxycycline
	penicillamine
	tetracycline
magnesium salts	nitrofurantoin
	tetracycline
	aminoquinolines
	digoxin (Lanoxin)
	penicillamine
zinc	fluoroquinolones
	tetracycline

APPENDIX 5: RECOMMENDED DIETARY ALLOWANCE CHART

FOOD AND NUTRITION BOARD, NATIONAL ACADEMY OF SCIENCES—NATIONAL RESEARCH COUNCIL RECOMMENDED DIETARY ALLOWANCES,[a] Revised 1989

Designed for the maintenance of good nutrition of practically all healthy people in the United States

Category	Age (years) or Condition	Weight[b] (kg)	(lb)	Height[b] (cm)	(in)	Protein (g)	Fat-Soluble Vitamins Vitamin A (μg RE)[c]	Vitamin D (μg)[d]	Vitamin E (mg α-TE)[e]	Vitamin K (μg)
Infants	0.0–0.5	6	13	60	24	13	375	7.5	3	5
	0.5–1.0	9	20	71	28	14	375	10	4	10
Children	1–3	13	29	90	35	16	400	10	6	15
	4–6	20	44	112	44	24	500	10	7	20
	7–10	28	62	132	52	28	700	10	7	30
Males	11–14	45	99	157	62	45	1,000	10	10	45
	15–18	66	145	176	69	59	1,000	10	10	65
	19–24	72	160	177	70	58	1,000	10	10	70
	25–50	79	174	176	70	63	1,000	5	10	80
	51+	77	170	173	68	63	1,000	5	10	80
Females	11–14	46	101	157	62	46	800	10	8	45
	15–18	55	120	163	64	44	800	10	8	55
	19–24	58	128	164	65	46	800	10	8	60
	25–50	63	138	163	64	50	800	5	8	65
	51+	65	143	160	63	50	800	5	8	65
Pregnant						60	800	10	10	65
Lactating	1st 6 months					65	1,300	10	12	65
	2nd 6 months					62	1,200	10	11	65

FOOD AND NUTRITION BOARD, NATIONAL ACADEMY OF SCIENCES—NATIONAL RESEARCH COUNCIL RECOMMENDED DIETARY ALLOWANCES,[a] Revised 1989

Designed for the maintenance of good nutrition of practically all healthy people in the United States

Category	Age (years) or Condition	Weight[b] (kg)	Weight[b] (lb)	Height[b] (cm)	Height[b] (in)	Pro-tein (g)	Vita-min C (mg)	Thia-min (mg)	Ribo-flavin (mg)	Niacin (mg NE)[f]	Vita-min B_6 (mg)	Folate (μg)	Vitamin B_{12} (μg)
Infants	0.0–0.5	6	13	60	24	13	30	0.3	0.4	5	0.3	25	0.3
	0.5–1.0	9	20	71	28	14	35	0.4	0.5	6	0.6	35	0.5
Children	1–3	13	29	90	35	16	40	0.7	0.8	9	1.0	50	0.7
	4–6	20	44	112	44	24	45	0.9	1.1	12	1.1	75	1.0
	7–10	28	62	132	52	28	45	1.0	1.2	13	1.4	100	1.4
Males	11–14	45	99	157	62	45	50	1.3	1.5	17	1.7	150	2.0
	15–18	66	145	176	69	59	60	1.5	1.8	20	2.0	200	2.0
	19–24	72	160	177	70	58	60	1.5	1.7	19	2.0	200	2.0
	25–50	79	174	176	70	63	60	1.5	1.7	19	2.0	200	2.0
	51 +	77	170	173	68	63	60	1.2	1.4	15	2.0	200	2.0
Females	11–14	46	101	157	62	46	50	1.1	1.3	15	1.4	150	2.0
	15–18	55	120	163	64	44	60	1.1	1.3	15	1.5	180	2.0
	19–24	58	128	164	65	46	60	1.1	1.3	15	1.6	180	2.0
	25–50	63	138	163	64	50	60	1.1	1.3	15	1.6	180	2.0
	51 +	65	143	160	63	50	60	1.0	1.2	13	1.6	180	2.0
Pregnant						60	70	1.5	1.6	17	2.2	400	2.2
Lactating	1st 6 months					65	95	1.6	1.8	20	2.1	280	2.6
	2nd 6 months					62	90	1.6	1.7	20	2.1	260	2.6

FOOD AND NUTRITION BOARD, NATIONAL ACADEMY OF SCIENCES—NATIONAL RESEARCH COUNCIL RECOMMENDED DIETARY ALLOWANCES,[a] Revised 1989

Designed for the maintenance of good nutrition of practically all healthy people in the United States

Category	Age (years) or Condition	Weight[b] (kg)	Weight[b] (lb)	Height[b] (cm)	Height[b] (in)	Protein (g)	Minerals Cal-cium (mg)	Phos-phorus (mg)	Mag-nesium (mg)	Iron (mg)	Zinc (mg)	Iodine (μg)	Sele-nium (μg)
Infants	0.0–0.5	6	13	60	24	13	400	300	40	6	5	40	10
	0.5–1.0	9	20	71	28	14	600	500	60	10	5	50	15
Children	1–3	13	29	90	35	16	800	800	80	10	10	70	20
	4–6	20	44	112	44	24	800	800	120	10	10	90	20
	7–10	28	62	132	52	28	800	800	170	10	10	120	30
Males	11–14	45	99	157	62	45	1,200	1,200	270	12	15	150	40
	15–18	66	145	176	69	59	1,200	1,200	400	12	15	150	50
	19–24	72	160	177	70	58	1,200	1,200	350	10	15	150	70
	25–50	79	174	176	70	63	800	800	350	10	15	150	70
	51+	77	170	173	68	63	800	800	350	10	15	150	70
Females	11–14	46	101	157	62	46	1,200	1,200	280	15	12	150	45
	15–18	55	120	163	64	44	1,200	1,200	300	15	12	150	50
	19–24	58	128	164	65	46	1,200	1,200	280	15	12	150	55
	25–50	63	138	163	64	50	800	800	280	15	12	150	55
	51+	65	143	160	63	50	800	800	280	10	12	150	55
Pregnant						60	1,200	1,200	300	30	15	175	65
Lactating	1st 6 months					65	1,200	1,200	355	15	19	200	75
	2nd 6 months					62	1,200	1,200	340	15	16	200	75

[a]The allowances, expressed as average daily intakes over time, are intended to provide for individual variations among most normal persons as they live in the United States under usual environmental stresses. Diets should be based on a variety of common foods in order to provide other nutrients for which human requirements have been less well defined. See text for detailed discussion of allowances and of nutrients not tabulated.

[b]Weights and heights of Reference Adults are actual medians for the U.S. population of the designated age, as reported by NHANES II. The median weights and heights of those under 19 years of age were taken from Hamill et al. (1979) (see pages 16–17). The use of these figures does not imply that the height-to-weight ratios are ideal.

[c]Retinol equivalents. 1 retinol equivalent = 1 μg retinol or 6 μg β-carotene.

[d]As cholecalciferol. 10 μg cholecalciferol = 400 IU of vitamin D.

[e]α-Tocopherol equivalents. 1 mg d-α tocopherol = 1 α-TE.

[f]1 NE (niacin equivalent) is equal to 1 mg of niacin or 60 mg of dietary tryptophan.

Reprinted with permission from *Recommended Dietary Allowances: 10th Edition.* Copyright © 1989 by the National Academy of Sciences. Courtesy of the National Academy Press, Washington, D.C.

Summary Table
ESTIMATED SAFE AND ADEQUATE DAILY DIETARY INTAKES OF SELECTED VITAMINS AND MINERALS[a]

| | | Vitamins | |
| | Age | Biotin | Pantothenic |
Category	(years)	(μg)	Acid (mg)
Infants	0–0.5	10	2
	0.5–1	15	3
Children and adolescents	1–3	20	3
	4–6	25	3–4
	7–10	30	4–5
	11 +	30–100	4–7
Adults		30–100	4–7

| | | Trace Elements[b] | | | | |
| | Age | Copper | Manganese | Fluoride | Chromium | Molybdenum |
Category	(years)	(mg)	(mg)	(mg)	(μg)	(μg)
Infants	0–0.5	0.4–0.6	0.3–0.6	0.1–0.5	10–40	15–30
	0.5–1	0.6–0.7	0.6–1.0	0.2–1.0	20–60	20–40
Children and	1–3	0.7–1.0	1.0–1.5	0.5–1.5	20–80	25–50
adolescents	4–6	1.0–1.5	1.5–2.0	1.0–2.5	30–120	30–75
	7–10	1.0–2.0	2.0–3.0	1.5–2.5	50–200	50–150
	11 +	1.5–2.5	2.0–5.0	1.5–2.5	50–200	75–250
Adults		1.5–3.0	2.0–5.0	1.5–4.0	50–200	75–250

[a]Because there is less information on which to base allowances, these figures are not given in main table of RDA and are provided here in the form of ranges of recommended intakes.

[b]Since the toxic levels for many trace elements may be only several times usual intakes, the upper levels for the trace elements given in this table should not be habitually exceeded.

APPENDIX 6: AMERICAN DIETETIC ASSOCIATION POSITION STATEMENT

The Recommended Dietary Allowances (RDAs) of the National Academy of Sciences (NAS) (1), which are the established standards for evaluation of dietary intakes of population groups, are set at levels that provide a substantial margin of safety, i.e., two standard deviations above the average needs. Evaluation of American diets, whether by government agencies (2,3) or researchers (4), indicates that although very few people consume 100% of the RDA for *all* nutrients, the vast majority meet at least their average needs (77% of the RDA) for all of the 14 nutrients for which data are available. A relatively small segment of the population with intakes more than two standard deviations below some RDA can be considered at potential nutritional risk; although this can be confirmed only on the basis of biochemical and/or clinical assessment of nutritional status.

Per capita data indicate that the US food supply is capable of providing recommended nutrient levels for the total population (5). However, dietary selection is quite variable and may not be adequate for some individuals because of social, cultural, and economic factors. Surveys consistently identify adolescent girls, individuals on limited incomes, pregnant and lactating women and the elderly as the groups most likely to have intakes less than recommended levels. Vitamins A and C, folate, and the minerals calcium, iron, and zinc are most likely to be consumed at suboptimal levels.

Nutrition education, fortification of staple food products, and nutrient supplements are three complementary approaches to enhancing the nutritional adequacy of at-risk segments of the population. Nutrition education concerning fortification and supplementation as they relate to an adequate diet is vital. Education may be offered at the point of purchase as a public health message or may be provided to individuals seeking information to benefit themselves. Food fortification is strictly a *public health* approach designed to increase the intake of a nutrient for a targeted population by increasing the quantity in the food supply. On the other hand, the use of dietary supplements is an *individual* approach. It is largely self-directed, although there is medical guidance for specific nutrients for vulnerable groups such as pregnant and lactating women, infants and young children, and those on low caloric intakes. Because the policy issues concerning both of these approaches are interrelated, this position paper addresses both food fortification and dietary supplements.

ENRICHMENT AND FORTIFICATION OF FOODS

Position Statement

It is the position of The American Dietetic Association that the US government establish a national policy on enrichment and fortification of the food supply that protects against nutrient insufficiencies and toxicities.

History

Historically, nutrient additions were undertaken as a public health measure to prevent the development of deficiency diseases in large segments of the population; for example, iodine was added to salt to prevent goiter and vitamin D was added to milk to prevent rickets (6). Restoration of nutrients lost during processing or the addition of nutrients to higher levels in cereal grain products to correct known nutrient shortfalls began in the 1940s. Nutrient additions have substantially supplemented the amount of thiamine; riboflavin; niacin; iron; iodine; and vitamins A, C, and D in the food supply (7), and have greatly reduced the prevalence of specific nutrient deficiencies in the population.

In January 1980, the Food and Drug Administration (FDA) established its position on food fortification in a policy statement (8). The policy is a series of voluntary guidelines that manufacturers are urged to follow if they elect to add nutrients to a manufactured or processed food, rather than regulations that would be legally binding. This document is also used by most states to establish their minimum regulation.

The premise underlying FDA's guidelines is that food fortification should provide a reasonable benefit without contributing to a nutritional imbalance in the diet and without misleading consumers into believing that consumption of the fortified food per se will ensure a complete or nutritionally sound diet (6). The agency's policy states that food fortification is appropriate to: (a) correct a dietary insufficiency recognized by the scientific community to exist and known to result in a nutritional deficiency disease; (b) restore such nutrient(s) to level(s) representative of the food before storage, handling, and processing; (c) balance the vitamin, mineral, and protein content of a food in proportion to its total caloric content (nutrient density); and (d) avoid nutritional inferiority in a food that replaces a traditional food in the diet.

FDA's policy does not encourage the indiscriminate addition of nutrients to foods nor consider it appropriate to fortify fresh produce, meat, poultry, or fish products, sugars, or snack foods, such as candies or carbonated beverages. However, food manufacturers have the option to add nutrients to enhance the marketability of a product so long as the content is accurately identified and the level considered safe.

Current and Changing Environment

The current environment for enrichment and fortification is much more complex than in earlier times. Large-scale nutrient-deficiency diseases have essentially disappeared in the Untied States, although deficiencies may occur in some subpopulations, for example, nursing home and hospital patients. The general interest in nutrients has shifted more to meeting the special dietary needs of specific subpopulations and to the putative roles of some nutrients and other food components in decreasing the risk for some chronic diseases and thereby establishing health claims for some nutrients. Under the Nutrition Labeling and Education Act of 1990 (NLEA) (9), FDA authorizes the use of health claims on labels or in the labeling of foods for certain relationships for which there is significant scientific agreement (e.g., calcium for osteoporosis and cholesterol and saturated fat for cardiovascular disease).

Additional factors constantly evolve that impinge on food fortication policy. In the future, there may be foods for specific purposes, and varying nutrient levels in foods could be recommended for specific populations. Already nutrient additions are specified for some foods (e.g., special requirements for infant formulas, increased nutrient density for very-low-calorie diets for weight control) and nutrient additions are made that focus on special needs of subpopulations (e.g., calcium for young women to achieve optimal bone mass). Furthermore, the shift in US demographics to a more ethnically heterogeneous population with increased numbers of older persons and single-person households has potential implications for food fortification. In addition, the increased use of food products and ingredients from outside the United States needs to be considered in the development of a policy on fortification. Advancing technology and increasing interest in food components will introduce additional policy considerations. Manufacturers and others are researching and developing food products based on the possible health effects of food components, for example, for reducing the risk of cancer.

There is also considerable interest in the potential health benefits that might be derived from intakes of nutrients in excess of known requirements. However, when major changes in nutrient additions are considered, it is often difficult to predict the outcome in terms of effects of increased consumption by various subpopulations. In addition, inadequate scientific data are available regarding the potential for unexpected nutrient interactions that may occur as a result of increased consumption of a specific nutrient or health effects in the long-term use of essential nutrients at levels far in excess of known human requirements.

A current example is high dietary intake of vitamin E or other fat-soluble antioxidants in the prevention of lipid peroxidation, which may have beneficial effects on some risk factors for heart disease (e.g., inhibiting oxidation of elevated low-density lipoproteins). However, the safety of long-term use of high levels of vitamin E has yet to be established. The general interest in nutrient intakes above required levels has triggered NAS to consider whether a second set of RDAs should be established for health promotion and disease prevention. ADA strongly endorses rigorous scientific evaluation of the issues involved before any new policy is developed.

DEVELOPMENT OF A SOUND POLICY

In this complex arena, it is essential that the federal government establish and enforce a national policy on food enrichment and fortification that will ensure safety and effectiveness in application for both domestic and imported food products and ingredients. Decisions regarding food enrichment

and fortification require careful analysis of data on health status and food consumption. Consideration must also be given to the need for monitoring the effects of increased consumption on persons in target and nontarget populations. When attempting to increase the intake of a specific nutrient in a small target population, fortification must be based on the ability to target the subgroup appropriately without causing unacceptably high levels of intake by other population groups. If a nutrient is added to a dietary staple to increase intake by young women, persons in the population who consume the greatest amount of the product will obviously achieve the greatest increase in intake. For example, the addition of calcium to orange juice is unlikely to be harmful to high consumers in the target population or in other population groups. In other cases, however, there may be potentially harmful effects in target and nontarget groups. For example, fortification of the general food supply with folic acid is currently under consideration for the purpose of increasing folate intakes in a subpopulation of women who may require increased levels of the vitamin before and during early pregnancy to reduce their risk of having an infant with a neural tube defect. However, at some level of folic acid intake, there is a health risk for individuals with marginal vitamin B-12 status, some of whom are in the target population, but the majority of whom are not. A determination of how best to work within the conflicting goals of increasing intake for some segments of the population while preventing excessive intakes by other segments represents the kinds of fortification issues that require careful scientific evaluation. Another approach to correcting this problem is providing nutrition education to the public for improving their nutrient intake.

In addition, with folic acid and other nutrients that may be added to foods, the total intake for individuals includes the amounts of the nutrient obtained from foods *and* the amounts consumed in dietary supplements. In determining food fortification policy, all dietary sources of the nutrient must be considered to assess the potential impact of a proposed fortification level on individuals. In addition, the nutritional status of the population must be monitored to determine whether particularly high intakes are being consumed by some subpopulations and whether there are possible health effects.

DIETARY SUPPLEMENTS

Position Statement
To assure the American public safe, nontoxic dietary supplements, it is the position of The American Dietetic Association that dietary supplements be regulated like foods and that all associated health claims be based on significant scientific agreement.

History
Food supplements in the form of food adjuncts such as garlic, licorice, and herbals have a long history in the practice of prescientific medicine, primarily for their purported pharmacologic properties. In contrast, the use of dietary supplements, primarily vitamins and minerals, is a phenomenon that has evolved during the last half century. This phenomenon reflects the advances in our knowledge of nutrition science, our capability of isolating and/or synthesizing vitamins and purifying mineral components, the growing recognition of the role of nutrients in health promotion and the prevention of some chronic diseases, and the growing trend for people to take responsibility for their own health.

As a result, there has been significant growth in the dietary supplement business in recent decades. The estimate for 1993 is that 60 million Americans spend $4 billion on products available by mail order, door-to-door sales, in health food stores, and virtually all groceries and pharmacies. Little information is available about either the users or levels of use of these products.

Regulation
Regulation of dietary supplements dates back to the passage of the Food, Drug, and Cosmetic Act of 1938 (10) when these products were considered to be "foods for special dietary purposes" and manufacturers and distributors were required to provide label information on their vitamin and mineral and other contents. The only safety consideration was that a food was regarded as adulterated if it contained an injurious substance; the burden of proof rested with FDA. A 1958 Food Additive Amendment (11) required a premarket evaluation of food additives with the processor responsible for data to establish safety. The Drug Amendment of 1962 (12) gave FDA the authority to remove from the market products sold as supplements that made drug claims without providing data to establish efficacy and safety for the intended use.

A 1973 attempt by FDA to establish maximum permissible potencies and nutritionally reasonable combinations for supplements was overturned in 1979 by Congressional passage of the Proxmire Amendment (13), which restricted FDA's authority to limit potency and composition of supplements except for reasons of safety or when marketed to children 12 years of age and younger. The NLEA requires nutrition labeling of dietary supplements like foods. Unlike drugs, foods (including supplements) do not have to have premarket approval or be proven effective in their use. The Dietary Supplement Act of 1992 (14) stayed FDA's actions on dietary supplements under NLEA, requiring separate regulations that were issued by FDA in January 1994 (15). The regulations provide general requirements for nutrition labeling for dietary supplements and require the same scientific standards for health claims for dietary supplements.

Concerns
For certain segments of the population identified at nutritional risk, supervised supplementation with specific nutrients, either through use of fortified foods targeted for that population or though dietary supplements is considered good public health policy. Such supplementation includes, for example, iron for infants and children over 6 months of age, iron for pregnant women, vitamin D for infants,

folate for women of childbearing age, and calcium for adolescent girls and young women.

However, many people self-prescribe supplements for various reasons, including concern about the adequacy of their own diet or of the food supply, a desire to be more healthy, or to treat or prevent an illness. This escalating, largely unsupervised, use of dietary supplements, which is often based on limited and subjective rather than objective information, raises safety and economic concerns.

Because there is no cap on the potency of dietary supplements, many high potencies (up to several hundred times the RDA) are promoted for a variety of reasons, many of which are unrelated to health benefits. Currently, promotion of antioxidants to provide protection against diseases such as cancer and heart disease is stimulating widespread use of vitamins A and C and beta-carotene. Vitamin E is being promoted and taken at levels that far exceed existing long-term safety evaluations. History is replete with comparable overzealous use of nutrient supplements, resulting in adverse rather than beneficial effects in sensitive individuals. For example, many people took nonphysiologically high doses of vitamin C in response to claims for the prevention of the common cold and of vitamin B-6 to alleviate the symptoms of premenstrual syndrome. It was only when high dosages of Vitamin C and B-6 became associated with significant clinical problems for many users that the issue came to the attention of health professionals, the Centers for Disease Control and Prevention, and the FDA.

Unfortunately, many marketing strategies for single dietary supplements do not assist consumers with objective information about their nutritional needs. Such marketing efforts are often carefully designed to stay within the letter of the law.

Development of a Sound Policy

ADA stresses the importance of a consuming a well-based diet to ensure adequate nutrient intake. However, some individuals have a potential need to use dietary supplements. For individuals to make appropriate decisions regarding dietary supplements, ADA urges the US government to establish regulations regarding health claims on dietary supplements and uniform labeling of such products. The policy must be based on significant scientific data to ensure the nutritional safety of individuals using dietary supplements.

ADA's Recommendations

ADA continues to favor obtaining adequate nutrients from a diet that reflects the *Dietary Guidelines for Americans* (16) and the dietary patterns in the Food Guide Pyramid (17). ADA also recognizes that under certain conditions both food fortification and dietary supplementation may have benefit for some of the US population. However, rigorous scientific analysis and evaluation of the benefits and risks are essential for development of food fortification and dietary supplement policies to safeguard national nutritional and health status.

A strongly enforced national food fortification policy that would ensure the nutritional safety of the food supply and the careful regulation of dietary supplements is essential. This policy must be based on significant scientific criteria that ensure safety of the food supply and provide a means to monitor health effects in the population.

ADA strongly urges the federal government to establish a comprehensive national policy on the enrichment and fortification of foods and ingredients, both domestic and imported. This policy would require supportive legislation to ensure that the responsible agencies have adequate authority and resources to enforce such policy. Federal authority is needed to ensure safe levels of nutrients used in enrichment and fortification. Similarly, regulation is needed regarding health claims and labeling of dietary supplements.

Implications for Practice

Nutrition education, one of the approaches to improving the nutrient intakes of the population, is one of ADA's mandates. As such, the Association and its members must take major responsibility for educating the public about food fortification and dietary supplement usage. To do that, ADA members need to be thoroughly informed about the issues and regulations surrounding nutrient additions to foods and dietary supplements. There is need, particularly, for continuing emphasis on public education about the proper interpretation and application of the RDA, education about nutritional evaluation of diets and dietary supplement usage, the appropriate use of food labeling information, and the nutritional impact of the use of dietary supplements and fortified foods.

References

1. Food and Nutrition Board. *Recommended Dietary Allowances.* 10th ed. Washington, DC: National Academy Press; 1989.

2. Life Sciences Office, Federation of American Societies for Experimental Biology. *Nutrition Monitoring in the Unites States—An Update Report on Nutrition Monitoring.* Washington, DC: US Depts of Agriculture and Health and Human Services; 1989. DHHS publication (PHS) 89–1255.

3. Block B, Sobar A F. Estimates of nutrient intake from a food frequency questionnaire: the 1987 National Health Interview Survey. *J Am Diet Assoc.* 1992; 92:969–977.

4. Wright H S, Guthrie H A, Wang M Q, Bernardo V. The 1987–8 Nationwide Food Consumption Survey: an update on the nutrient intake of respondents. *Nutr Today.* 1991; 26 (3):21–27.

5. Raper N R, Zizza C, Rourke J. *Nutrient Content of U.S. Food Supply, 1909–1988.* Washington, DC: US Dept of Agriculture; 1992. Home Economics Research Report No. 50.

6. Frattali, V P, Vanderveen, J E, Forbes, A L. The role of the Untied States government in regulating the nutritional value of the food supply. In: Karmas E, Harris R S, eds. *Nutritional Evaluation of Food Processing.* 3rd ed. New York, NY: Van Nostrand Reinhold; 1988:687–705.

7. Quick J A, Murphy E W. *The Fortification of Foods: A Review.* Washington, DC: US Government Printing Office; 1982. US Dept of Agriculture Handbook No. 598: 6.

8. Nutrient quality of foods: addition of nutrients. 45 (18) *Federal Register* 6314–6324.

9. Nutrition Labeling Education Act, Pub L No. 101-535, 104 Stat 2353.

10. *Federal Food, Drug, and Cosmetic Act, as Amended, and Related Laws.* Washington, DC: US Government Printing Office; 1990. HHS Publication No. (FDA) 89-1051.

11. Food Additives, Federal Food, Drug, and Cosmetic Act, USC §409 (IV).

12. Drugs and Devices, Federal Food, Drug, and Cosmetic Act, USC §501(A).

13. Vitamins and Minerals, Federal Food, Drug, and Cosmetic Act, USC §411 (IV).

14. Dietary Supplement Act, Pub L No. 102-571.

15. Dietary Supplement regulations. 59 (002) *Federal Register* 350–437.

16. *Dietary Guidelines for Americans.* 3rd ed. Washington, DC: US Dept of Agriculture; 1990. Home and Garden Bulletin No. 232.

17. *The Food Guide Pyramid.* Washington, DC: US Dept of Agriculture, Human Nutrition Information Service; 1992. Home and Garden Bulletin No. 252.

- ADA position on dietary supplements was adopted by the House of Delegates on October 24, 1993.
- ADA position on enrichment and fortification of foods was adopted by the House of Delegates on April 17, 1994.
- Recognition is given to the following for their contributions:
Authors:
Marilyn G. Stephenson, MS, RD; Helen A. Guthrie, PhD, DSc, RD

Reviewers:
Alfred E. Harper, PhD; Gil Leville, PhD; Christine Lewis, PhD, Rd; Nutrition Education for the Public dietetic practice group; Robert E. Olson, MD, PhD; Public Health Nutrition dietetic practice group; Sue Roberts, MS, RD

Reprinted courtesy of the American Dietetic Association.

APPENDIX 7: DIETARY SUPPLEMENT HEALTH AND EDUCATION ACT OF 1994

For Legislative History of Act, see Report for P.L. 103–417 in U.S.C.C. & A.N. Legislative History Section.

An Act to amend the Federal Food, Drug, and Cosmetic Act to establish standards with respect to dietary supplements, and for other purposes.

Be it enacted by the Senate and House of Representatives of the United States of America in Congress assembled.

SECTION 1. SHORT TITLE; REFERENCE; TABLE OF CONTENTS.

(a) SHORT TITLE.—This Act may be cited as the "Dietary Supplement Health and Education Act of 1994."

(b) REFERENCE.—Whenever in this Act an amendment or repeal is expressed in terms of an amendment to, or repeal of, a section or other provision, the reference shall be considered to be made to a section or other provision of the Federal Food, Drug, and Cosmetic Act.

(c) TABLE OF CONTENTS.—The table of contents of this Act is as follows:

SEC. 2. FINDINGS.

Congress finds that—

(1) improving the health status of United States citizens ranks at the top of the national priorities of the Federal Government;

(2) the importance of nutrition and the benefits of dietary supplements to health promotion and disease prevention have been documented increasingly in scientific studies;

(3)(A) there is a link between the ingestion of certain nutrients or dietary supplements and the prevention of chronic diseases such as cancer, heart disease, and osteoporosis; and

(B) clinical research has shown that several chronic diseases can be prevented simply with a healthful diet, such as a diet that is low in fat, saturated fat, cholesterol, and sodium, with a high proportion of plant-based foods;

(4) healthful diets may mitigate the need for expensive medical procedures, such as coronary bypass surgery or angioplasty;

(5) preventive health measures, including education, good nutrition, and appropriate use of safe nutritional supplements will limit the incidence of chronic diseases, and reduce long-term health care expenditures;

(6)(A) promotion of good health and healthy lifestyles improves and extends lives while reducing health care expenditures; and

(B) reduction in health care expenditures is of paramount importance to the future of the country and the economic well-being of the country;

(7) there is a growing need for emphasis on the dissemination of information linking nutrition and long-term good health;

(8) consumers should be empowered to make choices about preventive health care programs based on data from scientific studies of health benefits related to particular dietary supplements;

(9) national surveys have revealed that almost 50 percent of the 260,000,000 Americans regularly consume dietary supplements of vitamins, minerals, or herbs as a means of improving their nutrition;

(10) studies indicate that consumers are placing increased reliance on the use of nontraditional health care providers to avoid the excessive costs of traditional medical services and to obtain more holistic consideration of their needs;

(11) the United States will spend over $1,000,000,000,000 on health care in 1994, which is about 12 percent of the Gross National Product of the United States, and this amount and percentage will continue to increase unless significant efforts are undertaken to reverse the increase;

(12)(A) the nutritional supplement industry is an integral part of the economy of the United States;

(B) the industry consistently projects a positive trade balance; and

(C) the estimated 600 dietary supplement manufacturers in the United States produce approximately 4,000 products, with total annual sales of such products alone reaching at least $4,000,000,000;

(13) although the Federal Government should take swift action against products that are unsafe or adulterated, the Federal Government should not take any actions to impose unreasonable regulatory barriers limiting or slowing the flow of safe products and accurate information to consumers;

(14) dietary supplements are safe within a broad range of intake, and safety problems with the supplements are relatively rare; and

(15)(A) legislative action that protects the right of access of consumers to safe dietary supplements is necessary in order to promote wellness; and

(B) a rational Federal framework must be established to supersede the current ad hoc, patchwork regulatory policy on dietary supplements.

SEC. 3. DEFINITIONS.

(a) DEFINITION OF CERTAIN FOODS AS DIETARY SUPPLEMENTS.—Section 201 (21 U.S.C. 321) is amended by adding at the end the following:

"(ff) The term 'dietary supplement'—

"(1) means a product (other than tobacco) intended to supplement the diet that bears or contains one or more of the following dietary ingredients:

"(A) a vitamin;

"(B) a mineral;

"(C) an herb or other botanical;

"(D) an amino acid;

"(E) a dietary substance for use by man

to supplement the diet by increasing the total dietary intake; or

"(F) a concentrate, metabolite, constituent, extract, or combination of any ingredient described in clause (A), (B), (C), (D), or (E);

"(2) means a product that—

"(A)(i) is intended for ingestion in a form described in section 411(c)(1)(B)(i); or

"(ii) complies with section 411(C)(1)(B)(ii);

"(B) is not represented for use as a conventional food or as a sole item of a meal or the diet; and

"(C) is labeled as a dietary supplement; and

"(3) does—

"(A) include an article that is approved as a new drug under section 505, certified as an antibiotic under section 507, or licensed as a biologic under section 351 of the Public Health Service Act (42 U.S.C. 262) and was, prior to such approval, certification, or license, marketed as a dietary supplement or as a food unless the Secretary has issued a regulation, after notice and comment, finding that the article, when used as or in a dietary supplement under the conditions of use and dosages set forth in the labeling for such dietary supplement, is unlawful under section 402(f); and

"(B) not include—

"(i) an article that is approved as a new drug under section 505, certified as an antibiotic under section 507, or licensed as a biologic under section 351 of the Public Health Service Act (42 U.S.C. 262), or

"(ii) an article authorized for investigation as a new drug, antibiotic, or biological for which substantial clinical investigations have been instituted and for which the existence of such investigations has been made public,

which was not before such approval, certification, licensing, or authorization marketed as a dietary supplement or as a food unless the Secretary, in the Secretary's discretion, has issued a regulation, after notice and comment, finding that the article would be lawful under this Act.

Except for purposes of section 201(g), a dietary supplement shall be deemed to be a food within the meaning of this Act."

(b) EXCLUSION FROM DEFINITION OF FOOD ADDITIVE.—Section 201(s) (21 U.S.C. 321(s)) is amended—

(1) by striking "or" at the end of subparagraph (4);

(2) by striking the period at the end of subparagraph (5) and inserting "or"; and

(3) by adding at the end the following new subparagraph

"(6) an ingredient described in paragraph (ff) in, or intended for us in, a dietary supplement.".

(c) FORM OF INGESTION.—Section 411(c)(1)(B) (21 U.S.C. 350(c)(B)) is amended—

(1) in clause (i), by inserting "powder, softgel, gelcap," after "capsule,"; and

(2) in clause (ii), by striking "does not simulate and."

SEC. 4. SAFETY OF DIETARY SUPPLEMENTS AND BURDEN OF PROOF ON FDA.

Section 402 (21 U.S.C. 342) is amended by adding at the end the following:

"(f)(1) If it is a dietary supplement or contains a dietary ingredient that—

"(A) presents a significant or unreasonable risk of illness or injury under—

"(i) conditions of use recommended or suggested in labeling, or

"(ii) if no conditions of use are suggested or recommended in the labeling, under ordinary conditions of use;

"(B) is a new dietary ingredient for which there is inadequate information to provide reasonable assurance that such ingredient does not present a significant or unreasonable risk of illness or injury;

"(C) the Secretary declares to pose an imminent hazard to public health or safety, except that the authority to make such declaration shall not be delegated and the Secretary shall promptly after such a declaration initiate a proceeding in accordance with sections 554 and 556 of title 5, United States Code, to affirm or withdraw the declaration; or

"(D) is or contains a dietary ingredient that renders it adulterated under paragraph (a)(1) under the conditions of use recommended or suggested in the labeling of such dietary supplement.

In any proceeding under this subparagraph, the United States shall bear the burden of proof on each element to show that a dietary supplement is adulterated. The court shall decide any issue under this paragraph on a de novo basis.

"(2) Before the Secretary may report to a United States attorney a violation of paragraph (1)(A) for a civil proceeding, the person against whom such proceeding would be initiated shall be given appropriate notice and the opportunity to present views, orally and in writing, at least 10 days before such notice, with regard to such proceeding."

SEC. 5. DIETARY SUPPLEMENT CLAIMS.

Chapter IV (21 U.S.C. 341 et seq.) is amended by inserting after section 403A the following new section:

"DIETARY SUPPLEMENT LABELING EXEMPTIONS

"SEC. 403B. (a) IN GENERAL.—A publication, including an article, a chapter in a book, or an official abstract of a peer-reviewed scientific publication that appears in an article and was prepared by the author or the editors of the publication, which is reprinted in its entirety, shall not be defined as labeling when used in connection with the sale of a dietary supplement to consumers when it—

"(1) is not false or misleading;

"(2) does not promote a particular manufacturer or brand of a dietary supplement;

"(3) is displayed or presented, or is displayed or presented with other such items on the same subject matter, so as to present a balanced view of the available scientific information on a dietary supplement;

"(4) if displayed in an establishment, is physically separate from the dietary supplements; and

"(5) does not have appended to it any information by sticker or any other method.

"(b) APPLICATION.—Subsection (a) shall not apply to or restrict a retailer or wholesaler of dietary supplements in any way whatsoever in the sale of books or other publications as a part of the business of such retailer or wholesaler.

"(c) BURDEN OF PROOF.—In any proceeding brought under subsection (a), the burden of proof shall be on the United States to establish that an article or other such matter is false or misleading."

SEC. 6. STATEMENTS OF NUTRITIONAL SUPPORT.

Section 403(r) (21 U.S.C. 343(r)) is amended by adding at the end the following:

"(6) For purposes of paragraph (r)(1)(B), a statement for a dietary supplement may be made if—

"(A) the statement claims a benefit related to a classical nutrient deficiency disease and discloses the prevalence of such disease in the United States, describes the role of a nutrient or dietary ingredient intended to affect the structure or function in humans, characterizes the documented mechanism by which a nutrient or dietary ingredient acts to maintain such structure or function, or describes general well-being from consumption of a nutrient or dietary ingredient,

"(B) the manufacturer of the dietary supplement has substantiation that such statement is truthful and not misleading, and

"(C) the statement contains prominently displayed and in boldface type, the following: 'This statement has not been evaluated by the Food and

Drug Administration. This product is not intended to diagnose, treat, cure, or prevent any disease.'.

A statement under this subparagraph may not claim to diagnose, mitigate, treat, cure, or prevent a specific disease or class of diseases. If the manufacturer of a dietary supplement proposes to make a statement described in the first sentence of this subparagraph in the labeling of the dietary supplement, the manufacturer shall notify the Secretary no later than 30 days after the first marketing of the dietary supplement with such statement that such a statement is being made."

SEC. 7. DIETARY SUPPLEMENT INGREDIENT LABELING AND NUTRITION INFORMATION LABELING.

(a) MISBRANDED SUPPLEMENTS.—Section 403 (21 U.S.C. 343) is amended by adding at the end the following:

"(s) If—

"(1) it is a dietary supplement; and

"(2)(A) the label or labeling of the supplement fails to list—

"(i) the name of each ingredient of the supplement that is described in section 201(ff); and

"(ii)(I) the quantity of each such ingredient; or

"(II) with respect to a proprietary blend of such ingredients, the total quantity of all ingredients in the blend;

"(B) the label or labeling of the dietary supplement fails to identify the product by using the term 'dietary supplement', which term may be modified with the name of such an ingredient;

"(C) the supplement contains an ingredient described in section 201(ff)(1)(C), and the label or labeling of the supplement fails to identify any part of the plant from which the ingredient is derived;

"(D) the supplement—

"(i) is covered by the specifications of an official compendium;

"(ii) is represented as conforming to the specifications of an official compendium; and

"(iii) fails to so conform; or

"(E) the supplement—

"(i) is not covered by the specifications of an official compendium; and

"(ii)(I) fails to have the identity and strength that the supplement is represented to have; or

"(II) fails to meet the quality (including tablet or capsule disintegration), purity, or compositional specifications, based on validated assay or other appropriate methods, that the supplement is represented to meet."

(b) SUPPLEMENT LISTING ON NUTRITION LABELING.—Section 403(q)(5)(F) (21 U.S.C. 343(q)(5)(F)) is amended to read as follows:

"(F) A dietary supplement product (including a food to which section 411 applies) shall comply with the requirements of subparagraphs (1) and (2) in a manner which is appropriate for the product and which is specified in regulations of the Secretary which shall provide that—

"(i) nutrition information shall first list those dietary ingredients that are present in the product in a significant amount and for which a recommendation for daily consumption has been established by the Secretary, except that a dietary ingredient shall not be required to be listed if it is not present in a significant amount, and shall list any other dietary ingredient present and identified as having so such recommendation;

"(ii) the listing of dietary ingredients shall include the quantity of each such ingredient (or of a proprietary blend of such ingredients) per serving;

"(iii) the listing of dietary ingredients may include the source of a dietary ingredient; and

"(iv) the nutrition information shall immediately precede the ingredient information required under subclause (i), except that no ingredient identified pursuant to subclause (i) shall be required to be identified a second time."

(c) PERCENTAGE LEVEL CLAIMS.—Section 403(r)(2) (21 U.S.C. 343(r)(2)) is amended by adding after clause (E) the following:

"(F) Subclause (i) clause (A) does not apply to a statement in the labeling of a dietary supplement that characterizes the percentage level of a dietary ingredient for which the Secretary has not established a reference daily intake, daily recommended value, or other recommendation for daily consumption."

(d) VITAMINS AND MINERALS.—Section 411(b)(2) (21 U.S.C. 350(b)(2)) is amended—

(1) by striking "vitamins or minerals" and inserting "dietary supplement ingredients described in section 201(ff)";

(2) by striking "(2)(A)" and inserting "(2)"; and

(3) by striking subparagraph (B).

(e) EFFECTIVE DATE.—Dietary supplements—

(1) may be labeled after the date of the enactment of this Act in accordance with the amendments made by this section, and

(2) shall be labeled after December 31, 1996, in accordance with such amendments.

SEC. 8. NEW DIETARY INGREDIENTS.

Chapter IV of the Federal Food, Drug, and Cosmetic Act is amended by adding at the end the following:

"NEW DIETARY INGREDIENTS

"SEC. 413. (a) IN GENERAL.—A dietary supplement which contains a new dietary ingredient shall be deemed adulterated under section 402(f) unless it meets one of the following requirements:

"(1) The dietary supplement contains only dietary ingredients which have been present in the food supply as an article used for food in a form in which the food has not been chemically altered.

"(2) There is a history of use or other evidence of safety establishing that the dietary ingredient when used under the conditions recommended or suggested in the labeling of the dietary supplement will reasonably be expected to be safe and at least 75 days before being introduced or delivered for introduction into interstate commerce, the manufacturer or distributor of the dietary ingredient or dietary supplement provides the Secretary with information, including any citation to published articles, which is the basis on which the manufacturer or distributor has concluded that a dietary supplement containing such dietary ingredient will reasonably be expected to be safe.

The Secretary shall keep confidential any information provided under paragraph (2) for 90 days following its receipt. After the expiration of such 90 days, the Secretary shall place such information on public display, except matters in the information which are trade secrets or otherwise confidential, commercial information.

"(b) PETITION.—Any person may file with the Secretary a petition proposing the issuance of an order prescribing the conditions under which a new dietary ingredient under its intended conditions of use will reasonably be expected to be safe. The Secretary shall make a decision on such petition within 180 days of the date the petition is filed with the Secretary. For purposes of chapter 7 of title 5, United States Code, the decision of the Secretary shall be considered final agency action.

"(c) DEFINITION.—For purposes of this section, the term 'new dietary ingredient' means a dietary ingredient that was not marketed in the United States before October 15, 1994 and does not include and dietary ingredient which was marketed in the United States before October 15, 1994."

SEC. 9. GOOD MANUFACTURING PRACTICES.

Section 402 (21 U.S.C. 342), as amended by section 4, is amended by adding at the end the following:

"(g)(1) If it is a dietary supplement and it has been prepared, packed, or held under conditions that do not meet current good manufacturing practice regulations, including regulations requiring, when necessary, expiration date labeling, issued by the Secretary under subparagraph (2).

"(2) The Secretary may by regulation prescribe good manufacturing practices for dietary supplements. Such regulations shall be modeled after current good manufacturing practice regulations for food and may not impose standards for which there is no current and generally available analytical methodology. No standard of current good manufacturing practice may be imposed unless such standard is included in a regulation promulgated after notice and opportunity for comment in accordance with chapter 5 of title 5, United States Code."

SEC. 10. CONFORMING AMENDMENTS.

(a) SECTION 201.—The last sentence of section 201(g)(1) (21 U.S.C. 321(g)(1)) is amended to read as follows: "A food or dietary supplement for which a claim, subject to sections 403(r)(1)(B) and 403(r)(3) or sections 403(r)(1)(B) and 403(r)(5)(D), is made in accordance with the requirements of section 403(r) is not a drug solely because the label or the labeling contains such a claim. A food, dietary ingredient, or dietary supplement for which a truthful and not misleading statement is made in accordance with section 403(r)(6) is not a drug under clause (C) solely because the label or the labeling contains such a statement."

(b) SECTION 301.—Section 301 (21 U.S.C. 331) is amended by adding at the end the following: "(u) The introduction or delivery for introduction into interstate commerce of a dietary supplement that is unsafe under section 413."

(c) SECTION 403.—Section 403 (21 U.S.C. 343), as amended by section 7, is amended by adding after paragraph (s) the following "A dietary supplement shall not be deemed misbranded solely because its label or labeling contains directions or conditions of use or warnings."

SEC. 11. WITHDRAWAL OF THE REGULATIONS AND NOTICE.

The advance notice of proposed rulemaking concerning dietary supplements published in the Federal Register of June 18, 1993 (58 FR 33690–33700) is null and void and of no force or effect insofar as it applies to dietary supplements. The Secretary of Health and Human Services shall publish a notice in the Federal Register to revoke the item declared to be null and void and of no force or effect under subsection (a).

SEC. 12. COMMISSION ON DIETARY SUPPLEMENT LABELS.

(a) ESTABLISHMENT.—There shall be established as an independent agency within the executive branch a commission to be known as the Commission on Dietary Supplement Labels (hereafter in this section referred to as the "Commission").

(b) MEMBERSHIP.—

(1) COMPOSITION.—The Commission shall be composed of 7 members who shall be appointed by the President.

(2) EXPERTISE REQUIREMENT.—The members of the Commission shall consist of individuals with expertise and experience in dietary supplements and in the manufacture, regulation, distribution, and use of such supplements. At least three of the members of the Commission shall be qualified by scientific training and experience to evaluate the benefits to health of the use of dietary supplements and one of such three members shall have experience in pharmacognosy, medical botany, traditional herbal medicine, or other related sciences. Members and staff of the Commission shall be without bias on the issue of dietary supplements.

(c) FUNCTIONS OF THE COMMISSION.—The Commission shall conduct a study on, and provide recommendation for, the regulation of label claims and statements for dietary supplements, including the use of literature in connection with the sale of dietary supplements and procedures for the evaluation of such claims. In making such recommendations, the Commission shall evaluate how best to provide truthful, scientifically valid, and not misleading information to consumers so that such consumers may make informed and appropriate health care choices for themselves and their families.

(d) ADMINISTRATIVE POWERS OF THE COMMISSION.—

(1) HEARINGS.—The Commission may hold hearings, sit and act at such times and places, take such testimony, and receive such evidence as the Commission considers advisable to carry out the purposes of this section.

(2) INFORMATION FROM FEDERAL AGENCIES.—The Commission may secure directly from any Federal department or agency such information as the Commission considers necessary to carry out the provisions of this section.

(3) AUTHORIZATION OF APPROPRIATIONS.— There are authorized to be appropriated such sums as may be necessary to carry out this section.

(e) REPORTS AND RECOMMENDATIONS.—

(1) FINAL REPORT REQUIRED.—Not later than 24 months after the date of enactment of this Act, the Commission shall prepare and submit to the President and to the Congress a final report on the study required by this section.

(2) RECOMMENDATIONS.—The report described in paragraph (1) shall contain such recommendations, including recommendations for legislation, as the Commission deems appropriate.

(3) ACTION ON RECOMMENDATIONS.— Within 90 days of the issuance of the report under paragraph (1), the Secretary of Health and Human Services shall publish in the Federal Register a notice of any recommendation of Commission for changes in regulations of the Secretary for the regulation of dietary supplements and shall include in such notice a notice of proposed rulemaking on such changes to-

gether with an opportunity to present views on such changes. Such rulemaking shall be completed not later than 2 years after the date of the issuance of such report. If such rulemaking is not completed on or before the expiration of such 2 years, regulations of the Secretary published in 59 FR 395–426 on January 4, 1994, shall not be in effect.

SEC. 13. OFFICE OF DIETARY SUPPLEMENTS.

(a) IN GENERAL.—Title IV of the Public Health Service Act is amended by inserting after section 485B (42 U.S.C. 287c-3) the following:

"Subpart 4—Office of Dietary Supplements

"SEC. 485C. DIETARY SUPPLEMENTS.

"(a) ESTABLISHMENT.—The Secretary shall establish an Office of Dietary Supplements within the National Institutes of Health.

"(b) PURPOSE.—The purposes of the Office are—

"(1) to explore more fully the potential role of dietary supplements as a significant part of the efforts of the United States to improve health care; and

"(2) to promote scientific study of the benefits of dietary supplements in maintaining health and preventing chronic disease and other health-related conditions.

"(c) DUTIES.—The Director of the Office of Dietary Supplements shall—

"(1) conduct and coordinate scientific research within the National Institutes of Health relating to dietary supplements and the extent to which the use of dietary supplements can limit or reduce the risk of diseases such as heart disease, cancer, birth defects, osteoporosis, cataracts, or prostatism;

"(2) collect and compile the results of scientific research relating to dietary supplements, including scientific data from foreign sources or the Office of Alternative Medicine;

"(3) serve as the principal advisor to the Secretary and to the Assistant Secretary for Health and provide advice to the Director of the National Institutes of Health, the Director of the Centers for Disease Control and Prevention, and the Commissioner of Food and Drugs on issues relating to dietary supplements including—

"(A) dietary intake regulations;

"(B) the safety of dietary supplements;

"(C) claims characterizing the relationship between—

"(i) dietary supplements; and

"(ii)(I) prevention of disease or other health-related conditions; and

"(II) maintenance of health; and

"(D) scientific issues arising in connection with the labeling and composition of dietary supplements;

"(4) compile a database of scientific research on dietary supplements and individual nutrients; and

"(5) coordinate funding relating to dietary supplements for the National Institutes of Health.

"(d) DEFINITION.—As used in this section, the term 'dietary supplement' has the meaning given the term in section 201(ff) of the Federal Food, Drug, and Cosmetic Act.

"(e) AUTHORIZATION OF APPROPRIATIONS.— There are authorized to be appropriated to carry out this section $5,000,000 for fiscal year 1994 and such sums as may be necessary for each subsequent fiscal year.".

(b) CONFORMING   AMENDMENT.—Section 401(b)(2) of the Public Health Service Act (42 U.S.C. 281(b)(2)) is amended by adding at the end the following:

"(E) The Office of Dietary Supplements."

Approved October 25, 1994.

APPENDIX 8: THE NEW FOOD LABEL

Grocery store aisles are on their way to becoming avenues to *greater nutritional knowledge.*

The new food label will make it possible. Under new regulations from the Food and Drug Administration of the Department of Health and Human Services and the Food Safety and Inspection Service of the U.S. Department of Agriculture, the *food label will soon offer more complete, useful and accurate nutrition information than ever before.*

The purpose of food label reform is simple: to clear up confusion that has prevailed on supermarket shelves for years, to help consumers choose more healthful diets, and to offer an *incentive to food companies to improve the nutritional qualities of their products.*

Among key changes taking place are:

• nutrition labeling for almost all foods. Consumers now will be able to learn about the nutritional qualities of almost all of the products they buy.
• a new, distinctive, easy-to-read format that will enable consumers to more quickly find the label and the information they need to make healthful food choices
• information on the amount per serving of saturated fat, cholesterol, dietary fiber, and other nutrients that are of major health concern to today's consumers
• nutrient reference values, expressed as %Daily Values, that can help consumers see how a food fits into an overall daily diet
• uniform definitions for terms that describe a food's nutrient content—such as "light," "low-fat," and "high-fiber"—to ensure that such terms mean the same for any product on which they appear. These descriptors will be particularly helpful for consumers trying to moderate their intake of calories or fat and other nutrients, or for those trying to increase their intake of certain nutrients, such as fiber.
• claims about the relationship between a nutrient or food and a disease or health-related condition, such as calcium and osteoporosis, and fat and cancer. These will be helpful for people who are concerned about eating foods that may help keep them healthier longer.
• standardized serving sizes that make nutritional comparisons of similar products easier.
• declaration of total percentage of juice in juice drinks. This will enable consumers to know exactly how much juice is in a product.
• voluntary nutrition information for many raw foods.

NLEA

These and other changes are part of final rules published in the *Federal Register* in 1992 and 1993. FDA's rules implement the provisions of the Nutrition Labeling and Education Act of 1990 (NLEA), which, among other things, requires nutrition labeling for most foods (except meat and poultry) and authorizes the use of nutrient content claims and appropriate FDA-approved health claims.

Meat and poultry products regulated by USDA are not covered by NLEA. However, USDA's regulations closely parallel FDA's rules, summarized here.

Effective Dates

Some products bearing the new nutrition label are appearing now, although manufacturers have until May 8, 1994, to comply with FDA's mandatory nutrition labeling requirements. (They have until July 6, 1994, to comply with USDA's.)

FDA's deadline pertains only to foods labeled on or after May 8. It does not apply to products labeled before that date but not yet shipped in interstate commerce. Thus, consumers may still see the old nutrition label on some food packages after the May 8 deadline.

A few of the regulations went into effect earlier. A voluntary program for point-of-purchase information for fresh produce and raw fish has been available in many grocery stores since November 1991. And regulations pertaining to health claims and some aspects of ingredient labeling went into effect in May 1993.

Nutrition Labeling—Applicable Foods

The regulations call for nutrition labeling for most foods. In addition, they set up voluntary programs for nutrition information for many raw foods: the 20 most frequently eaten raw fruits, vegetables and fish each, under FDA's voluntary point-of-purchase nutrition information program, and the 45 best-selling cuts of meat, under USDA's program.

Although voluntary, FDA's program for raw produce and fish carries a strong incentive for retailers to participate. The program will remain voluntary only if at least 60 percent of a nationwide sample of retailers continue to provide the necessary information. (In a 1992 survey, FDA found that more than 70 percent of U.S. food stores were complying. A second survey will be done in 1994.)

Nutrition information also will be provided for some restaurant foods. The current regulations require nutrition information for foods about which health or nutrient-content claims are made on restaurant signs or placards. In June 1993, FDA proposed similar requirements for restaurant menu items with such claims. Under that proposal, restaurants would have to provide a "reasonable basis" for making claims. They would be given some flexibility in demonstrating that reasonable basis. For example, they could rely on recipes endorsed by medical or dietary groups.

Nutrition Labeling—Exemptions

Under NLEA, some foods are exempt from nutrition labeling. These include:

- food served for immediate consumption, such as that served in hospital cafeterias and airplanes, and that sold by food service vendors—for example, mall cookie counters, sidewalk vendors, and vending machines
- ready-to-eat food that is not for immediate consumption but is prepared primarily on site—for example, bakery, deli, and candy store items
- food shipped in bulk, as long as it is not for sale in that form to consumers
- medical foods, such as those used to address the nutritional needs of patients with certain diseases
- plain coffee and tea, some spices, and other foods that contain no significant amounts of any nutrients.

Food produced by small businesses also is exempt, under the NLEA amendments of 1993. The NLEA amendments provide for a system in which exemptions are based on the number of people a company employs and the number of units within a product line it makes yearly.

Under this system, the allowances for each factor are gradually lowered. In the first year following the law's full implementation (that is, May 9, 1994, to May 8, 1995), a food could be exempt from nutrition labeling if the company whose name appears on the label employs fewer than 300 full-time equivalent employees and makes fewer than

600,000 units of the product yearly. After May 1997, only businesses with fewer than 100 full-time equivalent employees producing fewer than 100,000 units within a product line for U.S. distribution could qualify for an exemption.

Almost all companies seeking an exemption will have to notify FDA that they meet the criteria. Those that do not are U.S. firms with fewer than 10 employees making fewer than 10,000 units of a food in a year.

Although these foods are exempt, they are free to carry nutrition information, when appropriate—as long as it complies with the new regulations. Also, they will lose their exemption if their labels carry a nutrient content or health claim or any other nutrition information.

Nutrition information about game meats—such as deer, bison, rabbit, quail, wild turkey, and ostrich—is not required on individual packages. Instead, it can be given on counter cards, signs, or other point-of-purchase materials. Because few nutrient data exist for these foods, FDA believes that allowing this option will enable game meat producers to give first priority to collecting appropriate data and make it easier for them to update the information as it becomes available.

Nutrition Panel Title

The new food label features a revamped nutrition panel. It has a new title, "Nutrition Facts," which replaces "Nutrition Information Per Serving." The new title signals that the product has been labeled according to the new regulations. Also, for the first time, there are requirements on type size, style, spacing, and contrast to ensure a more distinctive, easy-to-read label.

Serving Sizes

The serving size remains the basis for reporting each food's nutrient content. However, unlike in the past, when the serving size was up to the discretion of the food manufacturer, serving sizes now will be more uniform and will reflect the amounts people actually eat. They also must be expressed in both common household and metric measures.

FDA allows as common household measures: the cup, tablespoon, teaspoon, piece, slice, fraction (such as "¼ pizza"), and common household containers used to package food products (such as a jar or tray). Ounces may be used, but only if a common household unit is not applicable and an appropriate visual unit is given—for example, 1 oz (28g/about ½ pickle).

Grams (g) and milliliters (mL) are the metric units that will be used in serving size statements.

NLEA defines serving size as the amount of food customarily eaten at one time. The serving sizes that appear on food labels will be based on FDA-established lists of "Reference Amounts Customarily Consumed Per Eating Occasion."

These reference amounts, which are part of the regulations, are broken down into 139 FDA-regulated food product categories, including 11 groups of foods specially formulated or processed for infants or children under 4. They list the amounts of food customarily consumed per eating occasion for each category, based primarily on national food consumption surveys. FDA's list also gives the suggested label statement for serving size declaration. For example, the category "breads (excluding sweet quick type), rolls" has a reference amount of 50 g, and the appropriate label statement for sliced bread or roll is "__ piece(s) (__ g)" or, for unsliced bread, "2 oz (56 g/__ inch slice)."

The serving size of products that come in discrete units, such as cookies, candy bars, and sliced products, is the number of whole units that most closely approximates the reference amount. Cookies are an example. Under the "bakery products" category, cookies have a reference amount of 30 g. The household measure closest to that amount is the number of cookies that comes closest to weighing 30 g. Thus, the serving size on the label of a package of cookies in which each cookie weighs 13 g would read "2 cookies (26 g)."

If one unit weighs more than 50 percent but less than 200 percent of the reference amount, the serving size is one unit. For example, the reference amount for bread is 50 g; therefore, the label of a loaf of bread in which each slice weighs more than 25 g would state a serving size of one slice.

Certain rules apply to food products that are packaged and sold individually. If such an individual package is less than 200 percent of the applicable reference amount, the item qualifies as one serving. Thus, a 360-mL (12-fluid-ounce) can of soda is one serving, since the reference amount for carbonated beverages is 240 mL (8 ounces).

However, if the product has a reference amount of 100 g or 100 mL or more and the package contains more than 150 percent but less than 200 percent of the reference amount, manufacturers have the option of deciding whether the product can be one or two servings.

An example is a 15-ounce (420 g) can of soup. The serving size reference amount for soup is 245 g. Therefore, the manufacturer has the option to declare the can of soup as one or two servings.

Nutrition Information

There will be a new set of dietary components on the nutrition panel. The mandatory (underlined) and voluntary components and the order in which they must appear are:

- total calories
- calories from fat
- calories from saturated fat
- total fat
- saturated fat
- polyunsaturated fat
- monounsaturated fat
- cholesterol
- sodium
- potassium
- total carbohydrate
- dietary fiber
- soluble fiber
- insoluble fiber
- sugars

- sugar alcohol (for example, the sugar substitutes xylitol, mannitol and sorbitol)
- other carbohydrate (the difference between total carbohydrate and the sum of dietary fiber, sugars, and sugar alcohol if declared)
- protein
- vitamin A
- percent of vitamin A present as beta-carotene
- vitamin C
- calcium
- iron
- other essential vitamins and minerals

If a claim is made about any of the optional components, or if a food is fortified or enriched with any of them, nutrition information for these components becomes mandatory.

These mandatory and voluntary components are the only ones allowed on the nutrition panel. The listing of single amino acids, maltodextrin, calories from polyunsaturated fat, and calories from carbohydrates, for example, may not appear as part of the Nutrition Facts on the label.

The required nutrients were selected because they address today's health concerns. The order in which they must appear reflects the priority of current dietary recommendations.

Thiamine, riboflavin and niacin will no longer be required in nutrition labeling because deficiencies of each are no longer considered of public health significance. However, they may be listed voluntarily.

Nutrition Panel Format

The format for declaring nutrient content per serving also has been revised. Now, all nutrients must be declared as percentages of the Daily Values—the new label reference values. The amount, in grams, of macronutrients (such as fat, cholesterol, sodium, carbohydrates, and protein) still must be listed to the immediate right of each of the names of each of these nutrients. But, for the first time, a column headed "%Daily Value" will appear.

Requiring nutrients to be declared as a percentage of the Daily Values is intended to prevent misinterpretations that arise with quantitative values. For example, a food with 140 milligrams (mg) of sodium could be mistaken for a high-sodium food because 140 is a relatively large number. In actuality, however, that amount represents less than 6 percent of the Daily Value for sodium, which is 2,400 mg.

On the other hand, a food with 5 g of saturated fat could be construed as being low in that nutrient. In fact, that food would provide one-fourth the total Daily Value because 20 g is the Daily Value for saturated fat based on a 2,000-calorie diet.

Nutrition Panel Footnote

The %Daily Value listing carries a footnote saying that the percentages are based on a 2,000-calorie diet. Some nutrition labels—at least those on larger packages—will have these additional footnotes:

- a sentence noting that a person's individual nutrient goals are based on his or her calorie needs
- lists of the daily values for selected nutrients for a 2,000- and a 2,500-calorie diet.

An optional footnote for packages of any size is the number of calories per gram of fat (9), and carbohydrate and protein (4).

Format Modifications

In limited circumstances, variations in the format of the nutrition panel are allowed. Some are mandatory. For example, the labels of foods for children under 2 (except infant formula, which has special labeling rules under the Infant Formula Act of 1980) may not carry information about saturated fat, polyunsaturated fat, monounsaturated fat, cholesterol, calories from fat, or calories from saturated fat.

The reason is to prevent parents from wrongly assuming that infants and toddlers should restrict their fat intake, when, in fact, they should not. Fat is important during these years to ensure adequate growth and development.

The labels of foods for children under 4 may not include the %Daily Values for total fat, saturated fat, cholesterol, sodium, potassium, total carbohydrate, and dietary fiber. They may carry %Daily Values for protein, vitamins and minerals, however. These nutrients are the only ones for which FDA has set Daily Values for this age group.

Thus, the top portion of the "Nutrition Facts" panels of foods for children under 4 will consist of two columns. The nutrients' names will be listed on the left and their quantitative amounts will be on the right. The bottom portion will provide the %Daily Values for protein, vitamins and minerals. Only the calorie conversion information may be given as a footnote.

Some foods qualify for a simplified label format. This format is allowed when the food contains insignificant amounts of seven or more of the mandatory nutrients and total calories. "Insignificant" means that a declaration of zero could be made in nutrition labeling, or, for total carbohydrate, dietary fiber, and protein, the declaration states "less than 1 g."

For foods for children under 2, the simplified format may be used if the product contains insignificant amounts of six or more of the following: calories, total fat, sodium, total carbohydrate, dietary fiber, sugars, protein, vitamins A and C, calcium, and iron.

If the simplified format is used, information on total calories, total fat, total carbohydrate, protein, and sodium—even if they are present in insignficant amounts—must be listed. Other nutrients, along with calories from fat, must be shown if they are present in more than insignificant amounts. Nutrients added to the food must be listed, too.

Some format exceptions exist for small and medium-size packages. Packages with less than 12 square inches of available labeling space (about the size of a package of chewing gum) do not have to carry nutrition information unless a nutrient content or health claim is made for the product. However, they must provide an address or telephone number for consumers to obtain the required nutrition information.

If manufacturers wish to provide nutrition information on these packages voluntarily, they have several options:
(1) present the information in a smaller type size than that required for larger packages, or (2) present the information in a tabular or linear (string) format.

The tabular and linear formats also may be used on packages that have less than 40 square inches available for labeling and insufficient space for the full vertical format.

Other options for packages with less than 40 square inches of label space are:

• abbreviating names of dietary components
• omitting all footnotes, except for the statement that %Daily Values are based on a 2,000-calorie diet
• placing nutrition information on other panels readily seen by consumers.

A select group of packages with more than 40 square inches of labeling space is allowed a format exception, too. These are packages with insufficient vertical space (about 3 inches) to accommodate the required information. Some examples are bread bags, pie boxes, and bags of frozen vegetables. On these packages, the "Nutrition Facts" panel may appear horizontally, with footnote information appearing to the far right.

For larger packages in which there is not sufficient space on the principal display panel or the information panel to the right, FDA has proposed allowing nutrition information to appear on any label panel that is readily seen by consumers. The intent is to lessen the chances of overcrowding of information and to encourage manufacturers to provide the greatest amount of nutrition information possible.

For products that require additional preparation before eating, such as dry cake mixes and dry pasta dinners, or that are usually eaten with one or more additional foods, such as breakfast cereals with milk, FDA encourages manufacturers to provide voluntarily a second column of nutrition information. This is known as dual declaration.

With this variation, the first column, which is mandatory, contains nutrition information for the food as purchased. The second gives information about the food as prepared and eaten.

Still another variation is the aggregate display. This is allowed on labels of variety-pack food items, such as ready-to-eat cereals and assorted flavors of individual ice cream cups. With this display, the quantitative amount and %Daily Value for each nutrient are listed in separate columns under the name of each food.

Daily Value—DVs

The new label reference value, Daily Value, comprises two sets of dietary standards: Daily Reference Values (DRVs) and Reference Daily Intakes (RDIs). Only the Daily Value term will appear on the label, though, to make label reading less confusing.

As part of new regulations, DRVs are being introduced for macronutrients that are sources of energy: fat, carbohydrate (including fiber), and protein; and for cholesterol, sodium and potassium, which do not contribute calories.

DRVs for the energy-producing nutrients are based on the number of calories consumed per day. A daily intake of 2,000 calories has been established as the reference. This level was chosen, in part, because it approximates the caloric requirements for postmenopausal women. This group has the highest risk for excessive intake of calories and fat.

DRVs for the energy-producing nutrients are calculated as follows:

• fat based on 30 percent of calories
• saturated fat based on 10 percent of calories

- carbohydrate based on 60 percent of calories
- protein based on 10 percent of calories. (The DRV for protein applies only to adults and children over 4. RDIs for protein for special groups have been established.)
- fiber based on 11.5 g of fiber per 1,000 calories.

Because of current public health recommendations, DRVs for some nutrients represent the uppermost limit that is considered desirable. The DRVs for fats and sodium are:

- total fat: less than 65 g
- saturated fat: less than 20 g
- cholesterol: less than 300 mg
- sodium: less than 2,400 mg

Daily Value—RDIs

The RDI replaces the term "U.S. RDA," which was introduced in 1973 as a label reference value for vitamins, minerals and protein in voluntary nutrition labeling. The name change was sought because of confusion that existed over "U.S. RDAs," the values determined by FDA and used on food labels and "RDAs" (Recommended Dietary Allowances), the values determined by the National Academy of Sciences for various population groups and used by FDA to figure the U.S. RDAs.

However, the values for the new RDIs will remain the same as the old U.S. RDAs for the time being.

Nutrient Content Descriptors

The regulations also spell out what terms may be used to describe the level of a nutrient in a food and how they can be used. These are the core terms:
- *Free.* This term means that a product contains no amount of, or only trivial or "physiologically inconsequential" amounts of, one or more of these components: fat, saturated fat, cholesterol, sodium, sugars, and calories. For example, "calorie-free"

means fewer than 5 calories per serving and "sugar-free" and "fat-free" both mean less than 0.5 g per serving. Synonyms for "free" include "without," "no" and "zero."
- *Low.* This term could be used on foods that could be eaten frequently without exceeding dietary guidelines for one or more of these components: fat, saturated fat, cholesterol, sodium, and calories. Thus, descriptors would be defined as follows:

- *low fat:* 3 g or less per serving
- *low saturated fat:* 1 g or less per serving
- *low sodium:* 140 mg or less per serving
- *very low sodium:* 35 mg or less per serving
- *low cholesterol:* 20 mg or less and 2 g or less of saturated fat per serving
- *low calorie:* 40 calories or less per serving.
  Synonyms for low include "little," "few," and "low source of."
- *Lean and extra lean.* These terms can be used to describe the fat content of meat, poultry, seafood, and game meats.
- *lean:* less than 10 g fat, 4.5 g or less saturated fat, and less than 95 mg cholesterol per serving and per 100 g.
- *extra lean:* less than 5 g fat, less than 2 g saturated fat, and less than 95 mg cholesterol per serving and per 100 g.
- *High.* This term can be used if the food contains 20 percent or more of the Daily Value for a particular nutrient in a serving.
- *Good source.* This term means that one serving of a food contains 10 to 19 percent of the Daily Value for a particular nutrient.
- *Reduced.* This term means that a nutritionally altered product contains at least 25 percent less of a nutrient or of calories than the regular, or reference, product. However, a reduced claim can't be made on a product if its reference food already meets the requirement for a "low" claim.
- *Less.* This term means that a food, whether altered or not, contains 25 percent less of a nutrient or of calories than the reference food. For example,

pretzels that have 25 percent less fat than potato chips could carry a "less" claim. "Fewer" is an acceptable synonym.

• *Light.* This descriptor can mean two things:

First, that a nutritionally altered product contains one-third fewer calories or half the fat of the reference food. If the food derives 50 percent or more of its calories from fat, the reduction must be 50 percent of the fat.

Second, that the sodium content of a low-calorie, low-fat food has been reduced by 50 percent. In addition, "light in sodium" may be used on food in which the sodium content has been reduced by at least 50 percent.

The term "light" still can be used to describe such properties as texture and color, as long as the label explains the intent—for example, "light brown sugar" and "light and fluffy."

• *More.* This term means that a serving of food, whether altered or not, contains a nutrient that is at least 10 percent of Daily Value more than the reference food. The 10 percent of Daily Value also would apply to "fortified," "enriched" and "added" claims, but in those cases, the food must be altered. Alternative spelling of these descriptive terms and their synonyms are allowed—for example—"hi" and "lo"—as long as the alternatives are not misleading.

Other Definitions

The regulations also address other claims. Among them:

• *Percent fat free:* A product bearing this claim must be a low-fat or a fat-free product. In addition, the claim must accurately reflect the amount of fat present in 100 g of the food. Thus, if a food contains 2.5 g fat per 50 g, the claim must be "95 percent fat free."

• *Implied:* These types of claims are prohibited when they wrongfully imply that a food contains or does not contain a meaningful level of a nutrient. For example, a product claiming to be made with an ingredient known to be a source of fiber (such as "made with oat bran") is not allowed unless the product contains enough of that ingredient (for example, oat bran) to meet the definition for "good source" of fiber. As another example, a claim that a product contains "no tropical oils" is allowed—but only on foods that are "low" in saturated fat because consumers have come to equate tropical oils with high saturated fat.

• *Meals and main dishes:* Claims that a meal or main dish is "free" of a nutrient, such as sodium or cholesterol, must meet the same requirements as those for individual foods. Other claims can be used under special circumstances. For example, "low-calorie" means the meal or main dish contains 120 calories or less per 100 g. "Low-sodium" means the food has 140 mg or less per 100 g. "Low-cholesterol" means the food contains 20 mg cholesterol or less per 100 g and no more than 2 g saturated fat. "Light" means the meal or main dish is low-fat or low-calorie.

• *Standardized foods:* Any nutrient content claim, such as "reduced fat," "low calorie," and "light," may be used in conjunction with a standardized term if the new product has been specifically formulated to meet FDA's criteria for that claim, if the product is not nutritionally inferior to the traditional standardized food, and the new product complies with certain compositional requirements set by FDA. A new product bearing a claim also must have performance characteristics similar to the referenced traditional standardized food. If the product doesn't, and the differences materially limit the product's use, its label must state the differences (for example, not recommended for baking) to inform consumers.

• *Health:* FDA also has proposed defining the term "healthy." Under that proposal, "healthy" could be used to describe a food that is low in fat and saturated fat and contains no more than 480 mg sodium and no more than 60 mg cholesterol per serving. A final rule is expected in 1994.

'Fresh'

Although not mandated by NLEA, FDA also issued a regulation for the term "fresh." The agency took this step because of concern over the term's possible misuse on some food labels.

The regulation defines the term "fresh" when it is used to suggest that a food is raw or unprocessed. In this context, "fresh" can be used only on a food that is raw, has never been frozen or heated, and contains no preservatives. (Irridiation at low levels is allowed.) "Fresh frozen," "frozen fresh," and "freshly frozen" can be used for foods that are quickly frozen while still fresh. Blanching (brief scalding before freezing to prevent nutrient breakdown) is allowed.

Other uses of the term "fresh," such as in "fresh milk" or "freshly baked bread," are not affected.

Baby Foods

FDA is not allowing broad use of nutrient claims on infant and toddler foods. However, the agency may propose later claims specifically for these foods. The terms "unsweetened" and "unsalted" are allowed on these foods, however, because they relate to taste and not nutrient content.

Health Claims

Claims for seven relationships between a nutrient or a food and the risk of a disease or health-related condition will be allowed for the first time. They can be made in several ways: through third-party references, such as the National Cancer Institute; statements; symbols, such as a heart; and vignettes or descriptions. Whatever the case, the claim must meet the requirements for authorized health claims; for example, they cannot state the degree of risk reduction and can only use "may" or "might" in discussing the nutrient or food-disease relationship. And they must state that other factors play a role in that disease.

The claims also must be phrased so that consumers can understand the relationship between the nutrient and the disease and the nutrient's importance in relationship to a daily diet.

An example of an appropriate claim is: "While many factors affect heart disease, diets low in saturated fat and cholesterol may reduce the risk of this disease."

The allowed nutrient-disease relationship claims and rules for their use are:

• *Calcium and osteoporosis:* To carry this claim, a food must contain 20 percent or more of the Daily Value for calcium (200 mg) per serving, have a calcium content that equals or exceeds the food's content of phosphorus, and contain a form of calcium that can be readily absorbed and used by the body. The claim must name the target group most in need of adequate calcium intakes (that is, teens and young adult white and Asian women) and state the need for exercise and a healthy diet. A product that contains 40 percent or more of the Daily Value for calcium must state on the label that a total dietary intake greater than 200 percent of the Daily Value for calcium (that is, 2,000 mg or more) has no further known benefit.

• *Fat and cancer:* To carry this claim, a food must meet the descriptor requirements for "low-fat" or, if fish and game meats, for "extra lean."

• *Saturated fat and cholesterol and coronary heart disease (CHD):* This claim may be used if the food meets the definitions for the descriptors "low saturated fat," "low-cholesterol," and "low-fat," or, if fish and game meats, for "extra lean." It may mention the link between reduced risk of CHD and lower saturated fat and cholesterol intakes to lower blood cholesterol levels.

• *Fiber-containing grain products, fruits and vegetables and cancer:* To carry this claim, a food must be or must contain a grain product, fruit or vegetable and meet the descriptor requirements for "low-fat," and, without fortification, be a "good source" of dietary fiber.

• *Fruits, vegetables and grain products that contain fiber and risk of CHD:* To carry this claim, a food must be or must contain fruits, vegetables and grain products. It also must meet the descriptor requirements for "low saturated fat," "low-cholesterol," and "low-fat" and contain, without fortification, at least 0.6 g soluble fiber per serving.

• *Sodium and hypertension (high blood pressure):* To carry this claim, a food must meet the descriptor requirements for "low-sodium."

• *Fruits and vegetables and cancer:* This claim may be made for fruits and vegetables that meet the descriptor requirements for "low-fat" and that, without fortification, for "good source" of at least one of the following: dietary fiber or vitamins A or C. This claim relates diets low in fat and rich in fruits and vegetables (and thus vitamins A and C and dietary fiber) to reduced cancer risk. FDA authorized this claim in place of an antioxidant vitamin and cancer claim.

Folic Acid

On Jan. 4, 1994, FDA authorized the use of a health claim about the relationship between folic acid and the risk of neural tube birth defects for dietary supplements and for foods in conventional food form that are naturally high in folic acid. (In 1992, the U.S. Public Health Service had recommended that all women of childbearing age consume 0.4 mg folic acid daily to reduce their risk of giving birth to a child affected with a neural tube defect.) FDA plans to issue a final rule to allow the folic acid-neural tube defect claim for fortified foods, too.

Ingredient Labeling

As part of the rules, the list of ingredients will undergo some changes, too. Chief among them is a regulation that requires full ingredient labeling on "standardized foods," which previously were exempt. Ingredient declaration will now have to be on all foods that have more than one ingredient.

Also, the ingredient list will include, when appropriate:

• FDA-certified color additives, such as FD&C Blue No. 1, by name
• sources of protein hydrolysates, which are used in many foods as flavors and flavor enhancers
• declaration of caseinate as a milk derivative in the ingredient list of foods that claim to be non-dairy, such as coffee whiteners.

The main reason for these new requirements is that some people may be allergic to such additives and will now be better able to avoid them.

As required by NLEA, beverages that claim to contain juice now must declare the total percentage of juice on the information panel. In addition, FDA's regulation establishes criteria for naming juice beverages. For example, when the label of a multi-juice beverage states one or more—but not all—of the juices present, and the predominantly named juice is present in minor amounts, the product's name must state that the beverage is flavored with that juice or declare the amount of the juice in a 5 percent range—for example, "raspberry-flavored juice blend" or "juice blend, 2 to 7 percent raspberry juice."

Economic Impact

It is estimated that the new food label will cost FDA-regulated food processors between $1.4 billion and $2.3 billion over the next 20 years. The benefits to public health—measured in monetary terms—are estimated to well exceed the costs. Potential benefits include decreased rates of coronary heart disease, cancer, osteoporosis, obesity, high blood pressure, and allergic reactions to food.

Obtaining Regulations
and Related Information

Reprints of the Jan. 6, 1993 (the major portion of the regulations), and April 1 and 2, 1993, *Federal Register* documents on FDA's food labeling rules can be ordered by calling the National Technical Information Service at (703) 487-4650. Ask for #PB-93-139905. The cost is $91.

The Jan. 6 document also can be downloaded from the National Agricultural Library's electronic bulletin board, Agricultural Library Forum (ALF). The electronic bulletin board can be accessed 24 hours a day, seven days a week. The telephone numbers are (301) 504-6510, (301) 504-5111, (301) 504-5496, and (301) 504-5497. For assistance, call the FDA/USDA Food Labeling Education Information Center at (301) 504-5719.

Copies of the technical amendments published in the Aug. 18, 1993, *Federal Register* can be ordered free by calling FDA at (202) 205-5251.

The January and April 1993 documents also are included in the April 1, 1993, edition of the *Code of Federal Regulations,* which is available from the Government Printing Office (Title 21, Parts 100–169) for $21. This may be ordered by calling (202) 783-3238.

Also, FDA has available free copies of *Food Labeling, Questions and Answers,* a 53-page booklet that gives general guidance on the regulations. To order (one copy only), write to: Industry Activities Staff (HFS-565), Food and Drug Administration, 200 C St., S.W., Washington, DC 20204. Send two self-addressed adhesive labels.

Public Education

To help consumers get the most from the new food label, FDA and USDA have embarked on a food labeling education campaign. The campaign's purpose is to increase consumers' knowledge and effective use of the new food label and help them in making accurate and sound dietary choices in accordance with the Dietary Guidelines for Americans.

The campaign involves participation from consumer, trade and health groups, as well as government agencies, working through the FDA/USDA-created National Exchange for Food Labeling Education (NEFLE).

APPENDIX 9: ILLNESSES AND INJURIES ASSOCIATED WITH THE USE OF SELECTED DIETARY SUPPLEMENTS

Products marketed as "dietary supplements" include a diverse range of products, from traditional nutrients, such as vitamins or minerals, to such substances as high-potency free amino acids, botanicals, enzymes, animal extracts, and bioflavanoids that often have no scientifically recognized role in nutrition.

There is currently no systematic evaluation of the safety of products marketed as dietary supplements. Dietary supplements routinely enter the marketplace without undergoing a safety review by FDA. Published studies on the safety of these products are extremely sparse. There is no systematic collection and review of adverse reaction reports for dietary supplements, as there is for drugs, and physicians rarely seek information about their patients' use of dietary supplements. Despite the lack of any system for gaining information about the risks of dietary supplements, an increased number of reports of adverse reactions to dietary supplement products has recently been recognized. Because of concern about these products. FDA has, in the last year, initiated an effort to collect and evaluate existing studies and case reports on safety problems associated with dietary supplements. As a result of that effort, FDA has begun to identify dietary supplements for which serious adverse reactions have been documented. A list of selected dietary supplements associated with serious safety problems follows. This list is not intended to include all hazardous ingredients in dietary supplements.

I. Herbals

Herbal and other botanical ingredients of dietary supplements include processed or unprocessed plant parts (bark, leaves, flowers, fruits, and stems), as well as extracts and essential oils. They are available in a variety of forms, including water infusions (teas), powders, tablets, capsules, and elixirs, and may be marketed as single substances or in combination with other materials, such as vitamins, minerals, amino acids, and non-nutrient ingredients. Although data on the availability, consumer use, and health effects of herbals are very limited, some herbal ingredients have been associated with serious adverse health effects.

A. Chaparral *(Larrea tridentata)*

Chaparral, commonly called the creosote bush, is a desert shrub with a long history of use as a traditional medicine by Native Americans. Chaparral is marketed as a tea, as well as in table, capsule, and concentrated extract form, and has been promoted as a natural antioxidant "blood purifier," cancer cure, and acne treatment. At least six cases (five in the United States and one in Canada) of acute non-viral hepatitis (rapidly developing liver damage) have been associated with the consumption of chaparral as a dietary supplement. Additional cases have been reported and are under investigation. In the majority of the cases reported thus far, the injury to the liver resolves over time, after discontinuation of the product. In at least two patients, however, there is evidence that chaparral consumption causes irreversible liver damage. One patient suffered terminal liver failure requiring liver transplant.

Most of these cases are associated with the consumption of single ingredient chaparral capsules or tablets; however, a few of the more recent cases appear to be associated with consumption of multi-ingredient products (capsules, tablets or teas) that contain chaparral as one ingredient. Chemical analyses have identified no contaminants in the products associated with the cases of hepatitis. Products from at least four different distributors and from at least two different sources have been implicated thus far.

After FDA's health warning, many distributors of chaparral products voluntarily removed the products from the market in December of 1992. Some chaparral products remain on the market, however, and other distributors who removed their products from the market are seeking to clarify the status of these products.

B. Comfrey (*Symphytum officinale* (common comfrey), *S. asperum* (prickly comfrey), or *S. X uplandicum* (Russian comfrey))

Preparations of comfrey, a fast-growing leafy plant, are widely sold in the United States as teas, tables, capsules, tinctures, medicinal poultices, and lotions. Since 1985, at least seven cases of hepatic veno-occlusive disease—obstruction of blood flow for the liver with potential scarring (cirrhosis)—including one death, have been associated with the use of commercially available oral comfrey products.

Comfrey, like a number of other plants (e.g., *Senecio* species), contains pyrrolizidine alkaloids. The toxicity of pyrrolizidine alkaloids to humans is well-documented. Hepatic veno-occlusive disease, following ingestion of pyrrolizidine alkaloid-containing products, has been documented repeatedly throughout the world. Hepatic veno-occlusive disease is usually acute and may result in fatal liver failure. In less severe cases, liver disease may progress to a subacute form. Even after apparent recovery, chronic liver disease, including cirrhosis, has been noted. Individuals who ingest small amounts of pyrrolizidine alkaloids for a prolonged period may also be at risk for development of hepatic cirrhosis. The diagnosis of pyrrolizidine alkaloid-induced hepatic veno-occlusive disease is complex, and the condition is probably underdiagnosed.

The degree of injury caused by pyrrolizidine alkaloid-containing plants, like comfrey, is probably influenced by such factors as the age of the user, body mass, gender, and hepatic function, as well the total cumulative dose ingested and the type of exposure (i.e., whether exposure was to leaves or roots, infusions or capsules). Infants in general appear to be particularly susceptible to adverse effects of exposure to pyrrolizidine alkaloids: there are reports of infants developing hepatic veno-occlusive disease following acute exposure of less than one week. Transplacental pyrrolizidine poisoning has been suggested by the occurrence of hepatic disease in the newborn infant of a woman who consumed herbal tea during pregnancy.

Although liver damage is the major documented form of injury to humans from pyrrolizidine alkaloid-containing herbals, animal studies suggest that their toxicity is much broader. Animals exposed to pyrrolizidine alkaloids have developed a wide range of pulmonary, kidney and gastrointestinal pathologies. Pyrrolizidine alkaloid-containing plants, including comfrey, have also been shown to cause cancer in laboratory animals.

Four countries (the United Kingdom, Australia, Canada, and Germany) have recently restricted the availability of products containing comfrey, and other countries permit use of comfrey only under a physician's prescription.

C. Yohimbe (*Pausinystalia yohimbe*)

Yohimbe is a tree bark containing a variety of pharmacologically active chemicals. It is marketed in a number of products for body building and "enhanced male performance." Serious adverse effects, including renal failure, seizures and death, have been reported to FDA with products containing yohimbe and are currently under investigation.

The major identified alkaloid in yohimbe is yohimbine, a chemical that causes vasodilation, thereby lowering blood pressure. Yohimbine is also a prescription drug in the United States. Side effects are well recognized and may include central nervous system stimulation that causes anxiety attacks. At high doses, yohimbine is a monoamine osidase (MAO) inhibitor. MAO inhibitors can cause serious adverse effects when taken concomitantly with tyramine-containing foods (e.g., liver, cheeses, red wine) or with over-the-counter (OTC) products containing phenylpropanolamme, such as nasal decongestants and diet aids. Individuals taking yohimbe should be warned to rigorously avoid these foods and OTC products because of the increased likelihood of adverse effects.

Yohimbe should also be avoided by individuals with hypotension (low blood pressure), diabetes, and heart, liver or kidney disease. Symptoms or overdosage include weakness and nervous stimulation followed by paralysis, fatigue, stomach disorders, and ultimately death.

D. Lobelia (*Lobelia inflata*)

Lobelia, also known as Indian tobacco, contains pyridine-derived alkaloids, primarily lobeline. These alkaloids have pharmacological actions similar to, although less potent than, nicotine. There have been several reported cases of adverse reactions associated with consumption of dietary supplements containing lobelia.

Depending on the dose, lobeline can cause either autonomic nervous system stimulation or depression. At low doses, it produces bronchial dilation and increased respiratory rate. Higher doses result in respiratory depression, as well as sweating, rapid heart rate, hypotension, and even coma and death. As little as 50 milligrams of dried herb or a single milliliter of lobelia tincture has caused these reactions.

Because of its similarity to nicotine, lobelia may be dangerous to susceptible populations, including children, pregnant women, and individuals with cardiac disease. Lobelia is nevertheless found in dietary supplement products that are marketed for use by children and infants, pregnant women, and smokers.

E. Germander (*Teucrium* genus)

Germander is the common name for a group of plants that are contained in medicinal teas, elixirs and capsules or tablets, either singly or in combination with other herbs, and marketed for the treatment of obesity and to facilitate weight loss.

Since 1986, at least 27 cases of acute nonviral hepatitis (liver disease), including one death, have been associated with the use of commercially available germander products in France. These cases show a clear temporal relationship between ingestion of germander and onset of hepatitis, as well as the resolution of symptoms when the use of germander was stopped. In 12 cases, re-administration of germander was followed by prompt recurrence of hepatitis. Recovery occurred gradually in most cases, approximately two to six months after withdrawal of germander. Analyses of these cases does not indicate a strong relationship between the dosage or duration of ingestion and the occurrence of hepatitis.

Although the constituent in germander responsible for its hepatic toxicity has not been identified, germander contains several chemicals, including polyphenols, tannins, diterpenoids, and flavonoids.

On the basis of the 27 French hepatitis cases, the French Ministry of Health has forbidden the use of germander in drugs. Its use has been restricted in other countries.

F. Willow Bark (*Salix* species)

Willow bark has long been used for its analgesic (pain-killing), antirheumatic, and antipyretic (fever-reducing) properties. Willow bark is widely promoted as an "aspirin-free" analgesic, including in dietary supplement products for children. Because it shares the same chemical properties and the same adverse effects as aspirin, this claim is highly misleading. The "aspirin-free" claim is particularly dangerous on products marketed, without warning labels, for use by children and other aspirin-sensitive individuals.

The pharmacologically active component in willow bark is "salicin," a compound that is converted to salicylic acid by the body after ingestion. Both willow bark and aspirin are salicylates, a class of compounds that work by virtue of their salicylic acid content. Aspirin (acetylsalicylic acid) is also converted to salicylic acid after ingestion.

All salicylates share substantially the same side effects. The major adverse effects include irritation of the gastric mucosa (a particular hazard to individuals with ulcer disease), adverse effects when used during pregnancy (including stillbirth, bleeding, prolonged gestation and labor, and low-birth-weight infants), stroke, and adverse effects in children with fever and dehydration. Children with influenza or chickenpox should avoid salicylates because their use, even in small doses, is associated with development of Reye syndrome, which is characterized by severe, sometimes fatal, liver injury. Salicylate intoxication (headache, dizziness, ringing in ears, difficulty hearing, dimness of vision, confusion, lassitude, drowsiness, sweating, hyperventilation, nausea, vomiting, and central nervous system disturbances in severe cases) may occur as the result of over-medication or kidney or liver insufficiency. Hypersensitivity, manifested by itching, bronchospasm and localized swelling (which may be life-threatening), can occur with very small doses of salicylates, and may occur even in those without a prior history of sensitivity to salicylates. Approximately 5 percent of the population is hypersensitive to salicylates.

G. Jin Bu Huan

Jin Bu Huan is a Chinese herbal product whose label claims that it is good for "insomnia due to pain," ulcer, "stomachic [sic] neuralgia, pain in shrunken womb after childbirth, nervous insomnia, spasmodic cough, and etc." Jin Bu Huan has been recently reported to be responsible for the poisoning of at least three young children (ages 13 months to 2½ years), who accidentally ingested this product. The children were hospitalized with rapid-onset, life-threatening bradycardia (very low heart rate), and central nervous system and respiratory depression. One child required intubation (assisted breathing). All three ultimately recovered, following intensive medical care.

Although the product label identified the plant source for Jin Bu Huan as *Polygala chinensis,* this appears to be incorrect since preliminary analyses indicate the presence of tetrahydropalmatine (THP), a chemical not found in *Polygala.* THP is found, however, in high concentrations in plants of certain *Stephania* species. In animals, exposure to THP results in sedation, analgesia, and neuromuscular blockade (paralysis). The symptoms of the three children are consistent with these effects.

An additional case of THP toxicity, reported in the Netherlands, appears to be associated with the same product, and is being investigated.

H. Herbal products containing *Stephania* and *Magnolia* species

A Chinese herbal preparation containing *Stephania* and *Magnolia* species that was sold as a weight-loss treatment in Belgium has been implicated recently as a cause of severe kidney injury in at least 48 women. These cases were only discovered by diligent investigations by physicians treating two young women who presented with similar cases of rapidly progressing kidney disease that required renal dialysis. Once it was determined that both these women had used the herbal diet treatment, further investigation of kidney dialysis centers in Belgium found a total of 48 individuals with kidney injury who had used the herbal product.

At the time that a report of these adverse effects was published in February 1993, 18 of the 48 women had terminal kidney failure that will require either kidney transplantation or life-long renal dialysis.

I. Ma huang

Ma huang is one of several names for herbal products containing members of the genus *Ephedra*. There are many common names for these evergreen plants, including squaw tea and Mormon tea. Serious adverse effects, including hypertension (elevated blood pressure), palpitations (rapid heat rate), neuropathy (nerve damage), myopathy (muscle injury), psychosis, stroke, and memory loss, have been reported to FDA with products containing Ma huang as ingredients and are currently under investigation.

The *Ephearas* have been shown to contain various chemical stimulants, including the alkaloids ephedrine, pseudoephedrine and norpseudoephedrine, as well as various tannins and related chemicals. The concentrations of these alkaloids depends upon the particular species of *Ephedra* used. Ephedrine and pseudoephedrine are amphetamine-like chemicals used in OTC and prescription drugs. Many of these stimulants have known serious side effects.

Ma huang is sold in products for weight control, as well as in products that boost energy levels. These products often contain other stimulants, such as caffeine, which may have synergistic effects and increase the potential for adverse effects.

II. Amino Acids

Amino acids are the individual constituent parts of proteins. Consumption of foods containing intact proteins ordinarily provides sufficient amounts of the nine amino acids needed for growth and development in children and for maintenance of health of adults. The safety of amino acids in this form is generally not a concern. When marketed as dietary supplements, amino acids are sold as single compounds, in combinations of two or more amino acids, as components of protein powders, as chelated single compounds, or in chelated mixtures. Amino acids are promoted for a variety of uses, including body-building. Some are promoted for claimed pharmacologic effects.

The Federation of American Societies for Experimental Biology (FASEB) recently conducted an exhaustive search of available data on amino acids and concluded that there was insufficient information to establish a safe intake level for any amino acids in dietary supplements, and that their safety should not be assumed. FASEB warned that consuming amino acids in dietary supplement form posed potential risks for several subgroups of the general population, including women of childbearing age (especially if pregnant or nursing), infants, children, adolescents, the elderly, individuals with inherited disorders of amino acid metabolism, and individuals with certain diseases.

At least two of the amino acids consumed in dietary supplements have also been associated with serious injuries in healthy adults.

A. L-tryptophan

L-tryptophan is associated with the most serious recent outbreak of illness and death known to be due to consumption of dietary supplements. In 1989, public health officials realized that an epidemic of eosinophilia-myalgia syndrome (EMS) was associated with the ingestion of L-tryptophan in a dietary supplement. EMS is a systemic connective tissue disease characterized by severe muscle pain, an increase in white blood cells, and certain skin and neuromuscular manifestations.

More than 1,500 cases of L-tryptophan-related EMS have been reported to the national Centers for Disease Control and Prevention. At least 38 patients are known to have died. The true incidence of L-tryptophan-related EMS is thought to be much higher. Some of the individuals suffering from L-tryptophan-related EMS have recovered, while other individuals' illnesses have persisted or worsened over time.

Although initial epidemiologic studies suggested that the illnesses might be due to impurities in an L-tryptophan product from a single Japanese manufacturer, this hypothesis has not been verified, and additional evidence suggests that L-tryptophan itself may cause or contribute to development of EMS. Cases of EMS and related disorders have been found to be associated with ingestion of L-tryptophan from other batches or sources of L-tryptophan. These illnesses have also been associated with the use of L-5-hydroxytryptophan, a compound that is closely related to L-tryptophan, but is not produced using the manufacturing process that created the impurities in the particular Japanese product.

B. Phenylalanine

A number of illnesses, including those similar to the eosinophilia myalgia syndrome (EMS) associated with L-tryptophan consumption, have been reported to FDA in individuals using dietary supplements containing phenylalanine. There are also published reports of scleroderma/scleroderma-like illnesses, which have symptoms similar to EMS, occurring in children with poorly controlled blood phenylalanine levels, as well as in those with phenylketonuria (PKU), a genetic disorder characterized by the inability to metabolize phenylalanine.

III. Vitamins and Minerals

Vitamin and mineral dietary supplements have a long history of use at levels consistent with the Recommended Dietary Allowances (RDA's) or at low multiplies of the RDA's, and are generally considered safe at these levels for the general population. Intakes above the RDA, however, vary widely in their potential for adverse effects. Certain vitamins and minerals that are safe when consumed at low levels are toxic at higher doses. The difference between a safe low dose and a toxic higher dose is quite large for some vitamins and minerals and quite small for others.

A. Vitamin A

Vitamin A is found in several forms in dietary supplements. Preformed vitamin A (vitamin A acetate and vitamin A palmitate) has well-recognized toxicity when consumed at levels of 25,000 International Units (IU) per day, or higher. (Beta-carotene does not have the potential for adverse effects that the other forms of vitamin A do, because high intakes of beta-carotene are converted to vitamin A in the body at much lower levels.) The RDA for vitamin A is 1,000 retinol equivalents (RE) for men, which is equivalent to 3,300 IU of preformed vitamin A, and 80 percent of these amounts for women.

The adverse effects associated with consumption of vitamin A at 25,000+ IU include severe liver injury (including cirrhosis), bone and cartilage pathologies, elevated intracranial pressure, and birth defects in infants whose mothers consumed vitamin A during pregnancy. Groups especially vulnerable to vitamin A toxicity are children, pregnant women, and those with liver disease caused by a variety of factors, including alcohol, viral hepatitis, and severe protein-energy malnutrition.

There are some studies that suggest vitamin A toxicity has occurred at levels of ingestion below 25,000 IU. In addition, the severity of the injuries that occur at 25,000 IU suggests that substantial, but less severe and less readily recognized, injuries probably occur at somewhat lower intakes. Most experts recommend that vitamin A intake not exceed 10,000 IU for most adults or 8,000 IU for pregnant and nursing women.

B. Vitamin B$_6$

Neurologic toxicity, including ataxia (alteration in balance) and sensory neuropathy (changes in sensations due to nerve injury), is associated with intake of vitamin B$_6$ (pyridoxine) supplements at levels above 100 milligrams per day. As little as 50 milligrams per day has caused resumption of symptoms in an individual previously injured by higher intakes. The RDA for vitamin B$_6$ is 2 milligrams. Vitamin B$_6$ is marketed in capsules containing dosages in the 100-, 200- and 500-milligrams range.

C. Niacin (nicotinic acid and nicotinamide)

Niacin taken in high doses is known to cause a wide range of adverse effects. The RDA for niacin is 20 milligrams. Niacin is marketed in dietary supplements at potencies of 250 mg, 400 mg, and 500 mg, in both immediate and slow-release formulations. Daily doses of 500 mg from slow-release formulations, and 750 mg of immediate-release niacin, have been associated with severe adverse reactions, including gastrointestinal distress (burning pain, nausea, vomiting, bloating, cramping, and diarrhea) and mild to severe liver damage. Less common, but more serious (in some cases life-threatening), reactions include liver injury, myopathy (muscle disease), maculopathy of the eyes (injury to the eyes resulting in decreased vision), coagulopathy (increased bleeding problems), cytopenia (decreases in cell types in the blood), hypotensive myocardial ischemia (heart injury caused by too low blood pressure), and metabolic acidosis (increases in the acidity of the blood and urine).

Niacin (nicotinic acid) is approved as a prescription drug to lower cholesterol. Many of the observed adverse reactions have occurred when patients have switched to OTC formulations of niacin, and particularly when they have switched from immediate-release formulations to dietary supplements containing slow-release niacin formulations without the knowledge of their physicians.

D. Selenium

Selenium is a mineral found in dietary supplement products. At high doses (approximately 800 to 1,000 micrograms per day), selenium can cause tissue damage, especially in tissues or organs that concentrate the element. The toxicity of selenium depends upon the chemical form of selenium in the ingested supplement and upon the selenium levels in the foods consumed. Human injuries have occurred following ingestion of high doses over a few weeks.

IV. Other Products Marketed as Dietary Supplements

A. Germanium

Germanium is a nonessential element. Recently, germanium has been marketed in the form of inorganic germanium salts and novel organogermanium compounds, as a "dietary supplement." These products are promoted for their claimed immunomodulatory effects or as "health-promoting" elixirs. Germanium supplements, when used chronically, have caused nephrotoxicity (kidney injury) and death. Since 1982, there have been 20 reported cases of acute renal failure, including two deaths, attributed to oral intakes of germanium elixirs. In surviving patients, kidney function has improved after discontinuation of germanium, but none of the patients have recovered normal kidney function.

One particular organogermanium compound, an azaspiran organogermanium, has been studied for its potential use as an anticancer drug. Forty percent of the patients in this study experienced transient neurotoxicity (nerve damage), and two patients developed pulmonary toxicity. Because of these side effects, medically supervised administration of this drug with monitoring for toxicity has been recommended for those using germanium chronically.

BIBLIOGRAPHY

Allaby, Michael, ed. *The Concise Oxford Dictionary of Botany.* New York: Oxford University Press, 1992.

American Dietetic Association. "Caffeine: How Much Is Too Much?" Special advertising section, *Time,* November 21, 1994.

———. "Positions of the American Dietetic Association: Enrichment and Fortification of Foods and Dietary Supplements." *Journal of the American Dietetic Association* 94(1994): 661–663.

American Journal of Dentistry 5(1992): 269.

American Medical Association. *AMA Drug Evaluations Subscription.* Chicago, 1992.

American Medical Association. "Caffeine Use Can Lead to Dependence." News release, Department of Science News, Chicago, October 4, 1994.

American Medical Association. "Consumption of Dark Green, Leafy Vegetables Could Lower Risk of Vision Disorder." News release. Department of Science News, Chicago, November 8, 1994.

American Medical Association. "Some Herbal Medications May Cause Liver Injury." News release. Department of Science News, Chicago: February 7, 1995.

Appel, L. J., E. R. Miller 3d, A. J. Seidler, and P. K. Whelton. "Does Supplementation of Diet with 'Fish Oil' Reduce Blood Pressure? A Meta-Analysis of Controlled Clinical Trials." *Archives of Internal Medicine* 153(1993): 1429–1438.

Barnett, Robert A. "Can Vitamins Save Your Life?" *Family Circle,* February 1, 1995: 24.

Bartlow, Stephanie. "Drink up! Water Is a Necessity." *The Ocean County Medical News Update,* vol. 1, no. 9, June 1994: 8.

Berkow, R., M. B. Fletcher, et al. *The Merck Manual of Diagnosis and Therapy.* 15th ed. Rahway, N.J.: 1987.

Bielory, L., and R. Gandhi. "Asthma and Vitamin C." *Annuals of Allergy* 73(1994): 89–96.

Bittman, Mark. "Eating Well: A Little Cooking Goes a Long Way for Vegetable Nutrients." *New York Times,* August 31, 1994: C4.

Bourre, Jean-Marie, M. D. *Brainfood: A Provocative Exploration of the Connection Between What You Eat and How You Think.* Boston: Little, Brown and Company, 1990.

Braunwald, E., K. J. Isselbacher, R. G. Petersdorf, et al., eds. *Harrison's Principles of Internal Medicine.* New York: McGraw-Hill, 1987.

Brody, Jane E. "Illness Raises Concern on Herbal Preparations." *New York Times,* February 8, 1995.

Brown, H., B. R. Cassileth, J. P. Lewis, and J. H. Renner. "Alternative Medicine—or Quackery?" *Patient Care,* June 15, 1994: 91.

Burg, Dale. "Eat Your Spinach." *New Woman,* February 1994: 144.

Burtis, W. J., L. Gay, K. L. Insogna, et al. "Dietary Hypercalcemia in Patients with Calcium Oxalate Kidney Stones." *American Journal of Clinical Nutrition* 60(1994): 424–429.

Butler, J. C., et al. "Measles Severity and Serum Retinol (Vitamin A) Concentration Among Children in the United States." *Pediatrics* 91(1993): 1176–1181.

"Buying Vitamins: What's Worth the Price?" *Consumer Reports,* September, 1994.

Canadian Pediatric Society—Société Canadienne de Pédiatrie. "Megavitamin and megamineral therapy in childhood." *Canadian Medical Association Journal* 143(1990): 1009–1013.

Carroll, L. "Iodine Supplements in Pregnancy May Prevent Cretinism." *Medical Tribune,* February 2, 1995.

Cataldo, Corinne, Linda DeBruyne, and Eleanor Whitney. *Nutrition and Diet Therapy.* 3rd ed. St. Paul: West Publishing Co., 1992.

Chopra, Deepak, M. D. *Perfect Health: The Complete Mind/Body Guide.* New York: Harmony Books, 1991.

Christoffel, K. "A Pediatric Perspective on Vegetarian Nutrition." *Clinical Pediatrics* 20(1981): 632–643.

"Chronic fatigue diets rebuked." *Medical Tribune,* March 1993.

Couturier, Lisa. "Protecting Our Fellow Creatures." *New Woman,* February 1994: 96.

"Cure It with Herbs." *First,* February 27, 1995: 43–47.

Dalsky, G. P. "Exercise: Its Effect on Bone Mineral Content." *Clinical Obstetrics and Gynecology* 30(1987): 820–32.

Davis, Adelle. *Let's Eat Right to Keep Fit.* New York: New American Library, Harcourt Brace Jovanovich, Inc., 1970.

Dickinson, A. *Benefits of Nutritional Supplements.* Washington, D.C.: Council for Responsible Nutrition, 1987.

"Don't Eliminate All Fat from Diet." Your Body: An Owner's Manual column. *Asbury Park Press,* May 10, 1994.

Dorland's Illustrated Medical Dictionary. 28th ed. Philadelphia: W. B. Saunders, 1994.

Drug Information for the Health Care Professional. 14th ed. Taunton, Massachusetts: Rand McNally, 1994.

Elmer-Dewitt, Philip. "Fat Times: What Health Craze? Thanks to Too Much Food and Too Little Sweat, Americans Are Heavier Than Ever." *Time,* January 16, 1995: 58.

Findlay, S. "Nutritional Bodyguards." *Fitness,* March–April 1993: 4–6.

"Fish Oil Reported to Offer No Benefit Against Restenosis." *Cardiology World News,* September 15, 1994: 7.

Forman, A. "Mining for minerals—Zinc Is Worth Its Weight in Gold." *Environmental Nutrition* 17 (1994): 1–6.

Fried, J. *Vitamin Politics.* Buffalo, N.Y.: Prometheus Books, 1984.

Friedman, Max. "Whatever Happened to Hemp?" *Vegetarian Times,* August 1994: 71.

Friend, T. "Zinc Levels May Offer New Theory on Alzheimer's." *USA Today,* September 2, 1994.

"Fruits, Vegetables Provide Folic Acid." Nutrition column. *Asbury Park Press,* February 8, 1994.

Fulder, Stephen. *The Tao of Medicine: Ginseng, Oriental Remedies, and the Pharmacology of Harmony.* New York: Destiny Books, 1980.

Futoryan, T. and B. A. Gilchrest. "Retinoids and the Skin." *Nutrition Reviews* 52(1994): 299–306.

Gapinski, J. P., J. V. Van Ruiswyk, G. R. Heudebert, and G. S. Schectman. "Preventing Restenosis with

Fish Oils Following Coronary Angioplasty. A Meta-analysis." *Arch Internal Medicine* 153(1993): 1595–1601.

Garrison, R. H., and E. Somer. *The Nutrition Desk Reference.* 2nd ed. New Canaan, Conn.: Keats Publishing, 1990.

Gilman, A. G., T. W. Rall, A. S. Nies, and P. Taylor, eds. *Goodman and Gilman's The Pharmacological Basis of Therapeutics.* 8th ed. New York: McGraw-Hill, 1990.

Golden, W. E. "Folic Acid for the Prevention of Neural Tube Defects." *Patient Outcomes* July–August 1994: 23–25.

Goldfarb, S. "Diet and Nephrolithiasis." *Annual Review of Medicine* 45(1994): 235–243.

Greenberg, E. R., Baren, J. A., Tosteson, T. D., et al. "A Clinical Trial of Antioxident Vitamins to Prevent Colorectal Adenoma." *New England Journal of Medicine* 331(1994): 141–147.

Gutfeld, G. and T. Hanlon. "Choosing Your Best Prostate Prescription." *Prevention,* June 1994: 80, 90–91.

Harrington, Geri. *Real Food, Fake Food and Everything in Between.* New York: Macmillan Publishing Company, Inc., 1987.

Harris, R. "Vitamins and Neural Tube Defects. Editorial." *British Medical Journal* 296(1988): 80–81.

Heinonen, O. P., and D. Albanes. "The Effect of Vitamin E and Beta Carotene on the Incidence of Lung Cancer and Other Cancers in Male Smokers." *New England Journal of Medicine* 330(1994): 1029–1035.

Hendler, S. S. *The Doctor's Vitamin and Mineral Encyclopedia.* New York: Simon and Schuster, 1990.

Herbert, V., and M. S. Subak-Sharpe, eds. *The Mt. Sinai School of Medicine Complete Book of Nutrition.* New York: St. Martin's Press, 1990.

Hertog, M. G. L., et al. "Dietary Antioxidant Flavonoids and Risk of Coronary Heart Disease: The Zutphen Elderly Study." *Lancet* 342(1993): 1007–1011.

Hoffman, F. A. "Micronutrient Requirements of Cancer Patients." *Cancer* 55(1 Suppl)(1985): 295–300.

Hrabak, D. "A Fish Oil Story: Omega-3's Return to Fight Heart Disease, Cancer." *Environmental Nutrition* 17(1994): 1–3.

Hunter, D. J., et al. "Prospective Study of the Intake of Vitamins C, E, A and the Risk of Breast Cancer." *New England Journal of Medicine* 329(1993): 234.

Hutchens, Alma R. *Indian Herbology of North America.* Boston: Shambhala, 1991.

Jancin, B. "Calcium for Osteoporosis: Little Help, Little Harm." *Family Practice News,* February 15, 1994.

Joslin Diabetes Center. "New Research Suggests Vitamin E May Prevent Vascular Complications." Press release. October 25, 1994.

Kanter, M. M., L. A. Nolte, and J. O. Holloszy. "Effects of an Antioxident Vitamin Mixture on Lipid Peroxidation at Rest and Post-exercise." *Journal of Applied Physiology* 74(1993): 965–969.

Kail, K. "Multivitamin-Mineral Complexes: Your Nutritional Insurance Policy." *Health Foods Business,* April 1992: 87–89.

Koop, C. Everett, M. D., *The Surgeon General's Report on Nutrition and Health.* Rocklin, Calif.: Prima Publishing and Communications, 1988.

Krause, Marie V., and Kathleen L. Mahan. *Food, Nutrition and Diet Therapy.* 6th ed. Philadelphia: W. B. Saunders Co., 1979.

Kritz, Fran. "Government Taking a Closer Look at Medicinal Plants." *Medical Tribune,* January 19, 1995.

Lad, Vasant. *Ayurveda: The Science of Self-Healing.* Wilmot, Wis.: Lotus Press, 1985.

Lefferts, L. Y. "Run, Radicals, Run." *Nutrition Action Health Letter* 20(1993): 4.

Lieberman, S., and N. Bruning. *The Real Vitamin & Mineral Book.* Garden City Park, N.Y.: Avery Publishing Group. 1990.

Liebman, B. "The Ultra Mega Vita Guide." *Nutrition Action Health Letter.* 20(1993): 7–8.

Lipkowitz, M. A., and T. Navarra. *Allergies A to Z.* New York: Facts On File, 1994.

"Lorenzo's Oil and Lymphocytopenia." *New England Journal of Medicine* 330(1993), no. 8: 577.

Lust, John. *The Herb Book.* New York: Bantam Books, 1974.

Lyons, A. S., and R. J. Petrucelli. *Medicine, An Illustrated History.* New York: Abradale Press, 1987.

Marcuard, S. P., L. Albernaz, and P. G. Khazanie. "Omeprazole Therapy Causes Malabsorption of Cyanocobalamin (Vitamin B_{12}). *Annals of Internal Medicine* 120(1994): 211.

Margen, S., and D. A. Ogar. "Low Calorie Carrot Jewel of a Vegetable." *Asbury Park Press,* September 6, 1994.

Matthews, Karen. "Fungal Tea Mushrooming as Health Fad." *Asbury Park Press,* February 7, 1995: B1.

McAdam, P. "Vitamin D Drug Enhances Psoriasis Therapy." *Medical Tribune,* April 7, 1994.

McAllister-Smart, Joanne. "Antioxidants for the Uninitiated." *Vegetarian Times,* April 1994: 26.

McCann, J. "Antioxidants Show Promise in Cancer Therapy." *Medical Tribune,* April 7, 1994.

McIntyre, Anne. *The Complete Women's Herbal: A Manual of Healing, Herbs and Nutrition for Personal Well-Being and Family Care.* New York: Henry Holt Co., 1994.

Medicine the Year in Review 1992. New York: Medical Tribune, 1993.

MidLife Women's Network. "Food, Fats & You." *Midlife Woman* 2(1992): 1–9.

Miller, L. "Twice-a-Day Dose of Vitamin C May Be Key." *USA Today,* October 18, 1994.

Mindell, E. *Vitamin Bible.* New York: Warner Books, 1991.

Morris, M. C., F. Sacks, and B. Rosner. "Does Fish Oil Lower Blood Pressure? A Meta-analysis of Controlled Trials." *Circulation* 88(1993): 522–533.

"Most Everyone Can Use a Modest Increase in Calcium, Says NIH." *Modern Medicine,* 16(1995): 11.

"National Institute of Health (NIH)." *World Book Encyclopedia.* Chicago: World Book-Childcraft International 14(1979): 40.

National Research Council. *Recommended Dietary Allowances.*

New Jersey Naturally. Resource Directory for Natural Living, Winter/Spring 1995. New York: City Spirit Publications.

"Nutrition." *The New Encyclopedia Britannica, Macropedia.* vol. 13. Chicago: Encyclopedia Britannica, Inc., 1974.

"Nutrition Checklist." Washington, D.C.: The Nutrition Screening Initiative, 1992.

Nutrition column. *Asbury Park Press.* February 28, 1994.

Olin, B. R., and S. K. Hebel, et al., eds. *Facts and Comparisons.* St. Louis: J. B. Lippencott Co., 1994.

Pauling, L., and C. Moertel. "A Proposition: Megadoses of Vitamin C Are Valuable in the Treatment of Cancer." *Nutrition Review* 44(1986): 28–32.

Physician's Desk Reference. Montvale, N.J.: Medical Economics, 1994.

"Powerful Ephedrine Eyed for Side Effects, Toxicity." *The Ocean County Medical News Update,* vol. 1, no. 9, June 1994: 16.

Pratt, Steven. "MSG—Is It Harmless or an 'Excitotoxin'?" *Asbury Park Press,* August 3, 1994: B1.

Prochaska, Hans, Annette Santamaria, and Paul Talalay. "The Rapid Detection of Inducers of Enzymes

That Protect Against Carcinogens." The Proceedings of the National Academy of Science, USA, vol. 89, March 1992: 2394–2398.

Quinn, E. Q. and J. R. Meese. "Pseudotumor Cerebri, a Review." *The Female Patient* 19(1994): 16–24.

Recker, R. R. "Common Misconceptions about Calcium Absorption." Lecture. *Gastroenterology Observer,* July–August, 1994.

Reid, Ian, M. D., Ruth Ames, N.Z.C.S., Margaret Evans, B.Sc., et al. "The Effect of Calcium Supplementation on Bone Loss in Post-Menopausal Women." *The New England Journal of Medicine,* 328(1993): 460–464.

Richer, S. P. "Is There a Prevention and Treatment Strategy for Macular Degeneration?" *Journal of the American Optometric Association* 64(1993): 838–850.

Rivlin, R. S. "Nutrition and Aging." Lecture, University of Medicine and Dentistry of New Jersey, Robert Wood Johnson Medical School. April 27, 1990.

Roberts, H. J.: "Vitamin E and Gynecomastia." letter. *Hospital Practice* 29(1994): 12.

Roche Biomedical Laboratories. *Directory of Services.* Stowe, Ohio: Lexi–Comp, 1991.

Rosenbaum, Michael E., M. D., and Dominick Bosco. *Super Fitness Beyond Vitamins: The Bible of Super Supplements.* New York: New American Library Books, 1987.

Rubenstein, E., and D. D. Ferdermanm, eds. *Scientific American Medicine.* New York: Scientific American, 1987.

"Salmonella Arizona Infections Associated with Ingestion of Rattlesnake Capsules." Archives of Internal Medicine, 149(1989): 701, 705.

Sambrook, P., et al. "Prevention of Corticosteroid Osteoporosis; a Comparison of Calcium, Calcitriol and Calcitonin." *New England Journal of Medicine* 328(1993): 1747–1752.

Schart, D. "Vitamins 101, How to Buy Them." *Nutrition Action Health Letter.* January/February 1993: 5–6.

Seddon, J. M., and C. H. Hennekens. "Vitamins, Minerals and Macular degeneration. Promising but Unproven Hypothesis." Editorial: comments. *Archives of Ophthalmology* 112(1994): 176–179.

Severo, Richard. "Linus C. Pauling Dies at 93; Chemist and Voice for Peace." *New York Times,* August 21, 1994: 1.

Shils, M. E., J. A. Olson, and M. Shike, eds. *Modern Nutrition in Health and Disease.* 8th ed. Philadelphia: Lea & Febiger, 1994.

Simpson, Glenn. "A Raid on Your Medicine Chest." *US Weekend,* February 18–20, 1994.

Somer, E. *The Essential Guide to Vitamins and Minerals.* New York: HarperPerennial, 1992.

Southgate, D. A., "Minerals, Trace Elements, and Potential Hazards." *American Journal of Clinical Nutrition* 45(supplement)(1987): 1256–1266.

Spiro, H. M. *Clinical Gastroenterology.* 2nd ed. New York: Macmillan, 1977.

Stähelin, H. B. "Vitamins and Cancer." *Recent Results in Cancer Research* 108(1988): 227–234.

Tadesco, L. Conversations between Myron Lipkowitz with a registered nutritionist. August 1994 to February 1995.

"Taking vitamins—Can They Prevent Disease?" *Consumer Reports,* September 1994; 561–564.

Thomas, Clayton L., ed. *Taber's Cyclopedic Medical Dictionary.* 17th ed. Philadelphia: F. A. Davis Company, 1993.

Tierra, Michael. *The Way of Herbs.* New York: Pocket Books, 1990.

Toufexis, A. "The New Scoop on Vitamins." *Time.* April 6, 1992: 54–59.

U.S. Code Congressional and Administrative News, 103rd Congress, no. 9, December 1994. St. Paul: West Publishing Co., 108-Stat. 4329.

U.S. Code Service, Food and Drugs, Sections 1–600. Rochester, N.Y.: The Lawyers Co-Operative Publishing Co., 1994, pp. 288–290.

U.S. Department of Health and Human Services/Public Health Service. "Lead Poisoning Associated with Use of Traditional Ethnic Remedies—California, 1991–1992." *Morbidity and Mortality Weekly Report,* vol. 42, no. 27, July 16, 1993.

U.S. Food & Drug Administration. "Folic acid-fortified food." *FDA Medical Bulletin* 24(1994): 9.

U.S. Food & Drug Administration. "The new food label." *FDA Medical Bulletin* 24(1994): 2–3.

Ulene, A. *Count Out Cholesterol.* New York: Alfred A. Knopf, 1989.

Ulene, A., and V. Ulene. *The Vitamin Strategy.* Berkeley, Calif.: Ulysses Press, 1994.

United States Pharmacopia. 22nd rev. ed. The United States Pharmacopeial Convention, Inc. Easton, Pa.: Mack Printing Co., 1990.

"Vitamin E and C Supplements Lower Risk of Coronary Death Among the Elderly." *Modern Medicine* 63(1995): 15.

"Vitamins and Minerals from A to Z Quiz." McMahon Co., 1993.

"Vitamins for Vision." *Nutrition Action Health Letter,* January/February 1994. Original Source; *Archives of Ophthalmology* 111(1993): 1246.

"Vitamins linked to immune system." *Asbury Park Press,* September 13, 1994: B3.

Wade, Nicholas. "Method and Madness: Believing in Vitamins." *New York Times Magazine,* May 22, 1994: 20.

Ward, Bernard. *Healing Foods from the Bible.* Boca Raton, Fla.: Globe Communications Corp., 1994.

Ward, John T. "Vitamin Craze." *Asbury Park Press,* April 3, 1994: B1.

Weiss, Gaea, and Shandoe Weiss. *Growing and Using the Healing Herbs.* Emmaus, Pa.: Rodale Press, 1985.

Whitehead R. G. "Vitamins, Minerals, Schoolchildren and IQ." Editorial. *British Medical Journal* 302(1991): 548.

York, E. "Diet, Exercise and Bone Mineral Content." Letter. *Annals of Internal Medicine* 102(1985): 418.

ABOUT THE AUTHORS

Tova Navarra graduated magna cum laude from Seton Hall University. She is a registered nurse, former health columnist for Copley News Service, and the author of several books, including *Wisdom for Caregivers; An Insider's Guide to Home Health Care; Playing It Smart: What to Do When You're on Your Own; Your Body: Highlights of Human Anatomy;* and *The New Jersey Shore: A Vanishing Splendor.* Senior author of *Therapeutic Communication* and coauthor of *Allergies A–Z,* as a freelance writer she has been published in the *New York Times,* the *American Journal of Nursing, Cancer Practice* and many other periodicals. Ms. Navarra is an M.P.A. candidate at Fairleigh Dickinson University. She lives in Monmouth County, New Jersey.

Myron A. Lipkowitz, R.Ph., M.D., is a family practitioner, allergist and registered pharmacist. He is the coauthor of *Allergies A–Z* and *Therapeutic Communication.* He has also lectured to professional and lay audiences and written professional articles. He lives and practices medicine in Howell, New Jersey.

John G. Navarra, Jr., J.D., is an attorney who teaches physics and general sciences at Monsignor Donovan High School in Toms River, New Jersey. He has also taught at Seton Hall Preparatory School, Christian Brothers Academy and Ocean County College. A coauthor of *Therapeutic Communication,* he has written articles for the *American Journal of Nursing,* the *Asbury Park Press* and other publications. He lives in Monmouth County with his wife, Tova, and his son, Johnny.

INDEX

This index is designed to be used in conjunction with the many cross-references within the A-to-Z entries. The main A-to-Z entries are indicated by **boldface** page references. The general subjects are subdivided by the A-to-Z entries. Tables are indicated by "t" following the page locator; the chronology by "c"; and glossary items by "g".

H